AF754121

HEALTH AND HUMAN DEVELOPMENT

ADVANCED CANCER. PAIN AND QUALITY OF LIFE

HEALTH AND HUMAN DEVELOPMENT

JOAV MERRICK - SERIES EDITOR –

NATIONAL INSTITUTE OF CHILD HEALTH
AND HUMAN DEVELOPMENT,
MINISTRY OF SOCIAL AFFAIRS, JERUSALEM

Adolescent Behavior Research: International Perspectives
Joav Merrick and Hatim A. Omar (Editors)
2007. ISBN: 1-60021-649-8

Complementary Medicine Systems: Comparison and Integration
Karl W. Kratky
2008. ISBN: 978-1-60456-475-4

Pain in Children and Youth
Patricia Schofield and Joav Merrick (Editors)
2008. ISBN: 978-1-60456-951-3

Challenges in Adolescent Health: An Australian Perspective
David Bennett, Susan Towns, Elizabeth Elliott and Joav Merrick (Editors)
2009. ISBN: 978-1-60741-616-6 (Hardcover)
2009. ISBN: 978-1-61668-240-8 (E-book)

Behavioral Pediatrics, 3rd Edition
Donald E. Greydanus, Dilip R. Patel, Helen D. Pratt and Joseph L. Calles, Jr. (Editors)
2009. ISBN: 978-1-60692-702-1 (Hardcover)
2009. ISBN: 978-1-60876-630-7 (E-book)

Health and Happiness from Meaningful Work: Research in Quality of Working Life
Søren Ventegodt and Joav Merrick (Editors)
2009. ISBN: 978-1-60692-820-2

Obesity and Adolescence: A Public Health Concern
Hatim A. Omar, Donald E. Greydanus, Dilip R. Patel and Joav Merrick (Editors)
2009. ISBN: 978-1-60456-821-9

Poverty and Children: A Public Health Concern
Alexis Lieberman and Joav Merrick (Editors)
2009. ISBN: 978-1-60741-140-6

Living on the Edge: The Mythical, Spiritual, and Philosophical Roots of Social Marginality
Joseph Goodbread
2009. ISBN: 978-1-60741-162-8

Alcohol-Related Cognitive Disorders: Research and Clinical Perspectives
Leo Sher, Isack Kandel and Joav Merrick (Editors)
2009. ISBN: 978-1-60741-730-9 (Hardcover)
2009. ISBN: 978-1-60876-623-9 (E-book)

Child Rural Health: International Aspects
Erica Bell and Joav Merrick (Editors)
2010. ISBN: 978-1-60876-357-3

Advances in Environmental Health Effects of Toxigenic Mold and Mycotoxins- Volume 1
Ebere Cyril Anyanwu
2010. ISBN: 978-1-60741-953-2

Children and Pain
Patricia Schofield and Joav Merrick (Editors)
2009. ISBN: 978-1-60876-020-6 (Hardcover)
2009. ISBN: 978-1-61728-183-9 (E-book)

Conceptualizing Behavior in Health and Social Research: A Practical Guide to Data Analysis
Said Shahtahmasebi and Damon Berridge
2010. ISBN: 978-1-60876-383-2

Chance Action and Therapy. The Playful Way of Changing
Uri Wernik
2010. ISBN: 978-1-60876-393-1

Adolescence and Chronic Illness. A Public Health Concern
Hatim Omar, Donald E. Greydanus, Dilip R. Patel and Joav Merrick (Editors)
2010. ISBN: 978-1-60876-628-4 (Hardcover)
2010. ISBN: 978-1-61761-482-8 (E-book)

Adolescence and Sports
Dilip R. Patel, Donald E. Greydanus, Hatim Omar and Joav Merrick (Editors)
2010. ISBN: 978-1-60876-702-1 (Hardcover)
2010. ISBN: 978-1-61761-483-5 (E-book)

International Aspects of Child Abuse and Neglect
Howard Dubowitz and Joav Merrick (Editors)
2010. ISBN: 978-1-60876-703-8

Positive Youth Development: Evaluation and Future Directions in a Chinese Context
Daniel T.L. Shek, Hing Keung Ma and Joav Merrick (Editors)
2010. ISBN: 978-1-60876-830-1 (Hardcover)
2010. ISBN: 978-1-61668-376-4 (E-book)

Positive Youth Development: Implementation of a Youth Program in a Chinese Context
Daniel T.L Shek, Hing Keung Ma and Joav Merrick (Editors)
2010. ISBN: 978-1-61668-230-9

Pediatric and Adolescent Sexuality and Gynecology: Principles for the Primary Care Clinician
Hatim A. Omar, Donald E. Greydanus, Artemis K. Tsitsika, Dilip R. Patel and Joav Merrick (Editors)
2010. ISBN: 978-1-60876-735-9

Understanding Eating Disorders: Integrating Culture, Psychology and Biology
Yael Latzer, Joav Merrick and Daniel Stein (Editors)
2010. ISBN: 978-1-61728-298-0

Advanced Cancer Pain and Quality of Life
Edward Chow and Joav Merrick (Editors)
2010. ISBN: 978-1-61668-207-1

Bone and Brain Metastases: Advances in Research and Treatment
Arjun Sahgal, Edward Chow and Joav Merrick (Editors)
2010. ISBN: 978-1-61668-365-8 (Hardcover)
2010. ISBN: 978-1-61728-085-6 (E-book)

Environment, Mood Disorders and Suicide
Teodor T. Postolache and Joav Merrick (Editors)
2010. ISBN: 978-1-61668-505-8

Social and Cultural Psychiatry Experience from the Caribbean Region
Hari D. Maharajh and Joav Merrick (Editors)
2010. ISBN: 978-1-61668-506-5 (Hardcover)
2010. ISBN: 978-1-61728-088-7 (E-book)

Narratives and Meanings of Migration
Julia Mirsky
2010. ISBN: 978-1-61761-103-2 (Hardcover)
2010. ISBN: 978-1-61761-519-1 (E-book)

Self-Management and the Health Care Consumer
Peter William Harvey
2011. ISBN: 978-1-61761-796-6

Sexology from a Holistic Point of View
Soren Ventegodt and Joav Merrick
2011. ISBN: 978-1-61761-859-8

Principles of Holistic Psychiatry: A Textbook on Holistic Medicine for Mental Disorders
Soren Ventegodt and Joav Merrick
2011. ISBN: 978-1-61761-940-3

HEALTH AND HUMAN DEVELOPMENT

ADVANCED CANCER. PAIN AND QUALITY OF LIFE

EDWARD CHOW
AND
JOAV MERRICK
EDITORS

Nova Science Publishers, Inc.
New York

Copyright © 2010 by Nova Science Publishers, Inc.

All rights reserved. No part of this book may be reproduced, stored in a retrieval system or transmitted in any form or by any means: electronic, electrostatic, magnetic, tape, mechanical photocopying, recording or otherwise without the written permission of the Publisher.

For permission to use material from this book please contact us:
Telephone 631-231-7269; Fax 631-231-8175
Web Site: http://www.novapublishers.com

NOTICE TO THE READER

The Publisher has taken reasonable care in the preparation of this book, but makes no expressed or implied warranty of any kind and assumes no responsibility for any errors or omissions. No liability is assumed for incidental or consequential damages in connection with or arising out of information contained in this book. The Publisher shall not be liable for any special, consequential, or exemplary damages resulting, in whole or in part, from the readers' use of, or reliance upon, this material.

Independent verification should be sought for any data, advice or recommendations contained in this book. In addition, no responsibility is assumed by the publisher for any injury and/or damage to persons or property arising from any methods, products, instructions, ideas or otherwise contained in this publication.

This publication is designed to provide accurate and authoritative information with regard to the subject matter covered herein. It is sold with the clear understanding that the Publisher is not engaged in rendering legal or any other professional services. If legal or any other expert assistance is required, the services of a competent person should be sought. FROM A DECLARATION OF PARTICIPANTS JOINTLY ADOPTED BY A COMMITTEE OF THE AMERICAN BAR ASSOCIATION AND A COMMITTEE OF PUBLISHERS.

Additional color graphics may be available in the e-book version of this book.

Library of Congress Cataloging-in-Publication Data

Advanced cancer : pain and quality of life / editors, Edward Chow, Joav Merrick.
p. ; cm.
Includes bibliographical references and index.
ISBN 978-1-61668-207-1 (hardcover)
1. Cancer--Palliative treatment. 2. Cancer pain. I. Chow, Edward. II. Merrick, Joav, 1950-
[DNLM: 1. Neoplasms--therapy. 2. Pain--therapy. 3. Bone Neoplasms--secondary. 4. Neoplasms--complications. 5. Palliative Care. 6. Quality of Life. QZ 266 A2432 2010]
RC271.P33A38 2010
616.99'406--dc22
2010001051

Published by Nova Science Publishers, Inc. † New York

Contents

Preface

An estimated 166,400 new cases of cancer will occur in Canada in 2008. Bone metastases unfortunately remain a common site of recurrence, with breast and prostate cancer patients representing a substantial proportion of this population. Metastatic bone disease is associated with significant morbidity and mortality. Pain is experienced by up to two thirds of patients. The prognosis for patients with bone metastases is highly influenced by tumor type, performance status, and the presence of extraosseous disease. The median survival has been significantly longer in breast cancer patients with a first relapse in the axial skeleton (24 months) versus patients with initial relapse in the liver (3 months) (2). Survival after diagnosis of bone metastases is influenced by the subsequent development of extraosseous metastatic sites: 1.6 years versus 2.1 years in patients with bone-only disease.

Chapter I - The use of psychodynamic-oriented techniques has successfully been used to manage pain in 75 cancer patients by the use of psychodynamic principles. Pain is a subjective phenomenon that varies much from patient to patient with the same type and stage of cancer. This well-known variance is from a depth-psychological perspective explained by pain being a negative interpretation of inner reality caused by the patients' sub-conscious conflicts. Therefore much pain can be relieved, when these conflicts are resolved in the therapy, which happens when the patient bonds to the therapist and in an intimate therapeutic relationship regain deeper insight in self and life, and a positive and relaxed attitude. The intimacy with the patient was reached by selective therapeutic touch, i.e. hugs, in a holistic philosophical framework, making the intervention a type of clinical holistic medicine. The basic principle was that of "clinical medicine" and healing by supported self-exploration. Patients in acute or chronic states appeared to be able to utilize the intervention for existential healing (what Antonovsky called "salutogenesis") only when the therapeutic relationship was close and positive. Their resistance to a positive transference was a defense that could be resolved with reflective techniques thereby facilitating the use of these interventions. The hierarchy of degree of pain relief seemed to be 1) chemical side effects of medication being coupled with a positive suggestions of pain relief (placebo), 2) Counterfocus of irritations and pain within the soma to reduce the intensity of the actual pain site (integration of inner conflicts), 3) Directed aggressive imagery to have the patient angry at his or her pain (self-expression) and 4) Relaxation and escape imagery (letting go of tensions and negative ideas and attitudes). Estimated from the case stories one in two was helped (NNT=2 for cancer pains).

Chapter II - The purpose of this chapter was to determine the effect of the "Power Over Pain" intervention, a structured educational intervention for nurses, patients and caregivers managing cancer-related pain in the home. Using a longitudinal design, 232 home care nurses, 50 patients, and 46 caregivers were randomly assigned to one of four intervention groups. The nurse receiving the intervention showed significant increases in pain-related knowledge and perception of control over pain and decreases in barriers to pain control. Patients receiving the intervention demonstrated a significant decrease in barriers to pain control and trends toward decreased pain and symptom distress and increased functional status related to pain, pain management knowledge, and perception of control over pain. Caregivers in dyads whose home care nurse received the intervention had significant improvement in perception of control over pain. Results suggest that the "Power Over Pain" intervention is effective for improving cancer pain management in the home.

Chapter III - Cancer is a global health problem and for many patients result in chronic pain. Unfortunately the treatment of cancer pain is often inadequate. Nurses are in the best position to facilitate effective pain management due to the time they spend with the patient experiencing pain. The researcher initiated the research to determine if nurses were aware of the problem of cancer pain in relation to other problems a cancer patient could experience and if nursing practice facilitated effective pain management. A contextual, exploratory and comparative descriptive study was performend. The target population was all nurses entering an oncology nursing learning programme at a univeristy of technology in South Africa. The sampling method was convenient (n=35) and the participation rate 97.2%. Self-reported data were gathered by means of a questionnaire. Data were analysed using descriptive statisitcs and content analyses. The study provided evidence that despite nurses' awareness of cancer pain they lacked knowledge and skills pertaining to the management of pain. Nursing practice did not facilitate effective pain management. Educational programmes focusing on all aspects of pain management are urgently required. Nurses should also be involved in research on cancer pain and its management to enable them to have evidence of their important role in caring for the patient.

Chapter IV - Cancer remains a major public health problem and the control of end-of-life pain continues to be a challenge even in the face of major advancements in pain control methodology. Both radiation oncologist and hospice professionals have shown a propensity for successfully managing that pain, but educational and reimbursement issues have prevented the two specialties from delivering coordinated, concurrent care. Further optimization of pain control for these patients will require increased collaboration between the two specialties and a willingness on the part of radiation oncologists to employ single fraction therapy for appropriate patients who have bone metastasis pain. This paper presents a short review of the history, barriers and collaborations between the two specialities

Chapter V - The purpose was to investigate the clinical benefits of combining radiation and bisphosphonates in bone metastases. Methods: A systematic search on Medline was conducted from 1950 to November 2008. Eligible studies included in-vitro cell studies, animal tumor models, and any human studies combining the use of radiotherapy and bisphosphonates. This search was limited to English publications only. Results: A total of 13 studies involving the combination of bisphosphonates and radiotherapy were identified. Three were in-vitro cell studies, two were animal tumor models, and eight were human studies. Both in-vitro cell studies and animal tumor models demonstrate significant synergistic effects when combining both therapies. There are only two human randomized trials comparing combination therapy to placebo and radiation, which showed greater long term benefits using combination treatment. Conclusion: Preliminary evidence suggests that patients with bone metastases may significantly benefit from concurrent treatment with both radiotherapy and bisphosphonates when compared with either treatment alone.

Chapter VI - The purpose was to assess the relationship between pretreatment symptoms and pain response following palliative radiotherapy for bone metastases. Methods: All patients with bone metastases treated with palliative radiotherapy were followed at baseline, then 1, 2 and 3 months after radiotherapy with the Edmonton Symptom Assessment System (ESAS). This scale includes pain, fatigue, nausea, depression, anxiety, drowsiness, appetite, sense of well being and shortness of breath. Patients were categorized as either a responder or non-responder according to the International Consensus Guidelines for palliative radiotherapy. Statistical analysis included both Wilcoxon rank-sum and one-way ANOVA analysis. Results were considered significant at the 0.5% critical level ($p < 0.005$) applying the Bonferroni statistical correction for multiple comparisons. Results: For the entire cohort of 518 patients, only nausea at baseline was found to significantly correlate with a pain response to radiation at month 3. No other symptoms at baseline were found to predict a pain response to radiation at months 1, 2 or 3. Conclusion: There are no ESAS symptoms that can accurately predict a patient's pain response to radiation. Patients who are symptomatic from their bone metastases should be treated with palliative radiotherapy irrespective of their baseline ESAS symptoms.

Chapter VII - The purpose of this chapter was to assess pain and other common symptoms using the Edmonton System Assessment scale (ESAS) in patients with bone metastases following palliative radiotherapy. Methods: All patients with bone metastases treated with palliative radiotherapy were followed at baseline, then 1, 2, 4, 8 and 12 weeks after radiotherapy with ESAS. This scale includes pain, tiredness, nausea, depression, anxiety, drowsiness, appetite, sense of well being and shortness of breath. A Chi-squared test was used to search for the association between response effect and ESAS change at different weeks. To evaluate the response effect on the ESAS symptoms over time, a general linear mixed model was performed. Results: For the entire cohort of 518 patients, pain, anxiety, appetite, drowsiness and overall sense of well being significantly improved from baseline to last follow-up. Tiredness was the only symptom which showed worsening following palliative radiation in all patients. When looking at responders and non-responders with respect to pain, the greatest number of symptoms with a significant difference between the two groups occurred at week 12. Also when comparing the significant differences between responder and non-responders from week 1 to 12 inclusive, all ESAS symptoms were significantly better in responders with the exception of shortness of breath. Conclusions: Palliative radiotherapy not only decreased pain at the radiated site in patients with bone metastases, but also improved many other symptoms in ESAS in conjunction with other systemic therapies.

Chapter VIII - Pain flare following palliative radiotherapy (RT) for painful bone metastases is well-recognized with incidence rates of 2-44% reported in the literature. Objective was to investigate the impact of pain flare on patients with bone metastases treated with external beam RT. Methods: A five-item 'Pain Flare Qualitative Questionnaire' was developed to assess the psychological and functional impacts of the pain flare phenomenon. Results: Thirteen patients with pain flare completed the interview. There were three males and 10 females. The median age was 59 years (range: 48-89). The majority of participants had primary breast (9/13) or prostate cancer (2/13). Pain flare severely impacted patients' functional activity and carried resulted in negative mood and isolation from family and friends due to unbearable pain. Breakthrough pain medications were not adequate to control the pain increase in more than three quarters of the interviewed patients. Prophylactic medication was preferred as opposed to management with breakthrough analgesia. Although patients felt the RT was worthwhile, there was hesitation to repeat the treatment if necessary due to the previously experienced flare effect. Conclusions: Pain flare is a common side effect following palliative RT for painful bone metastases. Based on our patient interviews, this even was debilitating and worrisome. Patients should be informed of this potential side effect and health care professionals should ensure patients are equipped with sufficient analgesia to manage this increase in metastatic bone pain. However, prevention of the pain flare as opposed to management with breakthrough pain medications was preferable in this study.

Chapter IX - The purpose of this chapter was to explore optimal definitions for partial response and pain progression in patients receiving palliative radiotherapy (RT) for painful bone metastases. Methods: Patients referred to the Rapid Response Radiotherapy Program (RRRP) for palliative RT from May 2003 to November 2007 were evaluated. The Brief Pain Inventory (BPI) evaluates worst, current, and average pain, as well as seven items of functional interference on an 11-point (0-10) numeric scale. The BPI was administered at baseline, 1- and 2-months following RT for all patients. Analgesic intake was collected and converted into an oral morphine equivalent dose (OMED). The total sum score of the BPI items was calculated at baseline and at subsequent follow-ups. The follow-up sum score was subtracted from the baseline sum score to determine the difference in the BPI sum score. Various cut-points for difference in worst pain score and percent change in analgesic intake were determined using multivariate analysis of variance (MANOVA). Results: A total of 400 patients were evaluated, 235 males and 165 females, with a median age of 68 years (range: 30-91). The median Karnofsky Performance Status (KPS) was 70 (range: 30-90). At baseline, the mean worst pain score and OMED were 7.4 and 102mg/day respectively. Worst pain scores significantly decreased at the 1- and 2-month follow-up. Thirteen statistically significant and clinically relevant cut-points were identified in patients with BPI improvement or deterioration at 1- and 2-month follow-up.

Conclusion: The present study was a preliminary analysis and further investigation is required to validate our initial findings.

Chapter X - Postoperative radiation therapy has been routinely administered following the orthopedic stabilization of impending and pathological fractures due to metastatic bone disease. There have been no randomized studies conducted to date to verify the benefits of this practice. Townsend et al (1,2) retrospectively reviewed the benefits of postoperative radiation therapy in 60 patients with pathological or impending pathologic fracture after 64 orthopedic stabilization procedures. They compared the outcomes of 35 patients treated with adjuvant postoperative radiation therapy versus 29 patients treated with surgery alone. The delivery of post-op radiation therapy resulted in more patients regaining normal use of their extremity (with or without pain) and fewer reoperations to the same site (1,2). This supports the benefits of postoperative radiation therapy in this setting. Unless patients have very limited survival, we recommend the referral of patients after the orthopedic stabilization for a radiation oncology consult.

Kyphoplasty, vertebroplasty and cementoplasty have gained popularity as minimally invasive surgical procedures in patients with bone metastases. Some patients have been treated with these procedures alone. There have been few comparative studies addressing the benefits of adjuvant post procedure radiation therapy. Gerszten et al (3) did report using a combined kyphoplasty and spinal radiosurgery treatment in 26 patients with histologically confirmed pathological fractures, and an improvement in pain was seen in 24 patients. We encourage more prospective or retrospective research in this expanding area. Until then, extrapolating the evidence of benefits of adjuvant postoperative radiation therapy from the one retrospective study following the open orthopedic stabilization, we recommend patients likewise be treated with post procedure radiation therapy after kyphoplasty, vertebroplasty, or cementoplasty, unless they have received prior radiation to that site.

Chapter XI - Recent advances in effective systemic treatment and supportive care have resulted in an improved prognosis for patients with bone metastases. As patients are living with their metastatic bone disease for longer, skeletal related events (SREs) are of increasing concern. An SRE is defined as one of the following: the need for palliative surgery or radiation therapy (RT) for pain relief or stabilization of an osseous lesion, pathological fracture, spinal cord compression (SCC), or hypercalcaemia. Given that the occurrence of an SRE is associated with a worsening patient mortality, successful management of bone metastases is essential for not only reducing skeletal complications and maximizing patient quality of life (QOL), but also for improved survival.

Chapter XII - Advanced cancer patients often present with multiple concurrent symptoms that may have synergistic effect on patient morbidity. Previous research in oncology has suggested that certain symptoms tend to occur together, stay relatively stable over time, and remain relatively independent of other symptoms, with or without a shared etiology. Research on the co-management of symptoms through the analysis of symptom clusters can improve palliative care in oncology. This literature review analyzes symptom cluster studies in metastatic cancer. Common advanced cancer symptoms are discussed to explore their relationship within a cluster. Methods: A literature search was conducted to identify studies on symptom clusters in advanced cancer. Additionally, studies analyzing conceptual issues, statistical modelling and physiological mechanisms of symptoms common to advance cancer were examined. Results: The literature review identified 11 relevant studies published between 1997 and 2008. Eight studies focussed on metastatic cancer while three studies investigated symptom clusters in oncology patients representing various disease stages. Discussion: Investigation of symptom clusters is complicated and is influenced by several conceptual, methodological and patient related factors. Studies reviewed differed in their definitions of symptom clusters, types of assessment questionnaires and statistical analyses.

Further research to explore the mechanisms underlying symptom clusters and the stability of clusters over time will validate research on this concept.

Chapter XIII - The purpose was to validate the meaningful change in pain scores in the treatment of bone metastases. Methods: Patients with bone metastases treated with external beam radiotherapy were asked to score their 'worst' pain on a scale of 0-10 before treatment (baseline), daily during treatment and for 10 days after completion of external beam radiation. Patients were also asked to indicate if their pain at the time of follow up was "worse", "the same", or "better" when compared to the pre-treatment level. The change in pain score was accompanied with patient perception. Results: One hundred and seventy-eight patients were evaluated in this study. There were 82 male and 96 female patients with the median age of 65.5 years. A total of 1431 pain scorings were obtained. Patients perceived an improvement in pain when their self-reported pain score decreased by at least two points. Conclusion: Our current study validates the previous finding of meaningful change in pain score as reduction of patient self reported pain score by at least two points. This finding of the meaningful change in pain scores supports the investigation-defined partial response in clinical trials and the international consensus endpoints.

Chapter XIV - The purpose of this chapter was to review the coordinated, multidisciplinary approach to the management and care of cancer patients with metastatic bone disease at the one-stop bone metastases clinic (BMC) at the Odette Cancer Centre. Patients with symptomatic bone metastases are referred to the BMC and assessed by a team consisting of specialists in various disciplines such as interventional radiology, orthopedic surgery, palliative medicine, and radiation oncology. At initial consultation, patient demographics, reasons for referral, and case disposition were recorded. From June 2006 to December 2008, a total of 254 patients with bone metastases were seen at the BMC. The median age was 64 years (range 29-94) and median KPS score was 70 (range 10-100). The majority of patients arrived from home (85%), while 5% of patients came from a hospital. Approximately 16% of patients had 2 or more reasons for referral, yielding a total of 295 reasons. Bone pain was the main reason for referral (69%), followed by a pathological fracture (10%) and impending fracture (8%). Out of 254 patients, only 240 case dispositions were recorded, with 3 patients receiving 2 treatment recommendations. Almost a third of patients (28%) received palliative radiation, 20% needed further investigation and/or imaging, 17% were referred to other support /specialist services such as palliative care or physiotherapy, and 15% of patients were offered surgery. A co-ordinated multidisciplinary clinic is useful in managing symptomatic bone metastases in cancer patients.

Chapter XV - To examine if there is a gender difference in Edmonton Symptom Assessment System (ESAS) symptoms in patients with advanced cancer. Methods: Consecutive advanced cancer patients referred for outpatient palliative radiotherapy at the Rapid Response Radiotherapy Program (RRRP) completed the ESAS prior to radiation treatment. Baseline demographics were obtained for each patient. Correlation between gender, demographics, and the ESAS items was calculated using univariate logistic regression analysis. Results: A total of 1,107 patients were referred to RRRP from January 1999 to January 2002 and July 2007 to October 2008. There were 601 (54%) male and 506 (46%) female patients. The median age was 69 years (range 21 – 95). Males were older (male median age=70 years; female median age=66 years; $p<0.0001$). The most common primary cancer sites were lung (32%), breast (22%), and prostate (21%). Females reported significantly higher mean scores (± SD) for tiredness (5.1 ± 3.0 versus 4.7 ± 3.0, p=0.027), nausea (1.6 ± 2.6 versus 1.1 ± 2.1, p=0.0004) and anxiety (3.4 ± 3.2 versus 2.7 ± 3.0, p=0.0017). Conclusions: There is a gender difference in certain symptom distress scores in patients with advanced cancer. Our findings should be validated in future studies.

Chapter XVI - To compare the clinician predicted survival (CPS) with the actual survival (AS) of patients with advanced cancer we asked participants to estimate the median survival as well as the upper and lower range of expected survival in whole months from the time of referral to the outpatient radiotherapy clinic for five real cases presented in the survey. Secondly, the participants were asked to rank the five most important prognostic factors they considered in answering the previous questions. Finally they were asked to provide some basic information concerning time spent in their field of expertise so one could compare and contrast the survival estimates according to different disciplines, and according to their years of experience. Results: The response rates to the survey from physicians, nurses and radiation therapists were 50%, 53% and 59% respectively. In general, the survival prediction from all disciplines was not accurate. The predictions tended to be optimistic in patients with short-lived survival (= 6 months) and pessimistic in patients with longer survival (= 9 months). There did not appear to be significant differences in the direction of survival prediction among the three disciplines. The accuracy of survival prediction did not depend on the experience of the health care professionals. Conclusions: Survival predictions are important, but, given the poor predictions of the clinicians, it is necessary to develop better predictive models for survival using clinical parameters rather than relying on intuition and clinical judgment alone.

Chapter XVII - The purpose of this chapter was to investigate the potential practice of referral to non-radiation oncology health care professions in patients with advanced cancer. Methods: Patients referred to the Rapid Response Radiotherapy Program (RRRP) for palliative radiotherapy between July 2007 and October 2008 were evaluated. Basic demographic information was collected for all patients including age, primary cancer site and Karnofsky Performance Status (KPS). The Edmonton Symptom Assessment System (ESAS) was completed by all patients prior to consultation with the health care team. The ESAS evaluates the intensity of nine symptoms on a scale of zero (minimum distress) to ten (maximum distress). As part of the analysis, the numeric scale was converted into a categorical scale of none (score 0), mild (score 1-4), moderate (score 5-6) and severe (score 7-10). Patients with moderate to severe pain, lack of appetite, anxiety or depression were identified as potential referrals to other health care professionals for the purpose of symptom management. Results: Approximately 50% of patients reported moderate to severe pain and lack of appetite, and would need referral for symptom management. About 30% experienced moderate to severe anxiety or depression, and would need to be referred for psychosocial intervention. Conclusion: Cancer symptoms are complex and a multidisciplinary approach should be taken to provide timely symptom management for palliative patients. This may pose a burden to our existing health care system.

Chapter XVIII - The Palliative Performance Scale (PPS) was developed in 1996 to modernize the Karnofsky Performance Scale (KPS), an established tool for measurement of patient performance status. Although the reliability of the KPS is well established, there has been little research done on the reliability of the PPS, despite its wide use in Canada. Furthermore, only limited research has been done correlating the PPS with other performance status tools such as the KPS. Purpose: To examine the correlation between the KPS and the PPS in patients with advanced cancer. Methods: KPS and PPS were recorded for 421 patients seen in the Rapid Response Radiotherapy Program (RRRP) at the Odette Cancer Centre in Toronto, Ontario, between July 2007 and March 2008. KPS and PPS scores of patients were then examined using the Pearson correlation. This study was approved by the research ethics board at Sunnybrook Health Sciences Centre. Results: Good overall correlation was observed between KPS and PPS of the patients enrolled in this study ($r = 0.87$). The correlation between KPS and PPS was higher when the performance status of the patient fell within the middle portion of the scales at 50-80 ($r>0.5$; $p< 0.05$). Conclusion: PPS showed good correlation with the well-established KPS and thus is a reliable measure of patient performance status.

Chapter XIX - Patient morbidity from metastatic spinal cord compression (MSCC) includes back pain, paralysis/paresis, limb weakness, sensory loss, and bowel/bladder sphincter compromise. The goal of treatment with either surgery radiation or combined treatment is to improve the patient's quality of life (QOL) through palliation of pain and neurological recovery. QOL measures are important endpoints which are not well developed and infrequently measured. Objective: To identify clinical studies for patients with MSCC where QOL has been reported as either a primary or secondary endpoint. Furthermore, our aim was to report the specific measurement tools employed to capture QOL. Methods: A systematic literature review was conducted using the Ovid MEDLINE(R) 1950 to October 2008 database, Ovid Health and Psychosocial Instruments 1985 to October 2007 database, and EMBASE(R) 1980 to October 2008. Results: Five studies were identified. Two of the five (40%) studies employed the Schedule for Evaluation of Individualized Quality of Life (SEIQoL-DW) tool to measure QOL. The Short Form 36 (SF36) Health Survey Questionnaire, the Pediatric Quality of Life Inventory (PedsQL) 4.0 Generic Core scale, and the Functional Assessment of Cancer Therapy (FACT-G) scales were generic QOL investigation tools that were used in the remaining three studies. Conclusions: Amongst the five studies that defined QOL as an endpoint, there was no consistency in the measure used. There appears to be no specific QOL survey tool for the MSCC population. Therefore, we identify the need to develop a tool specific for this population in order to generate meaningful data for future trials.

Chapter XX - Clinical trials in palliative care settings require reliable and brief quality-of-life (QOL) assessment tools in order to obtain valid results with minimal burden on participants. Traditionally, patients with bone metastases in clinical trials have completed general QOL instruments, which did not cover the key issues pertinent for this specific population. The EORTC QLQ-BM22 was developed to supplement the EORTC QLQ-C30 core questionnaire as a bone metastases specific qualify-of-life instrument with cross-culture relevance. Methods: One hundred and fourteen patients at the Odette Cancer Centre and Princess Margaret Hospital were enrolled. Patients completed the EORTC QLQ-BM22 questionnaire in person at baseline during their clinic appointment, and completed the follow-up BM22 questionnaire one week later by telephone. A follow-up report was completed at the time of the one week follow-up to record any changes in clinical conditions and/or treatments. Results: Employing a 95% confidence interval, an intraclass correlation coefficient (ICC) was used to assess agreement between the baseline and follow-up responses for each BM22 item. The ICC values (median = 0.80; range of 0.55-0.89) for the 22 items revealed 'moderate' (2 items), 'good' (10 items), and 'very good' (10 items) reliability. Conclusion: Based on the overall consistent agreement between the baseline and follow-up interview results, the EORTC QLQ-BM22 appears to be a reliable instrument for cancer patients with bone metastases.

Chapter XXI - The purpose of this chapter was to test the reliability of patient perceptions in important bone metastases quality of life (QOL) items. A secondary objective was to determine whether changes in disease progression or changes in treatment affected the reliability of their responses. Methods: Twenty seven patients were asked to complete the EORTC – QLQ BM61 Bone Metastases Module upon visiting the Odette Cancer Centre on two occasions between 2005 and 2008. Patients were asked to complete 61 items assessing quality of life, ranking each item on a scale of 1 to 4 based on their own experience, then indicating whether they would recommend inclusion on the final questionnaire for each item. Basic demographic information was collected from each patient on first and re-approaches, as well as information regarding patients' condition and treatment regimens. New complications and changes in therapies were recorded. Results: Patient perception of the important bone metastases QOL issues was overall reliable over time, but was found to be related to changes in treatment and complications of disease. Conclusion: The finding should be kept in mind when developing QOL measurement tools based on patient perceptions of generated QOL issues, and when assessing the reliability of QOL measurement tools over time.

Chapter XXII - Purpose was to shorten the 22-item bone metastases (BM22) quality of life (QOL) instrument tool for bone metastases patients with a low performance status. Methods: The BM22 was developed in patients with bone metastases from eight countries. It was divided into four scales: painful sites, pain characteristics, functional interferences, and psychosocial aspects. Differential item functioning (DIF), item response theory (IRT), and item information functions (IIFs) analyses were used to shorten the tool. A Bonferroni adjusted p-value of < 0.002 was considered statistically significant. Results: The data from four hundred and ninety four patients were analyzed in this study. There were 283 females (57%) and 211 males (43%). The median age was 62 years. The majority of patients had primary breast (46%), prostate (22%), or lung (12%) cancer. No significant DIF was found between translations of the questionnaire (62 patients) and the original English version (432 patients). Based on the IRT model and IIFs, eight items were removed from the original version. Both the shortened 14-item and the original 22-item versions predicted four scales with excellent agreement. Demographic group comparisons yielded the same conclusions on both the shortened and original versions with little or no loss of measurement efficiency. Conclusion: The BM22 can be condensed to 14 items, which may ease patient burden in completing baseline and follow-up quality of life assessments in future clinical trials.

Chapter XXIII - The spinal column is the most frequent site for skeletal metastases. Complications from spinal metastases include pain, neurological deficits, and mechanical instability – all of which may require treatment. Upper cervical metastases are rare when compared to its spinal counterparts, however when they do occur, because of anatomic characteristics of that region, instability or pathological fractures may be perceived as life-threatening. Although radiotherapy is considered the standard treatment for spinal metastases, it has a delayed effect on pain, and is not able to treat any mechanical instability a patient may have. We report a case where a breast cancer patient required surgical stabilization due to a severely destructive lesion in the upper cervical region.

Chapter XXIV - Approximately 33% of patients with renal cell cancer develop bone metastases, most of which tend to be osteolytic in nature. Renal cell cancer is known to have a limited response to chemotherapy and radiation. In the present study, we describe a patient with renal cell cancer suffering from painful bone metastases in the left humerus. Despite surgical fixation and repeated palliative radiotherapy, the disease progressed leading to intractable pain. With no further palliative systemic, orthopedic or radiation treatments to offer as a means of pain relief, a simple brace was given to the patient. Fortunately, such bracing provided satisfactory symptom relief.

Chapter XXV - We present a case of a 45 year-old premenopausal patient with breast cancer who developed multiple sites of bone metastases. She presented with severe pain in her right femur and hip with inability to weight-bear. Imaging demonstrated extensive lytic destruction of the femoral neck and acetabulum. A combined approach with right hip hemiarthroplasty to treat the high risk proximal femoral lesion, cementoplasty to stabilize the acetabular lesion and palliative radiation was used. The patient suffered minimal procedural morbidity and was discharged after a 2 day inpatient stay. She had significant pain relief and rapidly regained functional independence with full weight bearing.

Chapter XXVI - Metastatic disease to the bone is a common manifestation of breast cancer. A skeletally related event (SRE) may occur in up to two-thirds of patients with bone metastases. An SRE may include pathological fractures, severe pain, hypercalcemia, spinal cord compression, need for surgery and radiation treatment. This case report highlights the management for an impending pathological fracture that most frequently presents in the femur, a weight-bearing area. This case study presents a patient with an osteolytic lesion within the intertrochantic region of the right femur. She was offered prophylactic fixation of the right hip and femur and post-operative radiotherapy, but she refused surgical intervention. Given the heightened concern for an impending pathological fracture, we managed her using radiotherapy with Clodronate, a bisphosphonate to stabilize and promote bone growth in the metastatic area. Based on our case study, we confirm radiotherapy in addition to bisphophonates may help to stabilize an osteolytic impending fracture from breast histology if patient is not a surgical candidate or refuses surgery if offered.

Chapters XXVIII-XXX contain acknowledgments, a description of the editors of this book, and information about the Health and Human Develoment series.

In: Advanced Cancer. Pain and Quality of Life
Editors: E. Chow, J. Merrick, pp. 1
ISBN: 978-1-61668-207-1
© 2010 Nova Science Publishers, Inc.

Foreword

With advances in systemic therapy and supportive care, survival of patients with metastatic cancer has steadily improved over the past two decades. Optimal symptom management of these patients has thus become particularly important.

Quality of life research in this field, specifically qualitative and quantitative data that can drive evidence-based practice in palliative care however has remained in infancy. Granting agencies have only recently begun to increase resource allocation to fund palliative research.

The Odette Cancer Centre, the comprehensive cancer program of Sunnybrook Health Sciences Centre is a leading regional cancer centre in Toronto, Ontario, Canada. It is the sixth largest cancer centre in North America in terms of number of new cancer patients seen per year. The Department of Radiation Oncology at Sunnybrook is an academic unit fully affiliated with the University of Toronto. Palliative radiotherapy is one of the key research foci in the Department of Radiation Oncology.

Research in patients with advanced cancer is always challenging due to their illness and death resulting in high attrition rates. Palliative research has to be dynamic and flexible yet maintaining a high level of scientific vigor. The authors of this book are to be congratulated for their efforts in advancing palliative cancer research.

Professor C Shun Wong, MD, FRCPC
Professor, Department of Radiation Oncology, University of Toronto
Professor, Department of Medical Biophysics, University of Toronto
Head, Radiation Treatment Program, Odette Cancer
Chief, Department of Radiation Oncology, Sunnybrook Health Sciences Centre
Senior Scientist, Cell and Molecular Biology, Sunnybrook Health Sciences Centre
Odette Cancer Centre
2075 Bayview Avenue
Toronto, Ontario, Canada
Email: shun.wong@sunnybrook.ca
Website: http://www.dro.facmed.utoronto.ca/inab/fac/oncologists/wong.htm

In: Advanced Cancer. Pain and Quality of Life
Editors: E. Chow, J. Merrick, pp. 3-7
ISBN: 978-1-61668-207-1
© 2010 Nova Science Publishers, Inc.

Introduction

Advanced Cancer Pain and Quality of Life

Edward Chow, MBBS and Joav Merrick, MD, MMedSc, DMSc [*]

Department of Radiation Oncology, Odette Cancer Centre, Sunnybrook Health Sciences Centre, University of Toronto, Toronto, Ontario, Canada, National Institute of Child Health and Human Development, Office of the Medical Director, Division for Mental Retardation, Ministry of Social Affairs, Jerusalem and Kentucky Children's Hospital, University of Kentucky, Lexington, United States of America

An estimated 166,400 new cases of cancer will occur in Canada in 2008 (1). Bone metastases unfortunately remain a common site of recurrence (2), with breast and prostate cancer patients representing a substantial proportion of this population (3).

Metastatic bone disease is associated with significant morbidity and mortality. Pain is experienced by up to two thirds of patients (4-7). The prognosis for patients with bone metastases is highly influenced by tumor type, performance status, and the presence of extraosseous disease (2,8-10). The median survival has been significantly longer in breast cancer patients with a first relapse in the axial skeleton (24 months) versus patients with initial relapse in the liver (3 months) (2). Survival after diagnosis of bone metastases is influenced by the subsequent development of extraosseous metastatic sites: 1.6 years versus 2.1 years in patients with bone-only disease (2).

[*] Correspondence: Edward Chow MBBS, PhD, FRCPC, Department of Radiation Oncology, Odette Cancer Centre, Sunnybrook Health Sciences Centre, 2075 Bayview Ave, Toronto, Ontario, Canada M4N 3M5. E-mail: Edward.Chow@sunnybrook.ca

Skeletal related events

Advances in effective systemic treatment and supportive care have resulted in an improved prognosis for patients with bone metastases (11-13). As patients are living with their metastatic bone disease for longer, skeletal related events (SREs) are of increasing concern. An SRE is defined as one of the following: the need for palliative surgery or radiation therapy (RT) for pain relief or stabilization of an osseous lesion, pathological fracture, spinal cord compression (SCC), or hypercalcaemia.Since an SRE is associated with a worsening patient mortality (11,14-18), successful management of bone metastases is essential for not only reducing skeletal complications and maximizing patient quality of life (QOL), but also for improved survival.

However, reported incidences of SREs in the literature are often cited in clinical trial data from bisphosphonate studies (11). We therefore decided to explore SRE data in a large population of patients with bone metastases enrolled in an international study evaluating relevant quality of life (QOL) issues (19).

Our analysis of the prevalence of SREs was conducted in 365 Canadian and Australian patients with bone metastases. Patients were accrued from medical oncology clinics (61%), radiation oncology clinics (32%), inpatient units (5%), or in a pain/symptom management clinic (2%). Of the 365 patients the overall incidence of SREs was 244/365 (67%). At the time of interview, 52% of patients reported one, 10% reported two, and 4% reported three SREs. In this cohort of patients, the types of SRE were palliative RT (71%), pathological fracture (8%), nerve root/SCC (6%), need for surgery (5%), and hypercalcaemia (5%).

Given the predominance of SREs in this study, a number of management questions still remain pertaining to optimal time of initiation, duration, and type of bisphosphonate therapy. In the breast cancer setting, the American Society for Clinical Oncology (ASCO) practice guidelines (20) advises the initiation of bisphosphonates in women with obvious lytic disease on plain radiographs; or with an abnormal bone scan, normal radiographs but a CT or MRI scan showing bone destruction. Similarly in multiple myeloma, bisphosphonate therapy is introduced following radiographic evidence of lytic destruction to the bone cortex. In prostate cancer patients with significant bone loss, bisphosphonate therapy should be strongly considered regardless of hormonal status or systemic disease (15). Indications for bisphosphonate use in lung cancer remain controversial with respect to presentation of a clinically meaningful benefit when prognosis is generally limited (21).

Unanswered questions

Despite these recommendations, questions remain unanswered: a) what bisphosphonate regimen (agent, dose, frequency, and duration) is best; b) can integration of bisphosphonates in patients without documented bone metastases prevent future osseous involvement; c) how can their use be integrated with other bone-metastases specific treatments; d) and what is the cost-benefit evaluation in the palliative literature in terms of patient transportation to and from the cancer centre, toxicity, compliance, and cost-effectiveness. What is clear is that despite widespread use of BPs SREs remain common and we therefore need new strategies to optimize patient management (22-25).

Effective prevention of SREs in patients with bone metastases is essential to preservation of functioning and maintenance of QOL. While RT is effective for localized pain relief and remineralization of osseous lesions, systemic bisphosphonate therapy may inhibit tumor cell adhesion to bone, tumor growth, angiogenesis (26), and provide pain relief (27). Integration of bisphosphonate and RT may have a synergistic effect on metastatic bone lesions and potentially reduce the risk of SREs when used in combination (26). Moreover, investigation of targeted therapies may have more pronounced effect on management of metastatic bone disease.

Pain remains an agonizing symptom in patients with advanced cancer and continues to be under-treated globally. As the trend is towards outpatient palliative care, improving cancer pain management in the home is vitally important and psychodynamic. Pain management involves many health care disciplines. The awareness of the nurses in cancer pain, the good working relationships between radiation oncologists and hospice professionals are crucial for optimal pain management.

Other than pain, patients with advanced cancer often present with multiple symptoms. Symptom clusters and gender difference need to be considered too. Patients and their family members often ask 'How long do I have to live?' They are often depressed and malnourished potentially requiring the advice from our psychosocial experts and dieticians. Spinal cord compression remains devastating to patients with terminal illness and is an emergency in radiation oncology. Timely management is crucial for the outcomes. Accurate prediction of patient survival, projected referral for health care services, quality of life in patients with spinal cord compression, appropriate use of a performance tool are important in end of life care. This book highlights some of the latest research in the area of pain in patients with advanced cancer and their quality of life.

References

[1] Canadian Cancer Society. Canadian Cancer Statistics 2008. 17 August 2008. Retrieved 12 October 2008 from <http://www.cancer.ca/Canada-wide/About%20cancer/Cancer%20statistics/Canadian%20Cancer%20Statistics.aspx?sc_lang=en>.

[2] Coleman RE. Clinical features of metastatic bone disease and risk of skeletal morbidity. Clin Cancer Res 2006;12(20 Suppl):6243-49.

[3] Coleman RE. Skeletal complications of malignancy. Cancer 1997;80(8 Suppl):1588-94.

[4] Mercadante S. Malignant bone pain: pathophysiology and treatment. Pain 1997;69(12):1-18.

[5] Janjan N. Bone metastases: approaches to management. Semin Oncol 2001;28(4 Suppl 11):28-34.

[6] Serafini AN. Therapy of metastatic bone pain. J Nucl Med 2001;42:895-906.

[7] Gralow J, Tripathy D. Managing metastatic bone pain: The role of bisphosphonates. J Pain Symp Manag 2007;33(4)462-72.

[8] Hansen BH, Keller J, Laitinen M, et al. Scandinavian Sarcoma Group Skeletal Metastasis Register. Survival after surgery for bone metastases in the pelvis and extremities. Acta Orthop Scand 2004;75:11-5.

[9] Katagiri H, Takahashi M, Wakai K, et al. Prognostic factors and a scoring system for patients with skeletal metastasis. J Bone Joint Surg Br 2005;87:698-703.

[10] van der Linden YM, Dijkstra SP, Vonk EJ, et al. Dutch Bone Metastasis Study Group. Prediction of survival in patients with metastases in the spinal column: results based on a randomized trial of radiotherapy. Cancer 2005;103:320-8.

[11] Lipton A. Treatment of bone metastases and bone pain with bisphosphonates. Supp Canc Ther 2007;4(2):92-100.

[12] Lipton A, Cook RJ, Major P, et al. Zoledronic acid and survival in breast cancer patients with bone metastases and elevated markers of osteoclast activity. Oncologist 2007;12:1035-43.

[13] Coleman RE. Metastatic bone disease: Clinical features, pathophysiology and treatment strategies. Cancer Treat Rev 2001;27:165-76.

[14] Hei YJ, Saad F, Coleman RE et al. Fractures negatively affect survival in patients with bone metastases from breast cancer [Abstract 6036]. 28th Annual San Antonio Breast Cancer Symposium; December 8-11, 2005.

[15] Saad F, Gleason D, Murray R, et al. Zoledronic acid provides long term reductions in skeletal morbidity for men with prostate cancer and bone metastases [Abstract 149]. American Society for Clinical Oncology Prostate Cancer Symposium; February 24-26, 2006.

[16] Theriault RL, Lipton A, Hortobagyi GN, et al. Pamidronate reduces skeletal morbidity in women with advanced breast cancer and lytic bone lesions: a randomized, placebo-controlled trial. Protocol 18 Aredia Breast Cancer Study Group. J Clin Oncol 1999;17:846–54.

[17] Oefelein MG, Ricchuti V, Conrad W, et al. Skeletal fractures negatively correlate with overall survival in men with prostate cancer. J Urol 2002;168:1005-7.

[18] Sugiura H, Yamada K, Sugiura T, Hida T, Mitsudomi T. Predictors of survival in patients with bone metastasis of lung cancer. Clin Orthop Relat Res 2008;466:729-36.

[19] Chow E, Hird A, Velikova G, et al. on behalf of the EORTC Quality of Life Group. Development of an EORTC disease-specific quality of life questionnaire module for patients with bone metastases. Eur J Cancer 2008 [e-pub ahead of print].

[20] Hillner BE, Ingle JN, Chlebowski RT, et al. American Society of Clinical Oncology 2003 update on the role of bisphosphonates and bone health issues in women with breast cancer. J Clin Oncol 2003;21(21):4042-57.

[21] Saba N, Khuri F. The role of bisphosphonates in the management of advanced cancer with a focus on non-small-cell lung cancer. Oncology 2005;68:18-22.

[22] Valdivielso JM, Fernandez E. Vitamin D receptor polymorphisms and diseases. Clinica Chimica Acta 2006;371(1-2):1-12.

[23] Simmons C, Ooi W, Dranitsaris G, et al. Phase II study of Vitamin D (10, 000 IU daily) supplementation in bisphosphonate-treated breast cancer patients with bone metastases [Abstract 176]. Breast Cancer Symposium; September 5-7, 2008.

[24] Masuda S, Jones G. Promise of vitamin D analogues in the treatment of hyperproliferative conditions. Mol Cancer Ther 2006;5(4):797–808.

[25] Lipton A, de Boer RH, Figueroa J, et al. Phase II study of denosumab in breast cancer patients with bone metastases naïve to intravenous bisphosphonate therapy: Extended efficacy and safety analysis [Abstract 266]. Breast Cancer Symposium; September 7-8, 2007.

[26] Ural AU, Avcu F, Baran Y. Bisphosphonate treatment and radiotherapy in metastatic breast cancer. Med Oncol 2008;25:350-5.

[27] Wong RKS, Wiffen PJ. Bisphosphonates for the relief of pain secondary to bone metastases. Cochrane Database Syst Rev 2002(2):002068.

Section One: Pain Management

In: Advanced Cancer. Pain and Quality of Life
Editors: E. Chow, J. Merrick, pp. 11-17
ISBN: 978-1-61668-207-1
© 2010 Nova Science Publishers, Inc.

Chapter I

Psychodynamic Pain Management for Cancer Patients

Frederick B. Levenson, MA, PhD, LP[1], Micah D. Levenson, LMSW[1], Søren Ventegodt, MD, MMedSci, EU-MSc-CAM[*2,3,4,5,6] and Joav Merrick, MD, MMedSci, DMSc[6,7,8,9]

[1]Private practice, Manhattan, New York, United States of America
[2]Quality of Life Research Center, Copenhagen, Denmark
[3]Research Clinic for Holistic Medicine and
[4]Nordic School of Holistic Medicine, Copenhagen, Denmark
[5]Scandinavian Foundation for Holistic Medicine, Sandvika, Norway and
[6]Interuniversity College, Graz, Austria
[7]National Institute of Child Health and Human Development
[8]Office of the Medical Director, Division for Mental Retardation, Ministry of Social Affairs, Jerusalem, Israel and
[9]Kentucky Children's Hospital, University of Kentucky, Lexington, United States

The use of psychodynamic-oriented techniques has successfully been used to manage pain in 75 cancer patients by the use of psychodynamic principles. Pain is a subjective phenomenon that varies much from patient to patient with the same type and stage of cancer. This well-known variance is from a depth-psychological perspective explained by pain being a negative interpretation of inner reality caused by the patients' sub-conscious conflicts. Therefore much pain can be relieved, when these conflicts are resolved in the therapy, which happens when the patient bonds to the therapist and in an intimate therapeutic relationship regain deeper insight in self and life, and a positive and relaxed attitude. The intimacy with the patient was reached by selective therapeutic touch, i.e. hugs, in a holistic philosophical framework, making the intervention a type of

* Correspondence: Søren Ventegodt, MD, MMedSci, EU-MSc-CAM, Director, Quality of Life Research Center, Classensgade 11C, 1 sal, DK-2100 Copenhagen O, Denmark. Tel: +45-33-141113; Fax: +45-33-141123; E-mail: ventegodt@livskvalitet.org

clinical holistic medicine. The basic principle was that of "clinical medicine" and healing by supported self-exploration. Patients in acute or chronic states appeared to be able to utilize the intervention for existential healing (what Antonovsky called "salutogenesis") only when the therapeutic relationship was close and positive. Their resistance to a positive transference was a defense that could be resolved with reflective techniques thereby facilitating the use of these interventions. The hierarchy of degree of pain relief seemed to be 1) chemical side effects of medication being coupled with a positive suggestions of pain relief (placebo), 2) Counterfocus of irritations and pain within the soma to reduce the intensity of the actual pain site (integration of inner conflicts), 3) Directed aggressive imagery to have the patient angry at his or her pain (self-expression) and 4) Relaxation and escape imagery (letting go of tensions and negative ideas and attitudes). Estimated from the case stories one in two was helped (NNT=2 for cancer pains).

Introduction

Psychodynamic pain management for these authors began with a realization that like beauty, pain is in the eye of the beholder. Pain can be viewed as a result of differentials of individual processing of irritation. One person's agony may be another's slight discomfort. In work with cancer patients for over thirty-five years, the first authors have witnessed many failed attempts at psychologically reducing pain (1). The superficiality of "think happy thoughts" does not serve this purpose well.

Certain techniques, which are almost always transference-based seem to achieve far better results. We will explore what has worked and what has not worked to ameliorate pain for patients suffering from allopathic medicine interventions and more rarely from the effects of neoplastic pressures. The subjects were 75 patients treated by the first author during the past 35 years.

What is pain?

From an existential perspective pain is caused by what is going against our will (2), or more philosophically put against our *purpose of life* (3-7). As our life mission is often repressed, most of us are not aware of the dynamics inside our self that causes pain. We therefore project the pain on physical organs or other structures in the material world. Pain comes in many qualities and degrees, as a consequence of the degree of responsibility the patient is able to assume, and the level of consciousness present. In principle, complete self-understanding leads to complete extinction of all pain and suffering, as already Lao Tse, Gautama Buddha and other wise men realized millennia ago. Psychodynamic psychotherapy is one road to self-exploration (8) and pain-relief now being used by many patients with chronic pain, often in combination with therapeutic touch. Pain relief in this way is highly efficient and in clinical holistic medicine (9-11) even severe pain can often be relieved in 10 or 20 sessions (12,13). In this paper we address the tools for relieving pain in psychodynamic psychotherapy without the use of therapeutic touch.

Counterfocus

The counterfocus technique began for the first author back in the 1960s. As a military recruit, he and his platoon were standing formation at rigid attention. Not even a blink was permitted. This unfortunate young man had a female of the Tabanus nigrovittatus persuasion (greenhead fly) alight to his right upper thigh. The lovely lady then proceeded to use her razor sharp mouth parts to bite through the tight fitted trousers and subsequent skin of the young recruit's leg. Reflexes overwhelmed reason and the right hand smacked the beast into insect heaven. Two rather large sergeants then smacked the young recruit just short of recruit heaven. "You are a rock; you feel nothing. Doing what you did in combat will get you and your comrades killed." The lesson was embedded forever even after the bruises healed.

The next time Tabanus nigrovittatus started munching on the first author's leg, arm, or back he picked another part of his anatomy that was in pain to focus upon. The next assault of the greenhead fly was met with a distraction to a painful canker sore on his lower front lip. The fly had her fill and the recruit avoided the wrath of his drill instructors. Previously he pictured pleasant thoughts, but this had little effect upon the pain of the bite. The Spanish moss hanging from the Magnolia tree was very pleasing to his eyes, but did nothing to adequately sooth the pain. Pleasant, soothing relaxation did little or nothing. Substitution of one lesser pain for another intense pain seemed to do the trick.

With cancer patients this author has instructed them to relax as thoroughly as possible and then move the pain to another area of the body. A left knee could be excruciating, but when pain was psychically created in the right knee a shift occurred. Pain in both seemed to abate. Willing pain away does not seem to work for most cancer patients. Relaxation seems inadequate. Shifting it to the healthy tissue merely by intense focusing on these tissues seems to have great value. The reader can experiment on oneself by focusing on one's left foot until it is uncomfortable or at least experiencing intense sensation – no need for an actual canker sore.

Relaxation and meditation as pain reducers seemed to be a logical intervention. Lamaze type breathing works for pain during childbirth so logically why not while battling cancer? The trouble is that childbirth is a miraculous moment that does not induce battle scenarios in most women. The caring, soothing intervention of the coach seems to transferentially replicate a maternal-infant bonding experience (14-18). These interventions do not place one in a psychic battleground; as a matter of fact it is just the opposite. The breathing puts the mother at a new focal point much like the canker sore for the fly bite. But does it really accomplish this as labor proceeds? For many women this counterfocus works. For many others it seems to have little or no effect on pain reduction. For a significant group, all the prior practice goes out the window as soon as labor gets intense.

For cancer patients, breathing exercises to control pain do not seem to have great efficacy. For many cancer patients breathing itself is very painful or labored at times. Letting one's mind float to a better place once breathing takes affect is, at times, impossible. Leaving the pain behind is easy for the non-sufferer to imagine, but close to impossible for the patient. It is almost comparable to telling a depressed patient to cheer up. Nonetheless, this author followed what others had reported as effective in this regard with little or no results with patients in extreme pain.

Directed anger

Helping the patient direct rage at the cancer enhances the ability to utilize a military visualization mode. The patient introjects the therapist into visualization by picturing their immune system as attacking soldiers or Marines who have some physical trait of the analyst. "All my Marines have green eyes and dark hair and they kill the cancer cells with no mercy." Patients introject the analyst on a cellular level (17,18).

Many combat veterans will report that they did heroic acts while seriously injured and felt no pain until it was over and the enemy was destroyed. Their wounds might have been devastating, but they felt no pain. This phenomenon can be harnessed by an enthusiastic analyst to help the patient. From the first author's experience the benefits, however, seem far less enduring than other techniques. To conjure up battle scenarios is not available to many patients' psyches. Getting angry at one's pain is short-term. Adreneric reactions seem to lack endurance and require impractical, frequent encouragement in combating pain. Maintaining a schedule of such aggressive imagery will help with visualization and should not ever be discouraged on the grounds that pain relief is temporary.

Medication

Perhaps the most effective pain management technique the first author has witnessed came with his first cancer patient's horrible suffering. She was a 28 year old woman suffering from a terrible metastatic breast carcinoma. Her body was riddled with cancer. The first author was called in by an oncologist to help her manage pain medication. He was fearful it would stop working, when she needed it. The risk then would be overdose. The question was never asked as to why an overdose would be bad considering her extremely negative prognosis.

After the first week of treatment, where she was obviously looking forward to contact with the therapist, the therapist asked the oncologist to switch the patient from Thorazine (used, in those days, to enhance pain medication) to Mellaril. The oncologist was asked to say that this was the therapist's idea. He cooperated. The patient was told that the new medication would tremendously relieve the pain once she experienced a metallic taste in her mouth. After two days of taking the Mellaril the metallic taste was reported. The pain almost totally disappeared. It never returned. The patient was in a positive transference and was positively suggestible (14-16).

Subsequent use of this technique showed it could be done, if the patient was in a positive transference (15,16). Even if the patient was only marginally suggestible it worked. Other drugs that induce a metallic taste were also utilized by other oncologists and this analyst. They all worked, when transferential conditions were right.

For patients who were immersed in a transference resistance or an obvious negative transference this intervention had to wait, until these dynamics were resolved (18). Even overtly skeptical patients were helped, if the therapeutic relationship was right. Medications were prescribed sometimes just for their side effect. The dosages were almost always sub-clinical, but the telltale metallic taste consistently showed up.

Taste and smell are chemically based. The physical senses of vision, audition, and the tactile sense are less primitive in theory. The chemical connects the infant to the mother. The chemical is thus the more powerful realm for the therapist to utilize for transferential purposes.

Discussion

The use of psychodynamic-oriented techniques has successfully been used to manage pain in 75 cancer patients treated by the first author over the past 35 years by the use of psychodynamic principles. Pain is a subjective phenomenon that varies much from patient to patient with the same type and stage of cancer. This well-known variance is from a depth-psychological perspective explained by pain being a negative interpretation of inner reality caused by the patient's sub-conscious conflicts. Therefore much pain can be relieved when these conflicts are resolved in the therapy, which happens when the patient bonds to the therapist and in an intimate therapeutic relationship regain deeper insight in self and life, and a positive and relaxed attitude. The intimacy with the patient was reached by selective therapeutic touch, i.e. hugs, in a holistic philosophical framework, making the intervention a type of clinical holistic medicine. The basic principle was that of "clinical medicine"and healing by supported self-exploration. Patients in acute or chronic states appear to be able to utilize the intervention for existential healing (what Antonovsky called "salutogenesis") (19,20) only when the therapeutic relationship is close and positive. Estimated from the case stories one in two was helped (NNT=2 for cancer pains).

Pain management has been shown to be successfully enhanced by the use of psychodynamic principles. Patients in acute or chronic states appeared to be able to utilize interventions, when the therapeutic relationship was positive. Their resistance to a positive transference was a defense that could be resolved with reflective techniques thereby facilitating the use of these interventions. The hierarchy of degree of pain relief seems to be 1) chemical side effects of medication being coupled with a positive suggestions (placebo) (14-16) of pain relief, 2) Counterfocus of irritations and pain within the soma to reduce the intensity of the actual pain site (integration of inner conflicts), 3) Directed aggressive imagery to have the patient angry at his or her pain (self-expression) (18) and 4) Relaxation and escape imagery (letting go of tensions and negative ideas and attitudes).

Acknowledgments

This paper is a part of the Open Source Protocol for Clinical Holistic Medicine (21). The Danish Quality of Life Survey, Quality of Life Research Center and the Research Clinic for Holistic Medicine, Copenhagen, was from 1987 till today supported by grants from the 1991 Pharmacy Foundation, the Goodwill-fonden, the JL-Foundation, E Danielsen and Wife's Foundation, Emmerick Meyer's Trust, the Frimodt-Heineken Foundation, the Hede Nielsen Family Foundation, Petrus Andersens Fond, Wholesaler CP Frederiksens Study Trust, Else and Mogens Wedell-Wedellsborg's Foundation and IMK Almene Fond. The research in quality of life and scientific complementary and holistic medicine was approved by the Copenhagen Scientific Ethical Committee under the numbers (KF)V. 100.1762-90, (KF)V. 100.2123/91, (KF)V. 01-502/93, (KF)V. 01-026/97, (KF)V. 01-162/97, (KF)V. 01-198/97, and further correspondence. We declare no conflicts of interest.

References

[1] Levenson FB. The causes and prevention of cancer. London: Sidgwick Jackson, 1985.

[2] Ventegodt S, Merrick J. Life mission theory VIII: A theory for pain. J Pain Manage 2008;1(1):5-10.

[3] Ventegodt S, Andersen NJ, Merrick J. Editorial: Five theories of human existence. ScientificWorldJournal 2003;3:1272-6.

[4] Ventegodt S. The life mission theory: A theory for a consciousness-based medicine. Int J Adolesc Med Health 2003;15(1):89-91.

[5] Ventegodt S, Andersen NJ, Merrick J. The life mission theory II: The structure of the life purpose and the ego. ScientificWorldJournal 2003;3:1277-85.

[6] Ventegodt S, Andersen NJ, Merrick J. The life mission theory V. A theory of the anti-self and explaining the evil side of man. ScientificWorldJournal 2003;3:1302-13.

[7] Ventegodt S, Flensborg-Madsen T, Andersen NJ, Merrick J. Life Mission Theory VII: Theory of existential (Antonovsky) coherence: a theory of quality of life, health and ability for use in holistic medicine. ScientificWorldJournal 2005;5:377-89.

[8] Ventegodt S, Andersen NJ, Kandel I, Merrick J. Formal errors in nonpharmaceutical medicine (CAM): Clinical medicine, mind-body medicine, body-psychotherapy, holistic medicine, clinical holistic medicine and sexology. Int J Adolesc Med Health 2009;21(2), in press.

[9] Ventegodt S, Kandel I, Merrick J. Principles of holistic medicine. Philosophy behind quality of life. Victoria, BC: Trafford, 2005.

[10] Ventegodt S, Kandel I, Merrick J. Principles of holistic medicine. Quality of life and health. New York: Hippocrates Sci Publ, 2005.

[11] Ventegodt S, Kandel I, Merrick J. Principles of holistic medicine. Global quality of life.Theory, research and methodology. New York: Hippocrates Sci Publ, 2005.

[12] Ventegodt S, Thegler S, Andreasen T, Struve F, Enevoldsen L, Bassaine L, Torp M, Merrick J. Clinical holistic medicine: Psychodynamic short-time therapy complemented with bodywork. A clinical follow-up study of 109 Patients. ScientificWorldJournal 2006;6:2220-38.

[13] Ventegodt S, Thegler S, Andreasen T, Struve F, Enevoldsen L, Bassaine L, Torp M, Merrick J. Clinical holistic medicine (mindful, short-term psychodynamic psychotherapy complemented with bodywork) in the treatment of experienced physical illness and chronic pain. ScientificWorldJournal 2007;7:310-6.

[14] Eibring E. Psychoanalysis and the dynamic psychotherapies. J Am Psychoanal Assoc 1954;2:745-70.

[15] Freud S. General introduction to psychoanalysis. New York: Liveright Publ, 1935.

[16] Greenson R. The technique and practice of psychoanalysis, Volume 1. New York: Int Univ Press, 1967.
[17] Kohut H. The analysis of the self. New York: Int Univ Press, 1971.
[18] Spotnitz H. Modern psychoanalysis of the schizophrenic patient. New York: Int Univ Press, 1954.
[19] Antonovsky A. Health, stress and coping. London: Jossey-Bass, 1985.
[20] Antonovsky A. Unravelling the mystery of health. How people manage stress and stay well. San Francisco: Jossey-Bass, 1987.
[21] Ventegodt S, Andersen NJ, Kandel I, Merrick J. The open source protocol of clinical holistic medicine. J Altern Med Res 2009;1(2), in press.

In: Advanced Cancer. Pain and Quality of Life
Editors: E. Chow, J. Merrick, pp. 19-32
ISBN: 978-1-61668-207-1
© 2010 Nova Science Publishers, Inc.

Chapter II

Improving Cancer Pain Management in the Home

April Hazard Vallerand, PhD, RN, FAAN*[*1], Susan M Hasenau, PhD, RN, NNP-BC[2] and Thomas Templin, PhD[1]

[1]Wayne State University College of Nursing, Detroit, Michigan

[2]Madonna University College of Nursing, Livonia, Michigan, United States of America

The purpose of this chapter was to determine the effect of the "Power Over Pain" intervention, a structured educational intervention for nurses, patients and caregivers managing cancer-related pain in the home. Using a longitudinal design, 232 home care nurses, 50 patients, and 46 caregivers were randomly assigned to one of four intervention groups. The nurse receiving the intervention showed significant increases in pain-related knowledge and perception of control over pain and decreases in barriers to pain control. Patients receiving the intervention demonstrated a significant decrease in barriers to pain control and trends toward decreased pain and symptom distress and increased functional status related to pain, pain management knowledge, and perception of control over pain. Caregivers in dyads whose home care nurse received the intervention had significant improvement in perception of control over pain. Results suggest that the "Power Over Pain" intervention is effective for improving cancer pain management in the home.

Introduction

For many patients with cancer, pain is a constant concern. The importance of proper pain assessment and treatment in patient care is recognized, yet studies show that actual progress in improving pain management remains slow. Numerous studies have revealed that pain tends to be underestimated and inadequately treated (1-3). Lack of education has been shown to be

* Correspondence: April Hazard Vallerand, PhD, Wayne State University College of Nursing, 5557 Cass Avenue Cohn Bldg. #364 Detroit, MI 48202 United States. E-mail: April.Vallerand@wayne.edu

a major barrier to adequate pain management (4). Additional educational programs on pain management are sorely needed. Surprisingly, few studies were found that targeted interventions for patients with cancer pain and their caregivers.

Wells and associates (4) utilized three groups in their study to determine if continued access to information after an educational intervention would improve pain control. Outcome measures in this study included knowledge and beliefs. While improvement was demonstrated, it was determined that the educational intervention itself was the cause of the improvement. Unfortunately, the sample size used (n=64) was too small for the anticipated effect size of the additional support. Miaskowski and associates (5) utilized a randomized clinical trial to test the PRO-SELF pain Control Program, developed by Dodd and colleagues (6). Outcome measures for this study were pain intensity and opioid analgesic intake. Pain intensity scores decreased significantly from baseline and the percentage of patients receiving appropriate analgesic prescriptions increased in patients receiving the intervention. Ward and colleagues (7) developed an individually tailored intervention to decrease patient-related barriers to cancer pain management. They hypothesized that patients receiving the intervention would have lower barriers scores, use more adequate analgesic medication, have lower analgesic side effect scores, have lower pain intensity scores, and experience less pain interference. In this study, although all participants experienced improvement in their pain management, no main effect for group on any of the dependent variables was found. Each of these studies used a randomized assignment and measured different outcomes. However, no study was found that measured outcomes for both patients and caregivers.

Pain is a symptom that is often managed by patients themselves or by their lay caregivers. In a review of interventions to overcome clinician- and patient-related barriers to pain management, Gunnarsdottir, Donovan, and Ward (8) found only one randomized controlled trial that aimed at patients and their caregivers. In that study, Given and colleagues (9) provided an 18-week supportive nursing intervention to decrease symptoms and found the group receiving the intervention reported fewer symptoms. Although the intervention group also reported less pain and fatigue, the differences did not reach significance. Unfortunately, the authors did not report outcomes related to the caregivers (9).

Pain-management-related education for nurses, patients, and caregivers is needed. While a number of educational programs have been presented regarding pain management, mastery of this content and its utilization in practice by nurses has not been achieved. In a study of cancer pain in a community setting, participation in an educational intervention improved physicians' and nurses' knowledge and attitudes regarding pain management but had minimal effect on the patients and caregivers (10). Bero and colleagues (11) suggested that passive dissemination of information is generally ineffective. In a systematic review of studies to provide the best evidence of effectiveness of different strategies to promote the implementation of research findings, they found that patient-mediated interventions and multifaceted interventions seem to be more effective than single interventions.

Recent changes in the delivery of healthcare services mean that numerous patients with pain, especially cancer-related pain, are being cared for in outpatient clinics or at home by family members and home care nurses rather than in inpatient settings. Because home care nurses often act as mediators between the physician and the patient and caregiver in the management of the patient's care, it is essential that they be knowledgeable about pain management (12). In order for nurses to improve their practice, especially in the area of pain management, two main factors are required: 1) nurses must be experts in pain management strategies, particularly in the area of pharmacologic options, and 2) nurses must have the communication skills to present viable options in an acceptable manner both to the physician and to the patient and/or caregiver (13). The purpose of this study was to determine the effect of the Power Over Pain intervention, a structured educational intervention directed at nurses and at patients and their caregivers on the management of pain and opioid-related side effects in home care patients with cancer. Included in the educational intervention was an emphasis on improving communication skills to advocate for needed changes in the analgesic regimen.

Our Study

To test the effectiveness of the "Power Over Pain" intervention, a longitudinal design was used. After approval was obtained from the appropriate institutional review boards, a sample of fourteen home care agencies were recruited and were randomly assigned to one of the four conditions: 1) nurses, patients, and caregivers received the intervention (NYPY), 2) nurses received the intervention; patients and caregivers did not (NYPN), 3) patients and caregivers received the intervention; nurses did not (NNPY), 4) neither nurses nor patients and caregivers received the intervention (NNPN) (see table 1). All nurses from a given agency were assigned to the same group to avoid crossover contamination. The longitudinal part of the design was different for nurses and patients/caregivers. For the primary tests of the intervention, nurse outcomes were assessed at baseline and end-of-session for both the beginning and advanced sessions (which was given 4-6 weeks after the beginning session), and at 3-months and 6-months after the advanced intervention session. Patients were assessed at 1-week (baseline), 2-weeks, 3-weeks, and 4-weeks and caregivers were assessed at 1-week (baseline) and 4-weeks. Table 2 presents a time schedule for the measurements taken for nurses, patients and caregivers. In addition to quantitative measurements, qualitative interviews were conducted with nurses, patients and caregivers. The results of this qualitative data are reported elsewhere (14, 15).

Table 1. Study Group Distribution

Study Condition	# of Agencies	# of Nurses	# of Patients	# of Caregivers
NYPY	4	49	14	14
NYPN	3	64	14	14
NNPY	3	56	12	10
NNPN	4	63	10	8

NYPY=Nurse Yes, Patient Yes; NYPN=Nurse Yes, Patient No; NNPY=Nurse No, Patient Yes; NNPN=Nurse No, Patient No (Related to receiving or not receiving the Educational Intervention)

Table 2. Schedule of Measurements Taken for Nurses, Patients, and Caregivers

	Nurse Intervention					Patient/Caregiver Intervention and Follow-up				Nurse Follow - Up	
Informant	Basic Session		2 Week Interval	Advanced Session		Week 1	Week 2	Week 3	Week 4	3 Month	6 Month
Nurse	Pre-test	Post-test		Pre-test	Post-test					*2nd qualitative interview for nurses.*	
Patient	Demo-1N PCS-1N BQ-1N KA-1N	------ PCS-2N BQ-2N KA-2N	*1st qualitative interview for nurses.*	------ PCS-3N BQ-3N KA-3N	------ PCS-4N BQ-4N KA-4N					--------- PCS-5N BQ-5N KA-5N	-------- PCS-6N BQ-6N KA-6N
	Recruit Patients (3 per nurse). *1st qualitative interview for patients*					Patient Session 1 Demo-1P PCS-1P BQ-1P PPQ-1 BPI-1 SDS-1	Patient Session 2 (Intervention Post) --------- --------- --------- --------- BPI-2 SDS-2	Patient Session 3 -------- -------- -------- -------- BPI-3 SDS-3	Patient Session 4 ---------- PCS-4P BQ-4P PPQ-4 BPI-4 SDS-4		
Patient	Recruit Caregivers (3 per Nurse) *1st qualitative interview for caregivers*					Caregiver Session 1 Demo-1C PCS-1C BQ-1C FPQ-1	Caregiver Session 2 Present for Educational Intervention	Caregiver Session 3	Caregiver Session4 PCS-4C BQ-4C FPQ-4		

Participants and setting

The home care setting was chosen because these nurses are knowledgeable in care of patients with many health problems. However, specific information regarding pain and symptom management may be lacking. Hospice nurses were excluded from this study based on the assumption that they had more training in pain and symptom management. Fourteen home care agencies were recruited to participate in the study and were randomly assigned to one of the four treatment groups defined. Two of the agencies were lost to the study during follow-up due to time constraints, leaving 12 agencies involving 232 nurses in the final sample. Nurses caring for patients with cancer pain were recruited from participating agencies to be in this study. Each nurse was asked to identify patients they cared for that met the inclusion criteria for this study: 18 years or older, cognitively intact, English-speaking, and experiencing cancer-related pain. Caregivers were identified by the patients who agreed to participate in the study as the person they defined as their caregiver. Data were collected in the patient's home by the principal investigator or a research assistant.

Nurses. The majority of the nurses participating in the study were female, Caucasian, married, and were registered nurses. The ages of the nurses ranged from 24 to 71 years with a mean of 44.22 years (SD = 8.59). Nurses identified themselves as having a Bachelor of Science (42.2%) or an Associate or Diploma degree (44.8%) in nursing. The majority of nurses reported having been in nursing for more than 5 years, with 8.5% reporting more than 20 years in nursing.

Patients and caregivers. There were 50 patients and 46 caregivers who participated in the study. Four of the designated caregivers were unable to be present for the data collection. The majority of the patients were female (52%), married (64%), Caucasian (70%) and were retired (50%). The patients' ages ranged from 36 to 88 with a mean age of 63.65 years (SD = 13.03). The majority of the patients were high school graduates with a mean education level of 12.82 years (SD = 2.55). Caregivers were primarily female (67.4%), married (71.7%), and Caucasian (65.2%). Sixty-six percent of the caregivers worked full time or part time and 15% were retired. Caregivers' ages ranged from 16 to 81 years with a mean of 55.39 years (SD = 14.95) and the majority of caregivers (71.7%) had graduated from high school.

Measures

Knowledge and attitudes. The Nurses' Knowledge and Attitudes Scale Regarding Pain (KAS) (16) was used to measure the nurse's knowledge and attitudes regarding pain management. This 39-item tool has been used extensively from 1987 to the present and was identified as discriminating between levels of expertise. Higher scores indicate higher levels of knowledge. Test-retest reliability was established ($r>.80$) by repeat testing in a continuing education class of staff nurses (N = 60). Internal consistency reliability was established (alpha > .70) with items reflecting both knowledge and attitude domains (16). The alpha for the current study was .75.

Patients' knowledge and experience. The Patient Pain Questionnaire (PPQ) (17), a 16 item linear analogue instrument, was used to measure the knowledge and experience of patients managing chronic cancer pain. The PPQ includes 9 items that measure knowledge about pain and 7 items that measure the patient's experience with pain. The instrument has established content validity (CVI>.90), construct validity (ANOVA, $p.<.05$), concurrent validity ($r>.60$, $p<.05$), and test/retest reliability ($r>.80$) (17). The alpha in the current study was .67.

Family caregivers' knowledge and experience. The Family Pain Questionnaire (FPQ) (18) is a 16-item linear analogue tool used extensively to measure knowledge and experience of a family caregiver managing chronic cancer pain. The instrument includes 9 items assessing knowledge of pain and 7 items assessing individuals' experiences with pain management with their loved ones. The instrument has established content validity (CVI>.90), construct validity (ANOVA, $p.<.05$), concurrent validity ($r>.60$, $p<.05$), factor analysis and test/retest reliability ($r>.80$) (18). For caregivers in the current study the alpha was .56.

Barriers to pain management. The Barriers Questionnaire (BQ) (19) was used to measure the nurses', patients' and caregivers' barriers to pain control. The original Barriers Questionnaire had 27 items that reflected two underlying concepts: beliefs affecting willingness to communicate about pain and beliefs that may interfere with the use of opioids to manage pain, such as a fear of addiction. Items were rated based on the extent of agreement, from 0 (do not agree at all) to 5 (agree very much). Lower scores on the BQ indicate fewer barriers to pain management. In a study of 270 cancer patients, the internal consistency (alpha) of the total scale was 0.89 (19), test-retest reliability was 0.90 (20), and the alphas for the subscales ranged from 0.52 to 0.91 (21). For this study, a shortened form of 17 items was used (22). Internal consistency was established at r = 0.84 (22). In the current study, the alpha for nurses was .75, for patients .78, and for caregivers .65.

Perceived control. Perceived control for nurses, patients and caregivers was measured by the Perceived Control Scale (PCS). Developed by Pellino and Ward (23), this instrument contains eight items that measure perceptions using a 7-point Likert scale where 1 is "extremely disagree" and 7 is "extremely agree". Lower numbers are indicative of higher perception of control over pain. A panel of experts established content validity of the original tool and Cronbach's alpha was 0.80 (23). For the present study, questions were modified, with permission, to relate to cancer pain. Questions were also reworded to apply to caregivers and nurses. In the current study, the alpha for nurses was .81, for patients .65, and for caregivers .67.

Pain. The Brief Pain Inventory (BPI) (24) was developed to assess pain in cancer patients and is short enough to be considered for routine clinical use with cancer patients. It consists of 0 to 10 numerical rating scales (NRS's) that ask the patient to rate the severity of their pain at its worst, least, average, and currently. The alpha for the Pain subscale was established at .85 (26) and was .81 for patients in the current study. Using 0 to 10 NRS's, with 0 representing "no interference" and 10 representing "interferes completely," the BPI also asks for ratings of how much pain interferes with mood, walking, other physical activity, work, social activity, relations with others, and sleep. This functional status subscale has an alpha of .93 (26) and for patients in this study the alpha was .89. The BPI also asks patients to draw the location of their pain on a pain drawing, and asks other questions about duration of pain relief and cause of pain. In addition, it provides a list of descriptors used to describe pain characteristics.

Symptom distress. The Symptom Distress Scale (SDS) developed by McCorkle and Young (25) was used to measure patients' symptom distress. The SDS is a self-rating instrument that evaluates 13 symptoms commonly experienced by patients with cancer: intensity and frequency of pain, intensity and frequency of nausea, outlook, appetite, insomnia, concentration, fatigue, bowel pattern, appearance, cough, and breathing with on a 1 to 5 rating scale with higher scores indicating increased symptom distress. The SDS has good psychometric properties with an alpha of .88 (26) and has been used to measure symptom distress in a variety of settings. In this current study, the alpha was .78

Procedure

Interventions for nurses. Nurses in the intervention group attended a series of two programs, called Power Over Pain (POP), designed to improve the management of pain and side effects in patients with cancer. At the start of the first program the study was explained and consent for participation was obtained from each nurse. Nurses then completed the demographic data questionnaire, PCS, BQ, and KAS. The first program was a 4 hour lecture/discussion covering misconceptions regarding analgesics (addiction, tolerance, dependence, and respiratory depression), pharmacologic management of pain, and management of analgesic side effects. The intervention also incorporated a focus on communication skills, including methods to communicate effectively with physicians regarding pain management needs of the patient, and methods of communicating with patients and caregivers regarding concerns about pain and its management. Nurses received a packet of information containing resources to help them manage pain and opioid-related side effects. At the completion of the program, nurses filled out posttest measures of the PCS, BQ, and KAS.

During the next 4-6 weeks nurses utilized the knowledge gained during the first program in caring for patients in their caseload. Dalton and colleagues (27) suggested that in order to implement new knowledge and achieve individualized goals for change, nurses must be allowed time to analyze the relationships between their beliefs about pain and the ways that they solve patient's pain problems. This 4-6 week period allowed the nurses to begin this change process.

Between the fourth and sixth week following the first POP session, nurses returned for the second POP session. At the beginning of this session, nurses were asked to complete the PCS, BQ, and KAS to determine any change in their previous scores. The second session of the educational intervention focused on the more advanced concepts of dose titration while managing side effects and emphasized communication and advocacy skills used in pain management. The session incorporated role-playing and assertiveness training to enhance the nurse's role as patient advocate to improve the communication between the nurse and the physician, and the nurse and the patient and caregiver. Nurses were asked to present specific examples from their patient caseload for feedback about communication difficulties. At the completion of the session, nurses were again asked to complete the PCS, BQ, and KAS to determine effects of the advanced intervention.

Approximately three months after and again at six months after the second POP nurse's session, nurses were contacted through their agencies and asked to complete the posttest measures (PCS, BQ, and KAS). The purpose of the 6-month posttest measures was two-fold: to look for latent changes and to determine durability of response.

Interventions for patients and caregivers. After obtaining informed consent from patients and their caregivers, the principal investigator or research assistant made weekly visits for the next four weeks. Patients completed a demographic data questionnaire, the PCS, BQ, PPQ, BPI, and SDS, and caregivers completed a demographic data questionnaire, the PCS, BQ, and FPQ during the initial visit. Table 3 includes the schedule of measurements taken for the patients and caregivers. Patients and caregivers were also provided with a packet of written materials reflecting the information to be discussed in the program and were asked to review this information prior to the second visit.

On the visits in weeks 2 and 3, patients were asked to complete the BPI and SDS. During the second visit, following the completion of the questionnaires, the principal investigator presented a 1-hour educational intervention to those patients and caregivers in the intervention group. The content of this POP program was similar to that received by the nurses, but presented at a level appropriate for the layman. Topics included the importance of pain management, misconceptions, analgesics, and side effect management. Ward and colleagues (28) suggested that for an educational program to be effective, patients and caregivers must be taught about erroneous beliefs and provided with information and skills related to coping with analgesic side effects.

During the week 4 visit, the patient completed the PCS, BQ, PPQ, BPI, and SDS. During this visit, caregivers were asked to complete the PCS, BQ and FPQ.

Analysis

Nurses. Participating nurses were measured for the primary outcomes of knowledge, barriers, and perceived control. Subject mortality was tracked as nurses frequently left or changed agencies and took vacation time during the study. Imputation of missing follow-up data was achieved indirectly by means of maximum likelihood in this general mixed linear model. Data analyses were performed in two ways. One analysis, intent to treat analysis (ITI), used all available data assuming missing at random. A second analysis omitted nurses from baseline who lacked either the three-month or six-month follow up. The strategy for selecting "mostly complete" cases did not completely eliminate the imbalance but the imbalance was substantially reduced except for the disproportionate drop in available nurses' data in the NNPY group at 6 months. Each outcome was analyzed separately using a 2 x 2 (x 4) general linear mixed model (GLMM) repeated measures with linear trends on time.

Patients and caregivers. Patients were seen weekly for four weeks for data collection on the outcome measures of pain, symptom distress, and interference from pain. The treatment of missing follow-up data depended on which of the two types of analyses were performed – intent to treat or per protocol. For the intent to treat analysis, maximum likelihood imputation of parameter estimates was achieved using all available data. The advantage of the intent to treat analysis is that it honors the randomization plan and provides the most secure basis for causal inference. The analysis makes the assumption however that data are missing completely at random or at least at random. An alternative to the intent to treat analysis that does not make this assumption used only cases that are complete. This per protocol analysis was used to examine the sensitivity of the intent to treat results to alternate missing value assumptions.

What We Found

Descriptive statistics for baseline variables for nurses

Baseline KAS was relatively high, 29.29 out of 39 for the intervention group and 26.70 for the control group. This may reflect the high level of experience of the study nurses or perhaps, due to the randomization at the agency level, it may reflect an agency specific emphasis on effective pain management. While the means are high, the potential range of the instrument (0 – 39) still allowed for demonstration of improvements in knowledge and attitudes regarding pain management. Similarly with the PCS, a mean of 5.36 in the intervention group and 4.42 in the control group with a range of 1 to 7 on the scale (higher scores meaning lower perception of control) allowed for demonstration of improvement in perceived control. The BQ subscales, on the other hand, with a possible range from 0 to 5, were already at the low end for two BQ subscales, indicating few barriers.

Nurse outcomes

Knowledge. The basic nurse intervention significantly increased nurses' knowledge relative to the control condition (F [1, 837] = 234.71; p = .000). The gain in knowledge persisted to the 6-month (24 weeks) retest period. The results were virtually identical when the nearly complete cases data was analyzed (Figure 1).

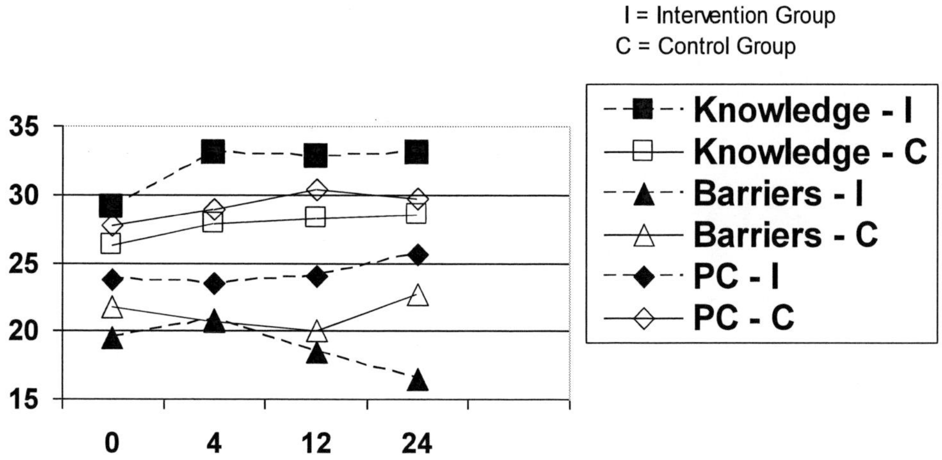

Figure 1. Outcomes for Nurses.

Barriers. The nurse intervention resulted in a significant reduction in perceived barriers (F[1,824] = 8.14; p = .004). The effect was larger at 6-months than 3-months. The results were the same in both the ITI and nearly complete case analysis.

Perceived control over pain. A significant reduction in the scores on the PCS (F [1,804] = 168.52; p = .000} reflecting an increased perception of control over pain also resulted from the nurse intervention. The effect was also larger at 6-months than 3-months.

Patient outcomes

Outcome measures for patients were analyzed from the four sessions when data was collected. Only one outcome, decrease in patient barriers, was significantly affected by either patient or nurse intervention. The patient intervention significantly reduced the number of perceived barriers from 24.5 (SD = 11.1) at week 1 to 17.8 (SD = 11.9) at week 4. Perceived barriers in the control group actually increased over the same interval. In both groups knowledge and perceived control increased, while pain, symptom distress, and interference from pain decreased, demonstrating a tendency for patients to improve in both the intervention and control condition (Figure 2).

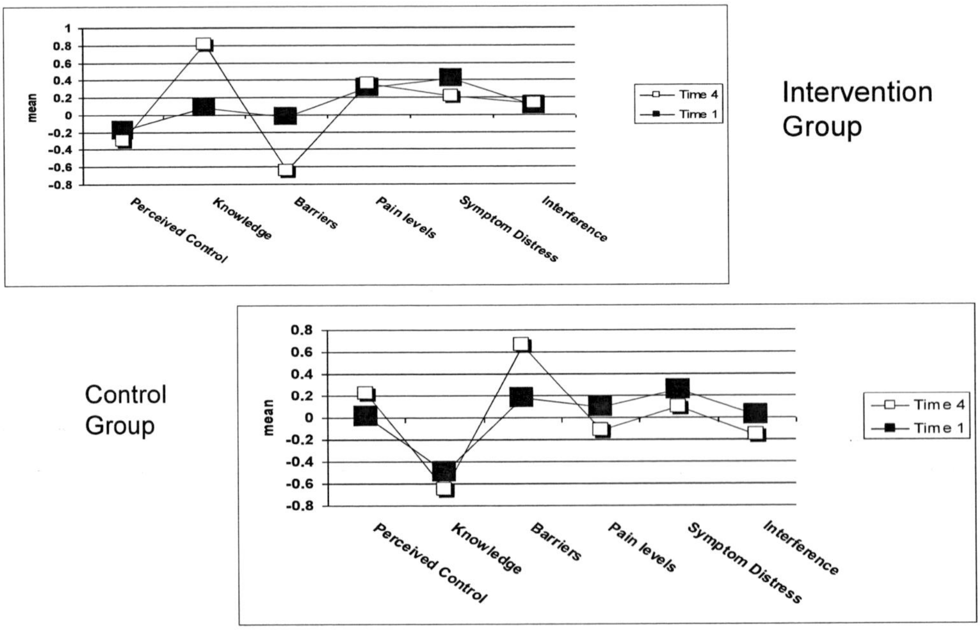

Figure 2. Outcomes of Patients (Z Scores)

Caregiver outcomes

Data from the caregivers was collected in the first week visit and at week 4. There was a significant effect of the nurse intervention on caregivers' perceived control (p=. 036). Caregivers of patients with nurses who received the intervention improved in perceived control over pain (3.87 [SD = .97] to 4.35 [SD = 1.24]; n = 28) relative to the control group (4.53 [SD = 1.42] to 4.00 [SD = 1.18]; n = 18). No other significant changes were seen (Figure 3).

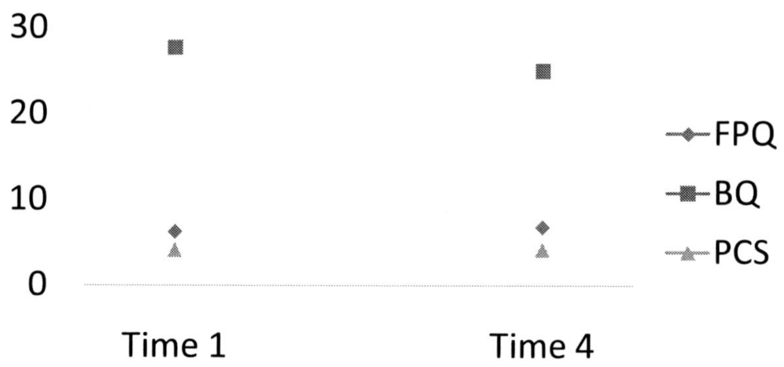

Figure 3. Outcomes for Caregivers.

Discussion

Pain remains an enormous problem for patients with cancer pain. Patients with cancer who were receiving home care in this study had mean worst pain scores of 7.76 (SD=2.44) on a 0 to 10 scale, indicating severe pain. Their reported mean average pain scores were 5.28 (SD=2.73), indicating moderate pain and they reported receiving approximately 50% relief of their pain with the modalities they were using for treatment. Symptom distress was also a problem for these patients with a mean symptom distress score of 1.81 (SD=.63) on a 0 to 4 scale. However, on this same scale, patients reported that pain caused a level of distress that was even higher than that of all symptoms. Patients reported a mean pain-related distress score of 2.56 (SD = 1.08), indicating that pain caused more distress than any other symptoms. This pain interfered at a moderate level in all activities of daily living with work, enjoyment of life, and walking being the activities with which pain most interfered. Although only 20% of the patients in this study were working, the interference of pain with enjoyment of life is striking and reflects the effects of pain on patients' quality of life

Patients receiving home care are cared for by home care nurses who may or may not have had any formal training in pain management. In addition, home care patients are under the care of physicians of various specialties, such as oncology, primary care, or family medicine, who may also be lacking in current knowledge of appropriate and effective pain management strategies. Therefore, homecare nurses must become experts in meeting the pain management needs of their patients. The Power Over Pain (POP) intervention for home care nurses proved to be an effective and durable mechanism for improving nurses' pain management abilities. Scores for nurses receiving the intervention resulted in significantly greater pain management knowledge and higher perceived control over pain, while scores on the Barriers Questionnaire demonstrated a significant decrease. These results were maintained throughout the six months of the study, indicating durability of the intervention.

The intervention for patients succeeded in significantly decreasing barriers to pain control. These barriers are often attitudinal barriers based on misconceptions or misinformation about pain and its management (29). These barriers, including fear of addiction, the belief that cancer pain is inevitable, and beliefs about communication with health care providers may cause patients to avoid the use of medications to control pain or keep from discussing their pain with their health care providers due to inaccurate beliefs. Decreasing barriers is essential to effective pain management. Although no other findings reached significance, all findings showed trends in the expected direction. Patients' pain and symptom distress scores decreased and their functional status, pain management knowledge, and perception of control over pain increased. The lack of significance of the findings may have been due to the small number of patients participating in the study.

The only significant finding for the sample of the caregivers was that caregivers whose nurses had received the POP intervention had greater perception of control over pain than caregivers whose nurses had not received the intervention. These findings may reflect the nurses' increased confidence in managing pain following the intervention and the effect of this increased confidence on the caregiver. From the analysis of the qualitative data from caregivers in this study (14), caregivers often feel powerless to affect the patient's pain. Seeing the nurse's confidence in their ability to manage the pain may have given the caregivers hope that they, too, would be able to manage the patient's pain.

Limitations

The major limitations in this study were the sample sizes for the patients and caregivers. The study was designed to enroll three patient/caregiver dyads identified by each nurse from his/her caseload. This expectation was not fulfilled primarily due to recent changes in home care regulations and reimbursement (HHRGs) issues that have dramatically changed the number of cancer patients referred to home care. Presently, Medicare patients must be homebound to receive home care and many agencies do not receive adequate reimbursement for services provided to cancer patients unless they have a co-morbid condition. This has led to patients being referred to home care and dying or going to hospice within days to weeks of admission, limiting the time in which a home care nurse can affect change. The referral pattern changes were severe enough to cause closure of the home care agency affiliated with the major cancer center in our area during this study. The stage of cancer of the patients was a common reason for patients not completing the study. Cancer patients referred to home care in late stages of the disease process were frequently unavailable for the four weeks of participation required for the study. Currently, many cancer patients are not receiving home care. They are followed in an outpatient setting, such as a clinic or doctor's office, increasing the responsibilities of the caregiver. Replication of the study in an outpatient setting would provide further data on the measures in this study.

Conclusions

The Power Over Pain intervention was effective in increasing home care nurses' knowledge regarding pain management and perception of control over pain, as well as decreasing barriers to pain control. The effects of the intervention were durable, maintaining their effects over the six months of the study. Home care patients who received the Power Over Pain intervention also had a significant decrease in their barriers to pain control. Although significant differences were not demonstrated in other variables, the most promising trends were observed in the expected direction, such as increases in knowledge regarding pain management and perception of control over pain. Most importantly, patients' pain levels and symptom distress decreased and functional status related to pain increased. Lastly, caregivers of home care cancer patients with pain whose nurses received the Power Over Pain intervention demonstrated significant improvement in perception of control over pain, suggesting that increasing nurses' perception of control over pain benefited the caregivers as well.

Based on these findings, the Power Over Pain intervention should be used to help nurses increase improve their care of cancer patients with pain. Further testing of the intervention in larger groups of patients and caregivers, and with other patient populations with pain is recommended.

Acknowledgment

Funded by the National Cancer Institute #1 K22 CA87713

References

[1] Green C, Anderson K, Baker T, et al. The unequal burden of pain: Confronting racial and ethnic disparities in pain. Pain Med 2003;4:277-94.

[2] Sterman E, Gauker S, Krieger J. Continuing education: A comprehensive approach to improving cancer pain management and patient satisfaction. Oncol Nurs Forum 2003;30:857-64.

[3] Vallerand AH, Hasenau S, Templin T, Collins-Bohler D. Disparities between black and white patients with cancer pain: The effect of perception of control over pain. Pain Med 2005;6:242-50.

[4] Wells N, Hepworth JT, Murphy BA, Wujcik D, Johnson R. Improving cancer pain management through patient and family education. J Pain Symptom Manage 2003;25:344-56.

[5] Miaskowski C, Dodd M, West C, et al.Randomized clinical trial of the effectiveness of a self-care intervention to improve cancer pain management. J Clin Oncol 2004;22:1713-20.

[6] Dodd M J, Miaskowski C. The PRO-SELF program: A self-care intervention program for patients receiving cancer treatments. Semin Oncol Nurs 2000;16:300-8.

[7] Ward SE, Donovan H S, Owen B, Grosen E, Serlin R. An individualized intervention to overcome patient-related barriers to pain management in women with gynecologic cancers. Res Nurs Health 2000;23:393-405.

[8] Gunnersdottir S, Donovan HS, Ward S. Interventions to overcome clinician-and-patient-related barriers to pain management. Nurs Clin North Am 2003;38:419-34.

[9] Given B, Given CW, McCorkle R, et al. Pain and fatigue management: Results of a nursing randomized clinical trial. Oncol Nurs Forum 2002;29:949-56.

[10] Elliott TE, Murray DM, Oken MM, et al. Improving cancer pain management in communities: Main results from a randomized controlled trial. J Pain Symptom Manage 1997;13:191-203.
[11] Bero LA, Grilli R, Grimshaw JM, Harvery E, Oxman AD, Thomson MA. Closing the gap between research and practice: An overview of systematic reviews of interventions to promote the implementation of research finding. BMJ 1998;317:465-8.
[12] Glajchen M, Bookbinder M. Knowledge and perceived competence of home care nurses in pain management: A national survey. J Pain Symptom Manage 2001;21:307-16.
[13] Vallerand AH, Riley-Doucet C, Hasenau SM, Templin T. Improving cancer pain management by homecare nurses. Oncol Nurs Forum 2004;31:809-16.
[14] Vallerand AH, Saunders M, Anthony M. Perception of control over pain by patients with cancer and their caregivers. Pain Manage Nurs 2007;8:58-63.
[15] Vallerand AH, Anthony M, Saunders M. Homecare nurses' perceptions of control over cancer pain. Home Healthc Nurse 2005;23:647-52.
[16] Ferrell BR, McCaffery M. Knowledge and attitudes survey regarding pain. Developed by authors, (http://prc.coh.org), 1987; revised 2008.
[17] Ferrell BR, Ferrell BA, Rhiner M, Grant M. Family factors influencing cancer pain management. Postgrad Med J 1991;67(suppl 2):S64-9.
[18] Ferrell BR, Rhiner M, Rivera LM. Empowering patients to control pain. Curr Issues Cancer Nurs1993;2:1-9.
[19] Ward SE, Goldberg N, Miller-McCauley V, et al. Patient-related barriers to management of cancer pain. Pain 1993;52:319-24.
[20] Ward SE, Gatwood J. Concerns about reporting pain and using analgesics. A comparison of persons with and without cancer. Cancer Nurs 1994;17:200-6.
[21] Berry PE, Ward SE. Barriers to pain management in hospice: A study of family caregivers. Hospice J 1995;10:19-33.
[22] Wells N, Johnson RL, Wujcik D. Development of a short version of the Barriers Questionnaire. J Pain Symptom Manage 1998;15:294-8.
[23] Pellino TA, Ward SE. Perceived control mediates the relationship between pain severity and patient satisfaction. J Pain Symptom Manage 1998;15:110-6.
[24] Cleeland CS, Syrjala KL. How to assess cancer pain. In: Melzack T, ed. Handbook of pain assessment. New York: Guilford, 1992:362-87.
[25] McCorkle R, Young K. Development of a symptom distress scale. Cancer Nurs 1978;1:373-8.
[26] Vallerand AH, Templin T, Haseanu SM, Riley-Doucet C. Factors that affect functional status in patients with cancer pain. Pain 2000;132:82-90.
[27] Dalton JA, Carlson J, Mann JD, Blau W, Bernard S, Youngblood R. An examination of nursing attitudes and pain management practices. Cancer Nurs 1998;1:373-8.
[28] Ward SE, Carlson-Dakes K, Hughes SH, Kwekkeboom KL, Donovan HS. The impact on quality of life of patient-related barriers to pain management. Res Nurs Health 1998;21:405-13.

Gunnarsdottir S, Serlin RC, Ward S. Patient-related barriers to pain management: The Icelandic Barriers Questionnaire II. J Pain Sympt Manage 2005;29:273-85.

In: Advanced Cancer. Pain and Quality of Life
Editors: E. Chow, J. Merrick, pp. 33-45
ISBN: 978-1-61668-207-1
© 2010 Nova Science Publishers, Inc.

Chapter III

Registered Nurse Awareness of and Practice Related to Cancer Pain

Johanna Elizabeth Maree, DCur (Pret) *

Adelaide Tambo School of Nursing Science,
Tshwane University of Technology, Pretoria, South Africa

Cancer is a global health problem and for many patients result in chronic pain. Unfortunately the treatment of cancer pain is often inadequate. Nurses are in the best position to facilitate effective pain management due to the time they spend with the patient experiencing pain. The researcher initiated the research to determine if nurses were aware of the problem of cancer pain in relation to other problems a cancer patient could experience and if nursing practice facilitated effective pain management. A contextual, exploratory and comparative descriptive study was performend. The target population was all nurses entering an oncology nursing learning programme at a univeristy of technology in South Africa. The sampling method was convenient (n=35) and the participation rate 97.2%. Self-reported data were gathered by means of a questionnaire. Data were analysed using descriptive statisitcs and content analyses. The study provided evidence that despite nurses' awareness of cancer pain they lacked knowledge and skills pertaining to the management of pain. Nursing practice did not facilitate effective pain management. Educational programmes focusing on all aspects of pain management are urgently required. Nurses should also be involved in research on cancer pain and its management to enable them to have evidence of their important role in caring for the patient.

* Correspondence: Professor Lize JE Maree, Adelaide Tambo School of Nursing Science, Tshwane University of Technology, Private Bag X680, Pretoria 0001, South Africa. Tel: +27 12 382 5285; Fax: +27 12 382 5033; E-mail: mareeje@tut.ac.za

Introduction

Cancer is a global health problem and one of the leading causes of death (1). One of the common problems of cancer is chronic pain (2). Pain relief, the right of every patient, was so important that the World Health Organization (WHO) in 1996 published recommendations on how cancer pain should be relieved. The recommendations of the WHO included the preferable route of administration as well as the drugs that should be used for pain management (3). The WHO's pain approach is relatively inexpensive and effective and if applied, can relieve the pain of approximately 90% of cancer patients (4). Unfortunately unrelieved cancer pain is still an international health problem (5) as 30 to 50% of cancer patients whilst treated with anti-neoplastic therapy and 60 to 90% patients with advanced disease experience chronic pain (6). When evaluating the level of pain control of cancer patients in an ambulatory care setting, it was found that 81% of patients were not adequately treated for pain and 75% were under-medicated (7). In a South African study conducted by Beck and Falkson (8) in 2001, it was found that 30 to 40% of cancer patients managed in active treatment centres experienced pain. No significant difference in the prevalence of pain was found between patients with advanced disease and those with earlier stage disease. Maree and Wright (9) found pain to be the biggest problem of cancer patients treated at two cancer centres in Tshwane, South Africa.

One of the reasons leading to the ineffective management of cancer pain is the lack of assessment. Assessment is the first step in determining the health needs of the patient and starts as soon as a nurse comes into contact with a patient (10). Unfortunately patients are not always invited to talk about their pain experience (11). According to Stromgen et al (12) it would be unlikely for any symptom to be treated, if it is not documented in the patient record. Assessment of and monitoring the intensity of pain is therefore crucial (13).

Due to the subjective nature of pain it is possible that others would inaccurately perceive the patient's pain (6). Assessment of pain refers to the communication between the assessor and the person experiencing the pain. An assessment tool to measure the pain is used to facilitate the communication (14). Of the total health care team, nurses spend more time with the patient in pain than any other team member. Nurses are therefore in the best position to evaluate the effectiveness of pain interventions and to advocate for changes when necessary (6). Nevertheless, the management of cancer pain needs an interdisciplinary approach. Xue et al (15) found that pain is more effectively managed by an interdisciplinary team than individual involvement of a single health care provider as the expertise of each member can contribute to effective management.

In South Africa, oncology nurses are extremely rare. In 2006 there were only 282 registered oncology nurses, which related to one oncology nurse for approximately every 39,400 patients with cancer (9). For a cancer patient to be nursed by an oncology nurse would be an extraordinary experience. Although the curricula of all pre-registration nursing learning programmes leading to registration at the South African Nursing Council as nurse has to include nursing of the patient with cancer (16,17), the practice of registered nurses regarding the management of cancer pain is not known. The research problem for the study was therefore: In relation to other problems that cancer patients can experience, are registered nurses entering an oncology nursing learning programme at a South African university of technology aware of the extent of cancer pain; what are their practice with regards to cancer pain and does their practice enhance effective pain management?

Our study

The overall purpose of the study was to explore registered nurses' knowledge of and practice regarding the management of cancer pain. The aims of the study were to explore whether registered nurses entering an oncology nursing learning programme at a South African university of technology were aware of the extent of cancer pain in relation to other symptoms cancer patients could experience. The study also attempted to compare the extent of cancer pain to other symptoms seen from the view of the patient and the nurse. The study further aimed to determine the practice of registered nurses and whether their practice enhanced effective management of cancer pain.

The research methods and design will be described in terms of the strategy and context, research design, population, data gathering and data analysis. The strategy for the study was exploratory and comparative descriptive. Exploratory research is designed to search for accurate information about the charateristics of specific groups or situations when little is known about the phenomenon.

A descriptive comparitive study allows the description in variables in two or more groups (18). Using an exploratory and descriptive comparitive strategy provided answers to whether registered nurses were aware of the problem of pain in relation to other symptoms experienced by patients; nursing practice regarding pain management and whether pain management practices enhanced effective pain management.

Research design

The research design for the study was a quatitative survey. Quantitative research allows precise measurement and quantification of phenomena. Direct questioning is used in a survey to obtain information about the activities, beliefs and preferences of people (19).

Research context

The research was contextual (18), implying that the results of the study are valid only for the situation in which the study was done. The context for the study was registered nurses entering an oncology learning programme at a univeristiy of technology in South Africa. The oncology nursing learning programm is a post registration learning programme and offered on a part time basis over two years. Students have to pass both theoretical and clinical nursing learning components to sucessfully complete the learning programme and be awarded a bacculaureate degree in oncology nursing. After completion, the students are registered at the South African Nursing Council as oncology nurse and can pracitice as oncology nurse.

Population

Burns and Grove (20), describe a population as all the elements (individuals, objects, events, or substances) that meet the sample criteria for inclusion in a study. The target population for the study was registered nurses entering an oncology nursing learning programme at an university of technology in South Africa. Only those willing to participate in the study were included. The sampling method was convenient. The sample size was 35 (n=35) and the participation rate 97.2%.

Data gathering

Self reported data were gathered using a questionnaire as data gathering instrument. Self-report is a data gathering method involving direct report of information by the person who is being studied. Self-report also gives access to information that is frequently difficult to gather by any other means (21). Using a questionnaire allows quesions to be presented in a consistent manner and lessens the opportunity for bias (22).

The questionnaire consisted of two sections. In section A, demographic data were gathered. In Section B, data regarding percieved patient problems, nursing practice and pain management practices were gathered. Section B was partially based on a questionnaire previously used in a study conducted by Maree and Wright (9). Section B contained both closed ended and open-ended questions. Open-ended question were used to give respondents the opportunity to motivate specific answers.

Data were gathered by the researcher on a day scheduled for lectures. Teaching and learning was specifically planned to allow respondents the opportunity to complete the questionnaire. Informed consent was obtained from each respondent before completion of the questionnaires commenced. No name of any respondent was entered onto the questionnaire to ensure anonymity and confidentiality.

Data analysis

Data were analyzed by means of descriptive statistics. Descriptive statistics summarise data to manageable portions and describes its various characteristics (18). The data were gathered in Excel spreadsheets and analysed using the SPSS version 14 program. Data gathered by means of open-ended questions were analysed using content analyses (23) during the examination of the data. A colour coding strategy (22) was used to code the data.

Validity and reliability

Validity refers to the ability of an instrument to measure what it is supposed to measure in an accurate manner. A valid instrument will truthfully reflect the concept which it is supposed to measure (18). Reliability can be described as the degree of consistency of the measure when repeatedly applied (23). Validity and reliability were assured as follows:

- The questionnaire was formulated and specifically planned to explore nurses' awareness of pain in relation to other problems cancer patients could experience and nursing practice with regards to the management of cancer pain.
- The questionnaire was partially based on a questionnaire used in a previous study (9). Permission to use the questionnaire was obtained.
- Data were collected at a venue and time specifically planned to collect data.
- The researcher is a registered nurse specialising in oncology nursing.
- The data analysis was done using SPSS version 14. Statistical analysis was done with the assistance of the statistical support division of the university of technology.

Ethical considerations

Conducting research ethically entails protecting the human rights of participants (22). The human rights of participants were protected by the fact that an information leaflet was handed to the participants explaining the purpose of the study and that they could withdraw from the study at any stage. With the information leaflet participants were assured that their responses would be regarded as confidential and they would not be disadvantaged during their study to become an oncology nurse. Anonymity was assured by numbering the questionnaires sequentially. Informed consent was obtained in writing from all participants.

Some of our findings

The majority of the respondents were Black and represented various cultural groups within the Black community in South Africa. Respondents also practiced in a variety of nursing sub-disciplines. The majority (94.3%; n=35) was female with 5.7% (n=35) male. Demographic characteristics are reflected in table 1.

Pain as problem of cancer patients

To explore if respondents realized the importance of pain in relation to other problems cancer patients could experience, respondents were given opportunity to select the ten most common problems of cancer patients. The list included 32 different problems representing the physical, psychosocial, spiritual and financial domains as well as a column for "other, please specify" should specific problems not be included. The problem of pain was identified by most participants (77.1%; n=35), followed by fear/anxiety (65.7%; n=35), weight loss (62.9%; n=35); depression (60.0%; n=35) and nausea and vomiting (57.1%; n=35). The comparison of the five most common problems reported by patients (9) to those indentified by the respondents is illustrated in table 2.

Table 1. Demographic characteristics (n=35).

Demographic characteristic	n	%
Cultural group		
South African Black	26	74.3
Non-South African Black	1	2.9
South African white	6	17.1
South African coloured	2	5.7
Age		
No answer	2	5.7
20 - 29	2	5.7
30 - 39	12	34.3
40 - 49	17	48.5
50 - 59	1	2.9
60 and older	1	2.9
Number of years practicing as registered nurse		
1 - 2	4	11.4
3 - 5	5	14.3
6 -10	8	22.9
11 - 15	10	28.6
16 to 20	5	14.3
More than 20	3	8.6
Number of years practicing in an oncology care setting		
None	12	34.3
1 - 2	11	31.4
3 - 4	4	11.4
5 - 7	4	11.4
8 - 10	2	5.7
More than 10	2	5.7
Current care setting employed at		
Specialized cancer care setting	19	54.3
Mixed with cancer patients in the majority	3	8.6
Mixed with cancer patients in the minority	7	20.0
Gynaecology	1	2.9
Stomatherapy	1	2.9
Other	3	8.6
Non practicing	1	2.9

Table 2. Comparison of the five most common problems reported by nurses (n=35) and patients (n=148)

Problem	Nurses (n=35)		Patients (n=148)(9)	
		%		%
Pain	1	77.1	1	77
Anxiety / fear	2	65.7	-	-
Weight loss	3	62.9	-	-
Depression	4	60.0	-	-
Nausea and vomiting	5	57.1	2	66
Weakness/fatigue/lack of energy	-	-	2	66
Dry and sore mouth	-	-	4	47
Thirst	-	-	5	41

To determine how important pain was, respondents were requested to list the ten identified problems according to their importance - one being the most important and 10 the least. Two (8%; n=35) of the respondents did not list the identified problems according to importance. However, for 52% (n=33) pain was the most important cancer related problem, 17.4% (n=33) rated it second, 4.3% (n=33) fourth, 13.0% (n=33) fifth, 8.7% (n=33) seventh, 4.3% (n=33) eighth and 8.7% (n=33) tenth. A higher percentage (87.5%, n=16) of participants practicing in other care settings recognized pain to be one of the 10 most common problems compared to 68.4% (n=19) practicing in specialized oncology care settings. The average importance of the five most commonly identified problems is reflected in table 3.

Table 3. Average importance of the five most commonly identified cancer related problems (n=33).

Problem	Importance
Pain	3.2
Anxiety / fear	3.4
Weight loss	5.6
Depression	4.1
Nausea and vomiting	3.7

Comparing the average importance of pain of participants practicing in specialized oncology care settings to those in other care settings, pain was more important to participants practicing in other care settings. Participants practicing in specialized oncology care settings considered pain to be fourth (4.3) (n=19) on the list of the ten most important problems compared to the 2.7 (n=16) of participants practicing in other care settings.

Nursing practice pertaining to the management of pain

To determine nursing practice, respondents were asked if pain was formally assessed and documented in the care setting where they practiced. Forty four percent (44%; n=34) of the respondents responded positively whilst the rest (54%; n=34) responded negatively. Slightly more than half (52.6%; n=19) of the respondents practicing in a specialized oncology care setting indicated that pain is formally assessed and documented. When asking respondents who indicated that pain was assessed and documented to identify the assessment tool they used only 26.7% (n=15) could name one. The numerical scale was the only assessment tool used and only applied in specialized cancer care settings. To explore how often pain was assessed, respondents were asked to identify the frequency pain assessment was conducted. The assessment tools used and frequency pain was assessed are summarized in table 4.

To explore views on assessment, respondents were asked if they were of the opinion that patient's problems would be addressed if no assessment was performed. Only 7.5% (n=35) indicated that problems would be addressed if not assessed. For the rest (92.5%; n=35) assessment was an essential component of problem management. To determine if oncology nurses influenced nursing practice respondents were asked if there were registered oncology nurses practicing in their specific care setting. More than half (58.8%; n=35) practiced with an oncology nurse, 34.3% (n=35) did not and 2.9% (n=35) were unsure. Oncology nurses were most commonly present in specialized cancer care settings (68.4%; n=19) and also present in the health care settings using the numerical scale to assess pain.

Table 4. Assessment tools used and frequency of pain assessment done (n=15).

Assessment tool	Frequency of pain assessment	n	%
None identified	None stated	3	20.0
None identified	As prescribed	1	6.7
None identified	4 hourly	3	20.0
Expression of the patient	4-houly	1	6.7
Assess efficacy of analgesic	4-hourly	2	13.3
Numerical scale	Weekly	1	6.7
Numerical scale	Every time when patient complains	1	6.7
Numerical scale	None stated	1	6.7
Numerical scale	4 hourly when patient complains	1	6.7
Assessment form	None stated	1	6.7

Respondents were also asked if they were of the opinion that cancer patients lie about the amount of pain they had, and if so, whether pain was over-reported or under-reported. Respondents were mostly (45.7%; n=35) of the opinion that cancer patients lie about cancer pain, whilst 40% (n=35) indicated that lies were not told and 14.3% (n=35) were unsure. Respondents were divided in terms of cancer patients lying about the amount of pain experienced as 50% (n=16) indicated that patients over-reported pain whilst the rest (50%; n=16) were of the opinion that patients under-reported cancer pain.

To determine respondent's involvement in pain management, two questions were asked. The first question determined the health professional that would know most about the problems cancer patients experienced. Respondents could choose between the nurse, doctor or other that had to be specified. Respondents were also asked to motivate their choice. The majority (94.3%; n=35) said the nurse would know most of patient's problems whilst 5.8% (n=35) indicated the doctor. When asking respondents to motivate their answer, 51.4% (n=35) responded that nurses spend most time with the patients. Other motivations included that nurses are "nearest" to patients (5.7%; n=35), patients "trust" and "rely" on nurses (5.7%; n=35) and that no language barrier exists between patients and nurses (2.9%; n=35). The second question explored if respondents were consulted on patient problems and to reflect their feelings about their situation. Respondents indicated that 42.9% (n=35) were consulted very often, 34.3% (n=35) sometimes, 11.4% (n=35) on rare occasions and 2.9% (n=35) not at all. Feelings about their particular situation were expressed as follows:

> "It makes me feel like I'm part of the team treating the oncology patient." # 29

> "It makes me feel that my opinion does not count and also that doctors know everything and they don't care that you know more about the patient. I assess the patient's needs and management can be based on those needs." # 16

To explore the pain management strategy used in the various care settings, respondents were asked if the WHO guidelines on the management of cancer pain were used. The biggest proportion of the respondents (45.7%; n=35) were not sure, whilst 14.3% (n=35) responded positively, 34.3% (n=35) negatively and 5.7% (n=35) preferred not to answer the question. Only 18.8% (n=19) of the respondents practicing in a specialized cancer care setting indicated that the WHO guidelines for pain management were followed, whilst 50% (n=16) were not sure and 31.3% (n=16) responded negatively.

To determine if the respondents had knowledge about the medication used for pain management, they were asked to identify the five drugs most commonly used. A total of 28 different drugs were mentioned of which six were neither analgesics nor analgesic adjuvants. Morphine (94.3%; n=35) was the most commonly used drug, followed by tramadol (48.6%; n=35), paracetamol (42.9%; n=35) and pethidine (28.6%; n=35). Five different nonsteriodal anti-inflammotory drugs were used. Of the analgesic adjuvants (24) no mention was made of any drug belonging to the anti-depressant, corticosteroid, anti-epileptic, antispasmodic, NMDA-receptor-channel blockers and bisphosphonate groups. Of the muscle relaxants, only diazepam (14.3%; n=35) was mentioned.

Discussion

The results of the study will be discussed in terms of the awareness of nurses of pain as problem of cancer patients followed by nursing practice.

Awareness of cancer pain

The study provides evidence that registered nurses are aware of the importance of pain as problem of cancer patients. Literature reflecting nurses awareness of cancer pain is scarce, however Bernardi, Catania and Tridello (25) found in 2007 that 30% of hospice nurses practicing in Italy underestimate cancer patients' pain. The awareness of nurses is however positive as awareness would facilitate nurses to prioritize pain management in all phases of cancer (26). According to Hemming and Maher (27) awareness of the extent of problems can assist nurses to focus their minds on the patient they encounter. It would be expected of nurses practicing in specialized cancer care settings to be more aware of the problem of pain than those practicing in other care settings, yet it was the opposite. The reason for this is not clear and Conner and Muir (28) remind us to ask patients to prioritize their symptoms as "our priorities may not be theirs".

Nursing practice pertaining to cancer pain

The study also provides evidence that nursing practice did not facilitate effective pain management. Despite the fact that nurses were aware of the importance of assessment and of the opinion that problems not assessed would not be managed, their practice demonstrated the opposite. Nurses lacked knowledge and skills of pain assessment as assessment could not have been conducted let alone properly done if the assessment tool and the frequency of the assessment could not be described. This finding is in contrast with the findings of McMillan et al (29) where nurses were most knowledgeable about asking patients about their pain and the study of Xue et al (15) describing nurses' expertise in pain assessment.

Assessment using the numerical scale was fruitless as the scale was only used on a weekly basis or for patients complaining of pain. Selecting the numerical scale was however positive as the numerical scale compared to the face scale, verbal rating scale and visual analogue scale was found to be the easiest for patients to understand and complete and also had the highest reliability value (30). Although the proper use of the numerical scale would have added to effective pain management, this scale only measures the severity of pain and does not explore pain in all its dimensions. Exploring only the physical dimension of pain can result in an incomplete and inappropriate pain regimen (31).

Nurses believed cancer patients lied about the amount of pain they experienced. This is not exceptional as Xue et al (15) found that 59% of medical oncology nurses and 49% of gynecologic oncology nurses believed that patients under-reported the amount of pain experienced. In the previous study nurses did not believe that cancer pain is over-reported. Attitudes towards pain however influence pain management. As it is believed that physicians who believe that the amount of pain experienced is over-reported are more likely to under treat pain (15) it is also possible for nurses to play down patient's pain which can result in ineffective management. Believing that cancer patients under-reported their pain did not change nursing practice. Pain was primarily assessed by means of the numerical scale only when patients complained. Patients experiencing pain and under-reported it by not complaining were excluded from the assessments.

A disturbing finding of the study was the fact that oncology nurses did not influence nursing practice to enable effective pain management. It would have been expected that in specialized cancer care settings where oncology nurses practiced, pain would have been assessed and recorded as an ongoing process. This was not the case and in terms of pain management, patients did not benefit from being nursed by an oncology nurse. Oncology nurses are not exclusively to be blamed as assessment of symptoms in palliative care is not the role of specialist nurses only but the role of every nurse (28).

Nurses considered them to be the health care professional knowing most of the cancer patient's problems. Except for Ger et al (6), Johnson (32) also agrees with this finding by quoting Solzhenitsyn: "How many adult human beings are there, now at this very minute, rushing about in mute panic wishing they could find a nurse, the kind person to whom they can pour out the fears they have deeply concealed?" Unfortunately nurses were not regarded as highly by other health care professionals. Nurses were not involved in the total management of the cancer patient. Twycross (24) states that palliative care is best delivered if it involves a group of people working together as a team. Twycross (24) also describes the core of the team as the doctor and the nurse. Nurses cannot expect to be regarded as a core member of the team or consulted if they lack knowledge and skills, do not teach and research and lacks leadership.

Nurses lacked knowledge of pain management. Not only were most not sure if the WHO step ladder approach was applied, they were also not sure of the medication used for pain management. This is not unique as various studies (25,29) found deficiencies in nurses knowledge of pain management. Lack of knowledge of pain management would not facilitate effective pain management as the nurse would not be able to fulfill her role as advocate for the patient if she does not know what to advocate for.

Limitations of the study

Due to its contextual nature the results could not be generalized and only be applied to the group of nurses registered for the learning programme in oncology nursing science at the specific university of technology in South Africa.

Recommendations for nursing practice

Educational programmes focusing on all aspects of pain management are urgently required should we want to relieve the pain and suffering cancer patients experience. Nurses should also be involved in research regarding pain and its management to enable them to have evidence of their important role in caring for the patient with cancer.

References

[1] World Health Organization. Cancer 2006. Accessed 2009 Mar 10. URL: http://www.who.int/mediacentre/factsheets/fs297/en/print.html.

[2] Sloan P, Van der Veer B, Snapp J, Johnson M, Sloan, DA. Cancer pain assessment and management recommendations by hospice nurses. J Pain Symptom Manage 1999;18:103-10.

[3] Farrer K. Pain control. In: Kinghorn S, Gamlin R. Palliative nursing: bringing comfort and hope. Edinburgh: Bailierre Tindall, 2000:13-33.

[4] World Health Organization. Palliative care 2008. Accessed 2009 Mar 10. URL: http://www.who.int/cancer/palliative/en/.

[5] Beck SL, Falkson G. Prevalence and management of cancer pain in South Africa. Pain 2001;94:75-84.

[6] Ger L, Chang C, Ho S, Lee M, Chiang H, Chao C, et al. Effects of a continuing education program on nurses' practices of cancer pain assessment and their acceptance of patients' pain reports. J Pain Symp Management 2004;27:61-71.

[7] Shvartzman P, Friger M, Shani A, Barak F, Yoram C, Singer Y. Pain control in ambulatory cancer patients - can we do better? J Pain Symptom Manage 2003;26:716-22.

[8] Beck S, Falkson G. Prevalence and management of cancer pain in South Africa. Pain 2001;94:75-84.

[9] Maree J, Wright S. Palliative care: a positive outcome for cancer patients? Curationis 2008;31:43-9.

[10] Travers E, Mitchell D. Strategic and global issues in palliative care. In: Kinghorn S, Gaines S. Palliative nursing: improving end-of-life care. Edinburgh: Elsevier, 2004:1-7.

[11] Van Dyk A, Small L, Zietman A. The pain experience and its management in cancer patients during hospitalisation (in Namibia). Health SA Gesondheid 2000;5:19-26.

[12] Stromgen A, Groenvold M, Pedersen L, Olsen A, Spile M, Sjorgen P. Does the medical record cover the symptoms experienced by cancer patients receiving palliative care? A comparison of the record and patient self-rating. J Pain Symptom Manage 2001;21:189-96.

[13] Reddy S, Rajagopal A, Gouondraj N. Palliative medicine - tutorial part 1. Pain Pract 2001;1:354-68.

[14] Duggleby W. The language of pain at the end of life. Pain Manage Nurs 2002:154-60.

[15] Xue Y, Schulman-Green D, Czaplinski C, Harris D, McCorkle R. Pain attitudes and knowledge among RNs, pharmacists, and physicians on an inpatient oncology service. Clin J Oncol Nurs 2007;11:687-95.

[16] Regulations relating to the approval of and the minimum requirements for the education and training of a nurse (general, psychiatric and community) and midwife leading to registration R. 425. SA Nursing Council, 1985.

[17] Regulations relating to the minimum requirements for a bridging course for enrolled nurses leading to registration as a general nurse or a psychiatric nurse R. 683. SA Nursing Council, 1989.

[18] Lo-Biondo Wood G, Harber J. Nursing research: methods and critical appraisal for evidence-based practice. St Louis: Mosby, 2006.

[19] Polit F, Beck C. Nursing research: generating and assessing evidence for nursing practice. 8th ed. Philadelphia: Lippincott Williams Wilkins, 2008.

[20] Burns N, Grove S. Understanding research: building an evidence-base. St Louis: Elsevier, 2007.

[21] Polit F, Beck C. Nursing research: principles and methods. Philadelphia: Lippincott, 2004.

[22] Burns N, Grove S. The practice of nursing research: conduct, critique, and utilization. 5 ed. St. Louis: Elsevier, 2005.

[23] Polit F, Beck C. Essentials of nursing research: methods, appraisal, and utilization. Philadelphia: Lippincott Williams Wilkins, 2006.

[24] Twycross R. Introducing palliative care. Oxon: Radcliffe, 2003.

[25] Bernardi M, Catania G, Tridello G. Knowledge and attitudes about cancer pain management: a national survey of Italian hospice nurses. Cancer Nurs 2007:E20-E6.

[26] Caraceni A, Brunelli C, Martini C, Zecca E, De Conno F. Cancer pain assessment in clinical trials. A review of the literature (1999-2002). J Pain Symptom Manage 2005;29:507-19.

[27] Hemming L, Maher D. Cancer pain in palliative care: why is management so difficult. Br J Community Nurs 2005;10:355.

[28] Conner A, Muir M. Managing symptoms: what can nurses do? A principle-based approach. In: Kinghorn S, Gaines S, eds. Palliative nursing: improving end of life care. Edinburgh: Elsevier, 2004.

[29] McMillan ST, M, Hagan S, Laughlin J, Tabler R. Knowledge and attitudes of nurses in veterans hospitals about pain management in patients with cancer. Oncol Nurs Forum 2000;27:1415-23.

[30] Gallasch C, Alexandre N. The measures of musculoskeletal pain intensity: a comparison of four methods. Rev Gaucha Enferm 2007;28:260-5.

[31] Metha A, Chan L. Understanding the concept of "total pain". J Hospice Palliat Nurs 2008;10:26-32.

[32] Johnson M. Overview of nursing developments in palliative care. In: Lugton J, Kindlen M. Palliative care: the nursing role. Edinburgh: Churchill Livingstone, 1999:1-26.

In: Advanced Cancer. Pain and Quality of Life
Editors: E. Chow, J. Merrick, pp. 47-51
ISBN: 978-1-61668-207-1
© 2010 Nova Science Publishers, Inc.

Chapter IV

The Relationship Factors between Radiation Oncologists and Hospice Professionals that Influence Cancer Pain Palliation

Stephen T. Lutz, MD*

Department of Radiation Oncology, Blanchard Valley Regional Cancer Center, Findlay, Ohio, United States of America

Cancer remains a major public health problem and the control of end-of-life pain continues to be a challenge even in the face of major advancements in pain control methodology. Both radiation oncologist and hospice professionals have shown a propensity for successfully managing that pain, but educational and reimbursement issues have prevented the two specialties from delivering coordinated, concurrent care. Further optimization of pain control for these patients will require increased collaboration between the two specialties and a willingness on the part of radiation oncologists to employ single fraction therapy for appropriate patients who have bone metastasis pain. This paper presents a short review of the history, barriers and collaborations between the two specialities

Introduction

Cancer remains a major public health problem, and the control of end-of-life pain continues to be a challenge even in the face of major advancements in pain control methodology. The dissemination of proper pain control education has not prevented some cancer patients from suffering debilitating pain because of their own fears about narcotic addiction or their

---

* ***Correspondence:*** Stephen T Lutz, MD, Department of Radiation Oncology, Blanchard Valley Regional Cancer Center, Findlay, Ohio 45840 United States. Tel: 419-423-3703; Fax: 419-427-0212; E-mail: slutz@bvha.org

physician's misunderstanding of appropriate pain medicine dosing (1). The most common cause of cancer pain is bony metastasis, and that pain may serve as a sensitive measure of disease activity. Additionally, patients with bone metastasis face the risk of other ominous effects of their disease such as pathologic fracture and spinal cord compression.

One study of referrals to an outpatient multidisciplinary bone metastasis pain clinic suggested that pain was the presenting symptom in 74% of those sent for evaluation (2). Twenty-three percent of patients rated their pain as severe, while 56% scored their pain as moderate. The patients' episodes of worst pain were described as severe by 78% and intolerable by 22% when measured in the day prior to consultation. Almost a quarter of these patients described their pain medicine regimens as ineffective, while nearly half said that their analgesic regimens provided relief that was only "good" (2).

Both radiation oncologists and hospice professionals are accustomed to managing patients with painful bony metastasis. Radiotherapy has been proven to be a safe, effective, and relatively inexpensive palliative intervention for end-of-life cancer patients with symptoms such as pain. Hospice programs provide efficient and timely pain relief for tens of thousands of cancer patients each year. Though these two specialties share in the care of a large population of cancer patients, in most instances that care is given in a sequential rather than concurrent fashion. Issues of physician education and Medicare reimbursement have acted to keep the pain control efforts of these two groups of specialists largely separated over time.

History of hospice care and pain management

The first hospice in the United States opened in 1974, and the overwhelming majority of the patients treated in early hospice settings had terminal cancer. The Medicare Hospice Benefit was defined in 1982 and specified that all end-of-life care be delivered by a certified hospice at a pre-determined per diem rate (3). The number of hospice programs in the US has since grown to greater than 4,500, and the percentage of non-cancer patients given hospice care has increased dramatically. Still, the absolute number of hospice patients with cancer continues to grow each year, and their need for pain relief is often one of the primary reasons that they are referred to hospice (4). The most common reimbursement scenario pays a hospice about $125 per day for providing all care to one patient, including interventions such as home nursing visits, hospital beds and necessary medications. That per diem must also be used to cover the costs of other palliative interventions, such as radiotherapy treatments.

Palliative radiotherapy and bone metastasis pain

More than a third of patients who receive radiotherapy do so with palliative goals and a significant percentage of patients treated with curative intent will eventually succumb to their cancer (5). The treatment of bone metastasis makes up the most common indication for palliative radiotherapy. Metastatic bone pain is relieved by radiotherapy at a rate of between two-thirds and three-quarters, with up to a third coming to enjoy complete relief. The first signs of pain relief most often begin within two weeks of the start of radiotherapy, while maximal pain relief is most often noted by 4-6 weeks after treatment is completed (6).

Radiation oncologists have historically prescribed a two week course dosed to deliver a total of 30 Gray in 10 treatments for painful bony metastasis, though several more recent randomized trials have proven that the rates of pain control are nearly identical following a single 8 Gray fraction (6,7). The delivery of a single fraction of radiotherapy decreases patient discomfort, transportation difficulties, and acute side effects when compared to a multi-fraction regimen. Single fraction radiotherapy has also been shown to be more cost effective than longer course treatment (8). Additionally, the cost for short course, uncomplicated radiotherapy may be less than the expense for ongoing analgesic use (9). Though the need for re-treatment to the same painful site may increase from about 10% to 20% following single fraction therapy as compared to a more prolonged course, the subsequent costs and inconvenience for re-treatment are not prohibitive.

Still, radiation oncologists in the United States have shown reluctance to prescribing single fraction radiotherapy, when compared to their counterparts in Canada and overseas (10). The principal factors that radiation oncologists report that they use in determining length of treatment course include patient prognosis, risk of spinal cord compression, and performance status. Other factors such as radiotherapy residency training, fear of long term side effects, and reimbursement rules may also inspire less use of single fraction palliative radiotherapy in the US.

Barriers dividing the specialties

The reluctance of radiation oncologists to prescribe single fraction therapy continues to serve as a point of contention between them and the hospice and palliative care community (11). The shift from payment per intervention to a per diem at the time of hospice admission has led to a behavior pattern where the more costly palliative interventions are finished prior to admission to the hospice team. These forces have created a short length of stay for cancer patients on the hospice service prior to death, numbering just greater than twenty days (12). Not surprisingly, those same interactions have caused a situation where nearly 90% of palliative care professionals believe that radiotherapy is important for palliation of cancer symptoms, but only between 1-3% of hospice patients receive radiotherapy (11,13).

The perception of the role of radiation oncologists varies greatly between these two groups of specialists. Nearly half of radiation oncologists would describe themselves as members of the "palliative care team", while less than ten percent of hospice professionals would see them that same way (14). Conversely, radiation oncologists often bond with their referring physicians by building a long term relationship, where treatment options are debated and consensus reached. The sequential pattern of end-of-life care by specialists has diminished the understanding by the radiotherapy community about many aspects of hospice including the delivery of care while paying heed to the economic construct of a per diem.

Collaborative initiatives

Several efforts have been initiated to increase collaboration between these two specialties on issues of education, research, and patient advocacy. There are currently about a dozen physicians who hold dual certification in both radiation oncology and hospice and palliative medicine. The American Board of Radiology (ABR) enthusiastically joined ten other medical specialties to co-sponsor the new hospice and palliative medicine subspecialty as recognized by the American Board of Medical Specialties (ABMS). One of the main roles of the new Hospice and Palliative board certified specialists will be to carry out assessment and management of pain and other symptoms in those facing the end of life. Those specialists will also be asked to enhance cost effective treatment and to collaborate care with a multi-disciplinary team.

The American Society for Radiation Oncology (ASTRO) has named an official liaison to the hospice and palliative medicine community and has also begun to increase palliative care educational opportunities through its national meeting and continuing medical education initiatives. The Centers for Medicare and Medicaid Services (CMS) has designated a specific reimbursement code for physician palliative care management. The National Hospice and Palliative Care Organization (NHPCO) and the American Academy of Hospice and Palliative Medicine have (AAHPM) have actively worked to make palliative radiotherapy education available for their membership.

Conclusions

While cancer pain remains an ongoing public health issue, both radiation oncologist and hospice professionals have shown a propensity for successfully managing that pain. Further optimization of pain control for these patients will require increased collaboration between the two specialties and willingness on the part of radiation oncologists to employ single fraction therapy for appropriate patients who have bone metastasis pain.

References

[1] Ward S, Berry P, Misiewicz H. Concerns about analgesics among patients and family caregivers in a hospice setting. Res Nurs Health 1996;19:205-11.

[2] Janjan A, Payne R, Gillis T, et al. Presenting symptoms in patients referred to a multidisciplinary clinic for bone metastases. J Pain Symptom Manage 1998;16:171-8.

[3] History of Hospice Care. National Hospice and Palliative Care Organization website. http://www.nhpco.org/i4a/pages/index.cfm?pageid=3285 most recently accessed June 3, 2008

[4] NHPCO Facts and Figures: Hospice Care in America November 2007 Edition. National Hospice and Palliative Care Organization Organization website. http://www.nhpco

.org/files/public/Statistics_Research/NHPCO_facts-and-figures_Nov2007.pdf most recently accessed June 3, 2008.

[5] Coia L, Hanks G, Martz K, et al. Practice patterns of palliative care for the United States 1984-1985. Int J Radiat Oncol Biol Phys 1988;14:1261-9.

[6] Wu J, Wong R, Johnston M, et al. Meta-analysis of dose-fractionation radiotherapy trials for the palliation of painful bone metastasis. Int J Radiat Oncol Biol Phys 2003;55:594-605.

[7] Hartsell W, Scott C, Bruener D, et al. Randomized trial of short- versus long-course radiotherapy for palliation of painful bone metastases. J Natl Cancer Inst 2005;97:798-804.

[8] Van den Hout W, van der Linden Y, Steenland E, et al. Single- versus multiple-fraction radiotherapy in patients with painful bone metastases: Cost utility analysis based on a randomized trial. J Natl Cancer Inst 2003;95:222-9.

[9] Macklis R, Cornelli H, Lasher J. Brief course of palliative radiotherapy for metastatic bone pain: A pilot cost-minimization comparison with narcotic analgesics. Am J Clin Oncol 1998;21:617-22.

[10] Fairchild A, Barnes E, Ghosh S, et al. International patterns of practice in palliative radiotherapy for painful bone metastasis: Evidence based practice? Int J Radiat Oncol Phys, in press.

[11] Lutz S, Spence C, Chow E, Janjan N, et al. Survey on use of palliative radiotherapy in hospice care. J Clin Oncol 2004;22:3581-6.

[12] National Hospice and Palliative Care Organization. NHPCO Facts and Figures: Hospice Care in America, November 2007 edition. www.nhpco.org/files /public/Statistics Research/NDS FY2007.pdf, most recently accessed April 12, 2008.

[13] Lutz S, Ashworth J, Spence C, et al. The use of radiotherapy in hospice patients: A population-based study from the National Hospice Outcomes Project [Abstract]. J Clin Oncol 2005;23 (Suppl. 16):8074.

[14] McCloskey S, Tao M, Rose C, et al. National survey of perspectives of palliative radiation therapy: role, barriers, and needs. Cancer J 2007;13:130-7.

Section Two: Palliative Radiotherapy

In: Advanced Cancer. Pain and Quality of Life
Editors: E. Chow, J. Merrick, pp. 55-68
ISBN: 978-1-61668-207-1
© 2010 Nova Science Publishers, Inc.

Chapter V

Bisphosphonates in Combination with Radiotherapy for the Treatment of Bone Metastases

Shaelyn Culleton, BSc(C), Amanda Hird, BSc(C), Janet Nguyen, BSc(C), Urban Emmenegger, MD, Sunil Verma, MD, Christine Simmons, MD, Elizabeth Barnes, MD, May Tsao, MD, Arjun Sahgal, MD, Cyril Danjoux, MD, Gunita Mitera, MRTT, MBA, Emily Sinclair, MRTT and Edward Chow, MBBS**

Rapid Response Radiotherapy Program, Department of Radiation Oncology and Division of Medical Oncology, Odette Cancer Centre, Sunnybrook Health Sciences Centre, University of Toronto, Toronto, Ontario, Canada

The purpose was to investigate the clinical benefits of combining radiation and bisphosphonates in bone metastases. Methods: A systematic search on Medline was conducted from 1950 to November 2008. Eligible studies included in-vitro cell studies, animal tumor models, and any human studies combining the use of radiotherapy and bisphosphonates. This search was limited to English publications only. Results: A total of 13 studies involving the combination of bisphosphonates and radiotherapy were identified. Three were in-vitro cell studies, two were animal tumor models, and eight were human studies. Both in-vitro cell studies and animal tumor models demonstrate significant synergistic effects when combining both therapies. There are only two human randomized trials comparing combination therapy to placebo and radiation, which showed greater long term benefits using combination treatment. Conclusion: Preliminary evidence suggests that patients with bone metastases may significantly benefit from

* Correspondence: Edward Chow, MBBS, PhD, FRCPC, Department of Radiation Oncology, Odette Cancer Centre, Sunnybrook Health Sciences Centre, 2075 Bayview Avenue, Toronto, ON M4N 3M5, Canada. Tel: 416-480-4998; Fax: 416-480-6002; E-mail: Edward.Chow@sunnybrook.ca

concurrent treatment with both radiotherapy and bisphosphonates when compared with either treatment alone.

Introduction

Skeletal metastases are a common and often debilitating complication of advanced cancer, with incidences ranging from 23 to 84% (1). Bone metastases can lead to skeletal related events (SREs), which cause significant morbidity, including hypercalcemia, pathological fractures, bone pain and spinal cord compression (1-6). On average, 45-75% of patients with bone metastases experience pain (7). In particular, patients with advanced breast, lung and prostate cancer are among those most commonly impacted by bone metastases (7), accounting for approximately 80% of all cases (8).

With advancements in systemic therapies, patients are now living longer with their diagnosis of bone metastases (8-11). Therefore, this cohort is at an increased risk for experiencing SREs, thereby making the prevention and management of these disease-related events of upmost importance. Two of the most prevalent treatments in managing and preventing adverse events and symptoms associated with bone metastases are radiotherapy (RT) and bisphosphonates (BPs) (12,13).

Radiotherapy is a well-established treatment for the palliation of symptomatic bone metastases (14). Approximately 50-80% of patients receive some pain relief, and approximately 20-30% of patients achieve complete pain relief (13-15). It also has been noted that RT is more effective at reducing incident pain than any analgesic regimen (13).

The most commonly prescribed doses of palliative RT for bone metastases are a single 8Gy fraction, 20Gy in five fractions, and 30Gy in 10 fractions (7,15-17). Palliative doses are considerably less than those used for curative intent, and as such, are usually associated with fewer side effects. Nevertheless, palliative RT not only reduces and often alleviates pain, but it also reduces the tumor burden. For bone metastases treated with RT, the consequence of suppression of progressive osteoclast activity serves to help irradiated bone restore integrity and enables osteoblastic repair. Even though the exact mechanisms of pain relief from RT are not yet fully understood, it is felt that complementary osteoclast inhibition by BPs and RT represents a rationale for the combined use of these two treatment modalities (14).

Since the 1980's, the use of BPs in managing bone metastases has been well established. BPs have a high affinity for bone minerals, allowing these molecules to congregate in areas of active bone destruction. Osteoclasts then take up these BPs and induce apoptosis and inhibit cell differentiation (18). This effect is even more pronounced in newer generation BPs modified with nitrogenous side chains (for example, zoledronic acid) (18). Large meta-analyses of randomized BP trials have shown that they significantly reduce SREs in breast and prostate cancer by 17% and 5.2%, respectively. In addition, both prostate and breast cancer trials have showed significant relief in metastatic bone pain. These effects are associated with an improvement in overall quality of life (6,10,11).

The mechanisms by which BPs suppress osteoclast and osteoblast activity are complex and encompasses various tumor factors, proteins and other molecules. Primarily, BPs act by suppressing both mature and precursor osteoclast cells, and provide physico-chemical protection from hypercalcemia by inhibiting calcium phosphate precipitation (6,14,19).

Bisphosphonates have proven effectiveness in managing both osteosclerotic and osteolytic lesions since both processes involve the hyperactivity of osteoclast cells (19,20).

Given that RT and BPs are effective in managing bone metastases, particularly with respect to the suppression of osteoclast activity, it is conceivable that combining these two treatments could enhance the overall effect of either treatment in isolation. Data has emerged from the literature within the last 10 years investigating this synergistic potential (21) and it is therefore the purpose of this review is to summarize relevant studies reporting the potential of this combined approach.

Our study

We conducted a systematic Medline (1950 to November 2008) and Cochrane Central Register of Controlled Trials (4th Quarter 2008) search. Search terms included combinations of "radiotherapy", "irradiation" "bone neoplasm" and "bisphosphonate". Secondary search terms included "zoledronic acid", "zoledronate", "etidronate", "clodronate", "pamidronate", "ibandronate" and "bone metastasis". The search results were manually reviewed, relevant literature was extracted and the references for all these publications were thoroughly examined for additional references.

Inclusion criteria

All studies involving the combination of BPs and palliative RT for the management of bone metastases were included. This criterion did not include in-vitro studies.

Exclusion criteria

Studies that were in a language other than English were not considered in our review.

What we found

We identified a total of 13 studies that combined both BPs and RT, three of which were in-vitro cell studies, and two of which studied combination therapy in animal tumor models. The remaining eight involved combination BP and RT treatment in humans.

Table 1. Summary of in-vitro studies

Author	Cell lines	Bisphosphonate (BP)	Total Dose of Radiation (RT)	BP + RT	Effect of BP + RT
Journe et al. [7]	MDA-MB-231 (Breast ER-)	Ibandronate (1-1,000μM)	1-15Gy	significantly reduced clongenic cell survival and increased apoptosis vs. RT, BP and control ($p<0.005$)	Synergistic effects observed irrespective of combined BP + RT dose or sequence
	MCF-7 (Breast ER+)			significantly reduced clongenic cell survival vs. RT, BP and control and increased apoptosis vs. control and BP ($p<0.005$)	Synergistic effects observed in low BP (1-3 μM) irrespective of RT dose or sequence
Algur et al. [18]	C4-2 (Androgen-independent prostate)	Zoledronic Acid (10-200 μM)	1-10Gy	significant reduction in cell viability vs. BP, RT, and control ($p<0.005$)	Synergistic effect of BP + RT is most obvious in lower BP doses (10-100 μM) irrespective of RT dose
	IM-9 (B-lymphoblastic Multiple Myeloma)			significant reduction in cell viability vs. BP, RT, and control ($p<0.005$)	
Ural et al. [3]	MCF-7 (Breast ER +)	Zoledronic Acid (0.1-100 μM)	2-8Gy	significant reduction in cell viability vs. BP, RT, and control ($p<0.005$)	Synergistic effects observed irrespective of combined BP + RT dose

BP = bisphosphonate; RT = radiotherapy

In-vitro cell studies

Three in-vitro studies combining both RT and BPs were identified. The main results of all three studies are summarized in table 1. All studies found a significant synergistic effect when the two treatments were combined, by means of a reduction in cell viability via induction of apoptosis (3,7,18). Only one study evaluated the effect of sequence and fractionation schedules on cell viability. This study found that although all sequences were effective (concurrent, BP before RT, or RT before BP), radiation delivered before BP was most effective, particularly in the ER-positive breast cancer cell line. This study also found no difference in cell response when comparing single or multi-fractionated radiation courses (7). Table 2 compares the results of cell viability data obtained by all three studies. Each study concluded that in a clinical situation, the combination of both RT and BPs may allow for a reduction in the dose of palliative RT delivered to a patient for their bone metastases. Interestingly, these data also support an advantage for the more potent BP, zoledronic acid, over ibandronate in the ER-positive breast cancer cell line.

Table 2. Percent cell viability compared to control

	Journe et al. [7*]		Algur et al. [18†]		Ural et al. [3‡]
	MDA-MB-231 (Breast ER-) (%)	MCF-7 (Breast ER+) (%)	C4-2 (androgen-independent prostate) (%)	IM-9 (B-lymphoblastic Multiple Myeloma) (%)	MCF-7 (Breast ER +) (%)
BP (100 μM)	91	62	35	20	37
RT (4 Gy)	60	62	74	22	64
BP (100 μM) + RT (4 Gy)	51	24	23	13	10

* Analysis was conducted after 160h at 37°C in 5% CO_2 atmosphere

† Analysis was conducted after 48.5h for the C4-2 cell line and 72.5h for the IM-9 cell line both at 37°C in 5% CO_2 atmosphere

‡ Analysis was conducted after 72h at 37°C in 5% CO_2 atmosphere

Animal tumor models

Two studies were identified that assessed the relationship between BPs and RT in animal tumor models. Primary results of those two studies have been summarized in table 3. In both studies, tumor cells that produced lytic metastases were injected into weight-bearing bones of rodents. Micro-computed tomography analysis was used in both studies to assess the microarchitecture, bone and/or tumor volume, bone density, trabecular number and trabecular separation of both normal and involved bone (1,5). These studies conclude that the combined administration of both BPs and RT may lead to improved mineralization and restabilization when compared with RT alone, and that early administration of BPs before RT was more beneficial than just RT alone (1,5).

Arrington et al (5) also reported on biomechanical testing on both normal and involved bone. In their analysis of the biomechanical properties in treated vs. normal bone, the combined BP and RT approach re-established strength and flexibility of the diseased bone to the equivalent level as that observed in normal bone. The outcome of all treatment schedules to normal bone was also compared, and only treatment with RT and BP was able to improve the microarchitecture of the involved bone to such an extent that it appeared very similar to normal bone under micro-computed tomography analysis. However, statistical analysis was not significant due to the small study population.

Krempien et al (1) also demonstrated that BPs delivered three days prior to RT had a significantly greater impact on bone remodeling and stabilization than concurrent administration of BPs and RT. Of note, both studies showed that RT alone was not able to quickly or completely remineralize and strengthen the involved bone, leaving the subjects at risk for a pathological fracture in the irradiated area.

Table 3. Summary of animal studies

Author	Total Number of Animals	Tumor Cell Variant	Bisphosphonate (BP)	Radiation (RT)	Groups	Bone Structure	Bone Density	Mechanical testing
Krempien et al. [1]	106	Walker 256B carcinosarcoma(lytic metastases) injected into proximal tibia	Clodronate (20mg/kg)	17 Gy	Group 1: RT treatment only (Day 7 post tumor injection) Group 2: Early BP + RT treatment (BP 3-6 days post tumor injection + RT (Day 7) Group 3: Concurrent BP (Days 7-10 post tumor injection) + RT (Day 7)	Group 2 showed significantly better bone preservation parameters* (p<0.001) vs. groups 1,3. Group 3 only had significantly less trabecular separation vs. Group 1 (P<0.02)	At 6 wks post tumor injection, there was a significant difference in bone density in Groups 1 and 3 vs. normal† (57.6% vs. 56.7% vs. 100% P<0.001). However there was no significant difference in Group 2 vs. normal† (88.1% vs 100%)	None preformed however better weight-bearing 3D trabecular microarchitecture in Group 2 vs. Groups 1 and 3.
Arrington et al. [5]	30	MDAMB-231 Breast cancer (lytic metastases) injected into distal femur	Zoledronic Acid (100μg/kg)	20 Gy	Group 1: No treatment Group 2: RT 3 weeks post tumor injection Group 3: RT 3 wks post tumor injection + BP given once weekly for 6 wks starting 3 days before RT.	BV‡ vs. normal for groups 1-3 (70% decrease (P<0.00009), 44% decrease (p<0.0107) and 15% increase (p<0.2602) respectively). Other bone parameters* showed no significant difference in Group 3 vs. Normal.	At 3 wks post tumor injection, Groups 1-3 vs. normal (15% decrease, 4% decrease, 14% increase) in bone density. At 6 wks, Group 2 had lower bone density vs. Group 3 (p< 0.005) and normal (P< 0.035).	No significant difference between groups 1 and 2 in mechanical testing§. Group 3 had no significant difference in mechanical testing§ vs. normal but was significantly better vs. Groups 1 and 2.

*Histomorphometric bone parameters include: bone area percent (= bone area/ tissue area x 100%), trabecular number and trabecular separation.

† Normal group received no injection of Walker 256B and no treatment

‡ Bone volume

§ Biomechanical testing includes: peak torque, energy to failure and initial stiffness of the intact limb through the knee joint.

Table 4. Summary of human studies

Author	Study Type	Population	Bisphosphonate (BP)	Radiation (RT)	Study Group(s)	Pain and analgesics	Skeletal Related Events (SREs)	Bone remodeling (assessed by X-ray or CT comparisons)
Kouloulias et al. [2, 25]	Open-labeled phase I/II Observational study	n=33 Breast cancer with lytic bone metastases	Disodium Pamidronate (180mg every 4 weeks)	30 Gy total dose with patients receiving 3Gy/day	RT and BP given concurrently	Pain scores decreased significantly from baseline to 6 mos*.	One patient had an SRE within 6 mos*. Skeletal complication-free survival was 17 mos*.	Significant bone healing and mineralization at 6 mos*.
Kouloulias et al. [23]	Randomized trial	n=42 Various solid tumors with lytic metastases	Disodium Pamidronate (180mg every 4 weeks)	30 Gy total dose with patients receiving 3Gy/day	Group 1: stepwise 90-180mg BP dose escalation (30mg every 4 wks) + concurrent RT	Patients had significantly reduced pain score in all groups at 6 mos* post baseline; most significant improvement noted in Group 2	Patients with BP had significantly delayed new bone metastases (p< 0.011)	Group 2 had greater recalcification vs. Group 1 (p<0.05) while Group 1 and 2 did significantly better than RT alone (P<0.05)
					Group 2: 180mg BP + concurrent RT			
					Group 3: RT only			
George et al. [22]	Randomized Phase II trial	n=40 Various solid tumors (except prostate or hematological ca) with bone metastases	Pamidronate dose	20Gy/5	Group 1: BP + RT 3 or more days later	No statistical significance between pamidronate vs. placebo in pain/analgesic scores at day 29 post BP	None reported	None reported
					Group 2: Placebo + RT 3 or more days later			
Kijima et al. [24]	Retrospective chart review	n=23 Renal cell with cancer with bone metastases	Zoledronic Acid (4mg every 3-4 weeks)	20-45Gy with patients receiving 1.8-2Gy/day	Group 1: RT only	None reported	In Group 1, 10/13 patients had an SRE vs. 1/10 patients in Group 2 (P<0.003) (skeletal event-free survival in Group 2 was 18.7 mos; not reached in Group 2)	6/10 patients in Group 2 had partial recalcification vs. 1/13 in Group 1 (p<0.019)
					Group 2: RT + BP concurrently			

Table 4. (continued)

Author	Study Type	Population	Bisphosphonate (BP)	Radiation (RT)	Study Group(s)	Pain and analgesics	Skeletal Related Events (SREs)	Bone remodeling (assessed by X-ray or CT comparisons)
Micke et al. [28]	Randomized Phase II trial	n=52 Various solid tumors with lytic metastases	Ibandronate	36-40 Gy	Group 1: 4mg BP + RT then 3mg every 28 days for 1 year	No significant difference in pain or analgesic scores in groups 1 vs. 2	None reported	No significant difference in recalcification rates in groups 1 vs. 2
					Group 2: 1mg BP + RT, 1mg days 8, 15 and 22; 3mg every 28 days for 1 year			
Vassiliou et al. [4]	Phase I observational study	n=45 Various solid tumors with bone metastases	Ibandronate (10 cycles of 6mg monthly)	30-40 Gy	RT + BP concurrently	Opioid use and pain scores decrease significantly at 3, 6, and 10 mos* vs. baseline. (P< 0.001)	At 10 months, 2 patients had an SRE	Significantly increased bone density at 3 mos* (19.8%), 6 (45.8%) and 10 (73.2%) vs. baseline. (p<0.001)
Vassiliou et al. [27]	Phase I observational study	n=52 Various solid tumors with bone metastases	Ibandronate (10 cycles of 6mg monthly)	30-40 Gy	Group 1: lytic metastases + concurrent BP + RT	In all groups pain and analgesic score significantly decreased at 3, 6, and 10 mos* vs. baseline. Greatest response occurred at 10mos* in Group 1 vs. baseline	None reported	Mean bone density for three groups were significant (p<0.05), highest increase in Group 1 at 10 mos*. Recalcification was noted in all groups.
					Group 2: mixed metastases + concurrent BP + RT			
					Group 3: sclerotic metastases + concurrent BP + RT			

* months

Human studies

At total of eight human studies involving the combination of BPs and RT were identified and are summarized in table 4. Only two of these studies were randomized, comparing a BP and RT arm with either RT and placebo or placebo alone (22,23). However, the randomized study done by George et al (22), which used a placebo arm, only followed patients for 29 days and the primary outcome only involved pain and analgesic scores. The majority of the studies are observational and the primary objectives of all studies have a variety of endpoints.

The most commonly prescribed doses of RT to treat bone metastases for the majority of these studies were within the range of 30-40Gy. Ibandronate and pamidronate were the BPs of choice in all studies, while a retrospective review by Kijima et al. evaluated zoledronic acid and RT (24). All studies that assessed long term pain and analgesic consumption noted a significant decrease from baseline in patients treated with both BP and RT (2, 4,23,25-27). Additionally, studies that reported bone remodeling found that mean bone density and recalcification rates significantly increased when compared to baseline scores (2,4,23,25,27).

The most compelling study of all those identified was a randomized trial done by Kouloulias et al (23). This study compared two different concurrent BP and RT schedules (high-dose BP versus dose escalated BP) to RT alone. Pain and analgesic scores were shown to significantly decrease in all groups, however high-dose BP and concurrent RT was noted to have the most significant improvement. Patients who received concurrent BP with RT had a significant delay in the development and incidence of new bony lesions when compared to the RT alone group ($p<0.011$). The high-dose BP and RT group also showed a significantly greater recalcification rate when compared to the RT alone group and dose escalation BP group ($p<0.05$). This study provided promising evidence regarding the benefits of using combination treatment to manage bone metastases. However, it was limited by its small study population.

Kijima et al (24) comparatively analyzed RT and combination BP treatment in a retrospective study. This report focused on advanced renal cell cancer patients who either received RT alone or concurrent zoledronic acid and RT for painful bone metastases. It was observed that significantly less patients treated with combination BP and RT experienced a SRE compared to those who just received RT ($p<0.003$). In addition, patients treated with combination therapy had achieved a significantly higher recalcification rate than those treated with RT alone ($p<0.019$). They concluded that based on these findings, prospective clinical trials should be established to investigate concurrent therapy in this population.

Human toxicities

No significant toxicities from combined treatments were reported in any of the studies apart from side effects commonly associated with the administration of BPs such as flu-like symptoms, myalgias and arthalgias (2, 4,23,27,28). The combination treatment was reportedly well tolerated among patients in two studies (4,27).

Discussion

Combined modality therapies have recently emerged in the management of the palliative cancer population. As patients with metastatic disease are living longer, quality of life is increasingly recognized as an important outcome. As such, more aggressive therapies for these patients aimed at more rapid and durable palliation of symptoms are emerging, analogous to strategies used in the curative cancer therapeutic approaches (29).

With respect to bone metastases, the combination of BPs and RT is being actively investigated to improve on exiting outcomes with either approach alone. The rationale is to take advantage of the commonalities in both RT and BP pain response pathways with respect to osteoclast suppression and tumor apoptosis (7,14).

In-vitro cell studies that combined both RT and BP have shown a significant synergistic effect (3,7,18). However, the exact mechanism is unknown. Ural et al (30,31) proposed that perhaps BPs have the ability to arrest cells in the M and G2 phase of the cell cycle, thereby increasing the proportion of tumor cells in the more susceptible phases of the cell cycle to RT. The outcome is increased apoptosis.

This is evident when considering data has shown that ibandronate alone had the ability to induce apoptosis in breast tumor cells to a slightly smaller degree than RT alone, however, the combination of both RT and ibandronate had an approximate doubling effect (7). In considering the three in-vitro studies presented in this review, a synergistic relationship between BPs and RT was concluded. Upon further study, this synergistic relationship could one day allow for BP or RT dose-reduction, which would subsequently result in lower treatment toxicities (3,7,18).

Although single or multi-fractionated RT regimens have been shown to be equally efficacious with minimal toxicity, a multi-fraction approach has shown significantly greater effectiveness in inducing remineralization of the bone and reducing re-treatment rates (16,32). Therefore a multi-fractionated course of RT with a BP could provide significantly greater benefits in terms of remineralization and reduced skeletal morbidity. However, human studies exploring BPs and either a single or multi-fractionated course of RT are needed to assess the potential benefits of a multi-fractionated course of RT.

Another factor that has shown to influence the efficacy of combined RT and BP treatment has been the order with which the treatments are scheduled. The one in-vitro cell study that assessed other alternatives to concurrent delivery found that RT given 3-6 days before BP administration had a greater synergistic effect than concurrent administration (7). Further exploration of different treatment schedules was assessed in animal tumor models. Both animal tumor model studies included at least one treatment arm which delivered BPs before RT (1,5). Krempien et al (1) found that BPs delivered 3-6 days before RT was significantly more effective than concurrent BP and RT. This study theorized that early BP administration helped to maintain the microarchitecture of the bone before RT was delivered, reducing the remodeling and chance of fractures in the irradiated area, which subsequently allowed for faster remineralization of the bone following RT (1). Overall, the animal tumor model suggests that early BP administration along with RT has significant benefits in bone remodeling and mechanical restoration within the irradiated area over RT alone. Both the no treatment and RT only groups in both animal tumor studies showed significantly decreased mineralization, bone density and mechanical testing when compared to normal bone (1,5). Though neither study evaluated BPs alone, BPs are not recommended as a first-line therapy for pain relief from bone metastases; RT is a recommended first-line treatment (6). Unfortunately, despite animal tumor model evidence that early BP administration before RT was of significant benefit, all of the published human studies (with one exception) chose to use concurrent (same-day) administration in their study protocols.

To examine how effective combined BP and RT was in human studies, pain scores and analgesic use, SREs, and recalcification rates were all used as determinates. When reviewing pain and analgesic scores of patients receiving combined RT and BPs, only four studies compared baseline and follow-up pain and analgesic scores. All four studies showed that pain scores significantly decreased at six month follow-up (2,4,23,25,27). Analgesic scores, reported only in studies by Vassiliou et al., showed a significant 61% decrease in opioid consumption by 10 month follow-up (4,27). This same study also showed a pain score reduction to zero in 70% of patients at three months and 80% at 10 months (4,27). In comparison, two large separate meta-analyses found that a complete pain reduction from RT alone occurred in only 32-33% of patients, and any response to RT occurred in 60% of patients (16,17,23). This suggests there may be a benefit with regards to pain reduction with combined BP and RT over RT alone, and this could be explored in further large randomized controlled trials. Only two studies were able to directly compare pain and/or analgesic scores of combined RT and BP to RT alone (22,23). Even though these two studies had contradictory findings with respect to pain relief from combination treatment, they both consisted of a small sample population of patients with varying solid tumor types, therefore the significance of these outcomes are somewhat limited.

Of all the eight human studies identified, only three reported SRE data. Two of these studies are observational studies and therefore comparisons are difficult to extrapolate. Nevertheless, one of these studies reported the event-free survival for 33 breast patients receiving 180mg pamidronate and RT was 17 months (2,25). When comparing this statistic to event-free survival of randomized pamidronate trials in breast cancer, the event-free survival was 11.9 months on average (11). However, the dose of pamidronate in the combined pamidronate and RT study was at least double that in pamidronate breast cancer trials (11). The only study that had detailed SRE data was a retrospective review of renal cell patients receiving either zoledronic acid plus RT verses RT alone for bone metastases. This study showed a significant difference in SREs between the two groups, strongly favouring the combination group (24).

With respect to the bone remodeling, five studies reported on recalcification rates following treatment using radiological imaging. All studies reported a significant increase in recalcification or bone density following combination treatment (2,4,23-25,27). Detailed recalcification rates by Vassiliou et al. showed that at 6 months, the average increased bone density was 45.8% from baseline and increased 73.2% at 10 months from baseline (4). In comparison, one of the only studies that evaluated the recalcification rate of lesions from various solid tumors treated with RT alone found that the recalcification rate of multi-fractionated courses at six months was approximately 73% (32). However, this particular study had a higher proportion of breast cancer patients than lung cancer patients when compared to Vassiliou et al (4,32). Patients with breast cancer have a higher response rate with respect to the remineralization to bone (77%) when compared with other primaries such as lung (27%) and renal cell (25%) (33).

Overall, all of the human studies evaluating the effectiveness of BPs and RT had very small patient populations (the largest study contained 52 patients), and the majority of them lacked randomization or a control arm. Though these studies suggest possible benefits from the combined treatment, the variability and subjectivity of all the studies are too great to draw any reasonable conclusions. Suffice to say, both RT and BPs are effective treatments in managing and treating painful bone metastases. This literature review shows that combining the two treatments does not show any added treatment toxicity, nor are either of the two treatments any less effective when combined (3,4,6,7,15,18,27).

Conclusions

We recommend further large randomized trials to evaluate the effectiveness of combining RT and BPs. We also suggest that further randomized studies assess concurrent versus pre-BP administration, as well as assess the potential benefits of using multi-fractionated RT in weight-bearing bones compared with a single fraction. Overall, both animal tumor models and in-vitro cell studies evaluating the use of combined RT and BPs suggest a synergistic effect that may be beneficial for patients with painful bone metastases (1,3,5, 7,18).

Acknowledgments

The studentship was funded by the Michael and Karyn Goldstein Cancer Research Fund. We also thank Stacy Lue, Candi Flynn, Jennifer Wong and Julie Napolskikh for their help. No conflict of interest declared.

References

[1] Krempien R, Huber PE, Harms W, Treiber M, Wannenmacher M, Krempien B. Combination of early bisphosphonate administration and irradiation leads to improved remineralization and restabilization of osteolytic bone metastases in an animal tumor model. Cancer 2003;98(6):1318-24.

[2] Kouloulias V, Matsopoulous G, Kouvaris J, Dardoufas C, Bottomley A, et al. Radiotherapy in conjunction with intravenous infusion of 180 mg of disodium pamidronate in management of osteolytic metastases from breast cancer: Clinical evaluation, biochemical markers, quality of life, and monitoring of recalcification using assessments of grey-level histogram in plain radiographs. Int J Radiation Oncology Biol Phys 2003;57(1):143-57.

[3] Ural AU, Avcu F, Candir M, Guden M, Ozcan MA. In vitro synergistic cytoreductive effects of zoledronic acid and radiation on breast cancer cells. Breast Cancer Res 2006;8(4):R52.

[4] Vassiliou V, Kalogeropoulou C, Christopoulos C, Solomou E, Leotsinides M, Kardamakis D. Combination ibandronate and radiotherapy for the treatment of bone metastases: Clinical evaluation and radiologic assessment. Int J Radiat Oncol Biol Phys 2007;67(1):264-72.

[5] Arrington SA, Damron TA, Mann KA, Allen MJ. Concurrent administration of zoledronic acid and irradiation leads to improved bone density, biomechanical strength, and microarchitecture in a mouse model of tumor-induced osteolysis. J Surg Oncol 2008;97(3):284-90.

[6] Wong R, Wiffen PJ. Bisphosphonates for the relief of pain secondary to bone metastases. Cochrane Database Syst Rev 2002(2):002068.

[7] Journe F, Magne N, Chaboteaux C, Kinnaert E, Bauss F, Body J. Sequence- and concentration-dependent effects of acute and long-term exposure to the bisphosphonate ibandronate in combination with single and multiple fractions of ionising radiation doses in human breast cancer cell lines. Clin Exp Metastasis 2006;23(135):137-47.

[8] Falkmer U, Jarhult J, Wersall P, Cavallin-Stahl E. A systematic overview of radiation therapy effects in skeletal metastases. Acta Oncol 2003;42(5-6):620-33.

[9] Jasmin C, Capanna R, Coleman RE, Coia LR, Saillant G, eds.Textbook of bone metastases. Hoboken, NJ: Wiley, 2005.

[10] Yuen KK, Shelley M, Sze WM, Wilt T, Mason MD. Bisphosphonates for advanced prostate cancer. Cochrane Database Syst Rev 2006(4):006250.

[11] Pavlakis N, Stockler M. Bisphosphonates for breast cancer.update in cochrane database syst rev. Cochrane Database Syst Rev 2002(1):003474 and 2005;(3):CD003474.

[12] Ross J, Saunders Y, Edmonds P, Patel S, Broadley K, Johnston S. Systematic review of bisphosphonates on skeletal morbidity in metastatic cancer. BMJ 2003;327:469.

[13] McQuay HJ, Collins SL, Carroll D, Moore RA. Radiotherapy for the palliation of painful bone metastases. Cochrane Database Syst Rev 2000(2):001793.

[14] Hoskin PJ. Bisphosphonates and radiation therapy for palliation of metastatic bone disease. Cancer Treat Rev 2003;29(4):321-7.

[15] Chow E, Harris K, Fan G, Tsao M, Sze W. Palliative radiotherapy trials for bone metastases: A systematic review. J Clin Oncol 2007;25(11):1423-36.

[16] Sze W, Shelley M, Held I, Mason M. Palliation of metastatic bone pain: Single fraction versus multifraction radiotherapy. Cochrane Database Syst Rev 2004;(2):CD004721.

[17] Wu J, Wong R, Johnston M, Bezjak A, Whelan T. Meta-analysis of dose-fractionation radiotherapy trials for the palliation of painful bone metastases. Int J Radiat Oncol Biol Phys 2003;55(3):594-605.

[18] Algur E, Macklis R, Hafeli U. Synergistic cytotoxic effects of zoledronic acid and radiation in human prostate cancer and myeloma cell line. Int J Radiat Oncol Biol Phys 2005;61(2):535-42.

[19] Fleisch H. The role of bisphosphonates in breast cancer: Development of bisphosphonates. Breast Cancer Res 2002;4:30-4.

[20] Adami S. Bisphosphonates in prostate carcinoma. Cancer 1997;80:1674-9.

[21] Ural AU, Avcu F, Baran Y. Bisphosphonate treatment and radiotherapy in metastatic breast cancer. Med Oncol 2008;25:350-5.

[22] George R, Hephzibah J, John S. Does pamidronate enhance the analgesic effect of radiotherapy? A randomized trial. Palliat Med 2007;21(8):719-20.

[23] Kouloulias EV, Kouvaris RJ, Antypas C, Mystakidou K, Matsopoulos G, Uzunoglu CN, Moulopoulos A, Vlahos JL. An intra-patient dose-escalation study of disodium pamidronate plus radiotherapy versus radiotherapy alone for the treatment of osteolytic metastases. monitoring of recalcification using image-processing techniques. Strahlentherapie Onkologie 2003;179(7):471-9.

[24] Kijima T, Fujii F, Suyama T, Okudo Y, Yamamoto S, Masuda H, Yonese J, Fukui I. Radiotherapy to bone metastases from renal cell carcinoma with or without zoledronate. BJU Int 2009;103(5):620-4.

[25] Kouloulias V, Dardoufas C, Kouvaris J, Antypas C, Sandilos P, Matsopoulos G, Vlahos L. Use of image processing techniques to assess effect of disodium pamidronate in conjunction with radiotherapy in patients with bone metastases. Acta Oncol 2002;41(2):164-9.

[26] Kouloulias V, Kouvaris J, Mystakidou K, Varela M, Kokakis J, Pistevou-Gombaki K, Balafouta M, Gennatas C, Vlahos L. Duration of bisphosphonate treatment: Results of a non-randomised study in patients previously treated with local irradiation for bone metastases from breast cancer. Curr Med Res Opin 2004;20(6):819.

[27] Vassiliou V, Kalogeropoulou C, Giannopoulou E, Leotsinidis M, Tsota I, Kardamakis D. A novel study investigating the therapeutic outcome of patients with lytic, mixed and sclerotic bone metastases treated with combined radiotherapy and ibandronate. Clin Exp Metastasis 2007;24:169-78.

[28] Micke O, Berning D, Schafer F, Bruns F, Willich N. Combination of ibandronate and radiotherapy in metastatic bone disease - final results of a randomized phase II trial. Eur J Cancer Suppl 2003;1(5):S150.

[29] Hillner B, Ingle J, Chlebowski R, Gralow J, Yee G, Janjan N, Cauley J, Blumenstein B, Albain K, Lipton A, Brown S. American society of clinical oncology 2003 update on the role of bisphosphonates and bone health issues in women with breast cancer. J Clin Oncol 2003;21(21):4042-57.

[30] Ural AU, Avcu F. Therapeutic role of bisphosphonate and radiation combination in the management of myeloma bone disease. Clin Cancer Res 2007;13(11):3432.

[31] Ural AU. Zoledronic acid sensitized tumor cells to radiation: In response to algur et al. Int J Radiat Oncol Biol Phys 2005;63(3):970.

[32] Koswig S, Budach V. Remineralization and pain relief in bone metastases after after different radiotherapy fractions (10 times 3 gy vs. 1 time 8 gy). A prospective study. Strahlentherapie Onkologie 1999;175(10):500-8.

[33] Weber W, Rosler HP, Doll G, Dostert M, Kutzner J, Schild H. [The percuaneous irradiation of osteolytic bone metastases—a course assessment]. Strahlentherapie Okologie 1992;168(5):275-80.

In: Advanced Cancer. Pain and Quality of Life
Editors: E. Chow, J. Merrick, pp. 69-76
ISBN: 978-1-61668-207-1
© 2010 Nova Science Publishers, Inc.

Chapter VI

Are Baseline ESAS Symptoms Related to Pain Response in Patients Treated with Palliative Radiotherapy for Bone Metastases?

Shaelyn Culleton, BSc (C), Jocelyn Pang, BSc (C), Liying Zhang, PhD, Roseanna Presutti, BSc (C), Janet Nguyen, BSc (C), Gunita Mitera, MRT (T), Emily Sinclair, MRT (T), Elizabeth Barnes, MD, May Tsao, MD, Cyril Danjoux, MD, Arjun Sahgal, MD and Edward Chow, MBBS* [*]

Rapid Response Radiotherapy Program, Department of Radiation Oncology, Odette Cancer Centre, Sunnybrook Health Sciences Centre, University of Toronto, Ontario, Canada

The purpose was to assess the relationship between pretreatment symptoms and pain response following palliative radiotherapy for bone metastases. Methods: All patients with bone metastases treated with palliative radiotherapy were followed at baseline, then 1, 2 and 3 months after radiotherapy with the Edmonton Symptom Assessment System (ESAS). This scale includes pain, fatigue, nausea, depression, anxiety, drowsiness, appetite, sense of well being and shortness of breath. Patients were categorized as either a responder or non-responder according to the International Consensus Guidelines for palliative radiotherapy. Statistical analysis included both Wilcoxon rank-sum and one-way ANOVA analysis. Results were considered significant at the 0.5% critical level ($p < 0.005$) applying the Bonferroni statistical correction for multiple comparisons. Results: For the entire cohort of 518 patients, only nausea at baseline was found to significantly correlate with a pain response to radiation at month 3. No other symptoms at baseline

* Correspondence: Edward Chow, MBBS, PhD, FRCPC, Department of Radiation Oncology, Odette Cancer Centre, Sunnybrook Health Sciences Centre, 2075 Bayview Avenue, Toronto, ON M4N 3M5, Canada. Tel: 416-480-4998; Fax: 416-480-6002; E-mail: Edward.Chow@sunnybrook.ca

were found to predict a pain response to radiation at months 1, 2 or 3. Conclusion: There are no ESAS symptoms that can accurately predict a patient's pain response to radiation. Patients who are symptomatic from their bone metastases should be treated with palliative radiotherapy irrespective of their baseline ESAS symptoms.

Introduction

Bone metastases are an unfortunate complication which occurs in approximately 50% of all cancer patients. The most common primary cancer sites which metastasize to bone are breast, prostate and lung carcinomas (1). Symptomatic metastatic bone lesions, which develop in about 50-70% of all patients with bone metastases, can be quite distressing in patients. Most often these patients will experience severe pain and can often have very serious skeletal complications. The most common skeletal related complications include pathological fractures (8-30%), hypercalcemia (10%), and spinal cord compression (5%) (1-4). Palliative radiation has been proven to be an effective treatment for symptomatic bone metastases, with 24% of all patients experiencing complete pain relief and up to 59% reporting some pain relief (2). This treatment is more effective at reducing incident pain than any other analgesic regimen, which is why palliative radiation is considered a first-line therapy for bone metastases (5,6).

Many patients who receive palliative radiotherapy for their painful bone metastases experience other common advanced cancer symptoms as well (7). Though pain from bone metastases may be the most distressing, these other symptoms may also have an effect on a patient's overall quality of life (QOL) and performance status. Some of the most common advanced cancer symptoms apart from pain are fatigue, dypsnea, depression, nausea and lack of appetite (7). It has been suggested that the presence of certain common advanced cancer symptoms prior to radiation may predict a patient's response. In a study by Kovner et al (8), which assessed 42 advanced cancer patients treated with palliative radiotherapy, higher levels of anxiety and depression prior to treatment showed a greater reduction in pain following treatment. Kovner et al (8) also mentioned that this pain reduction had a positive effect on patients' QOL and that this effect was noticed before any medical results were apparent.

The purpose of the present study is to determine if certain advanced cancer symptoms predict a response to radiation treatment by exploring the relationship between pre-RT symptoms and patient response to radiotherapy. To assess changes in symptoms during treatment, the Edmonton Symptom Assessment System (ESAS) was used before radiation (at baseline) and follow-up with advanced cancer patients receiving palliative radiation for bone metastases. This scale has been validated as an effective tool in monitoring common advanced cancer symptoms in the palliative population. This nine item questionnaire includes six symptoms related to physical well-being and three items related to psychological symptoms (9). Comparing ESAS symptoms from baseline to subsequent follow-ups will allow us to determine if the rating of symptoms prior to radiation predicts a patient's response to radiation treatment for bone metastases.

Our study

The Odette Cancer Centre (OCC) is one of two regional cancer centres providing radiotherapy in the Greater Toronto Area. The Rapid Response Radiotherapy Program (RRRP) at the OCC provides timely palliative radiation for symptomatic metastases. On initial consultation, patients with bone metastases were asked to rate the severity of symptoms they were experiencing using the ESAS. This 11-point visual analogue scale asks patients to rate nine of their symptoms from 0 (absence of symptom) to 10 (worst possible feeling of that symptom). Pain, tiredness, nausea, depression, anxiety, drowsiness, appetite, overall sense of well being and shortness of breath are the nine symptoms assessed through ESAS. This tool has been proven to be very indicative of a patient's current status and is noted for its quick and easy administration (9).

Patient demographics such as primary cancer site, age, Karnofsky Performance Status (KPS), analgesic intake and other sites of metastases were also recorded at the time of initial consultation. Radiation dosage and site of radiation were also recorded. The initial baseline assessment was completed before radiation treatment and follow-up interviews were conducted by telephone or in person at months one, two and three after the delivery of radiation treatment.

Statistical analysis

Response to radiation was determined by employing the International Consensus on Palliative Radiotherapy Endpoints. According to these endpoints, a complete response to radiation is defined as a pain score of zero with no concomitant increase in analgesic intake. Partial response is defined as either a pain reduction of two or more at the treated site without an increase in analgesic intake, or a reduction of analgesic intake of 25% or more with no increase in pain score. Patients who responded to radiation treatment are considered to have achieved either a complete or partial response (10).

Results were expressed as mean, standard deviation (SD), and median (range) for continuous variables, and proportion (%) for categorical variables. Mean and median values were calculated for ESAS scales in responders and non-responders at month one, month two and month three. To determine if baseline symptoms predicted response at consecutive months post radiation treatment, two statistical methods were employed. The Wilcoxon rank-sum test (non-parametric) and One-Way ANOVA test (parametric) were both used to search for a relationship between response rate (responders versus non-responders) and baseline ESAS scales. The Bonferroni statistical correction for multiple comparisons, in which the adjusted P-value is found by dividing 0.05 by the number of outcomes, was applied in this study (11). As there are nine items in the ESAS, results were considered significant at the 0.5% critical level ($p < 0.005$). The Statistical Analysis Software (SAS Institute, version 9.1 for Windows) was used for the analysis.

Table 1. Patient demographics

Sex	
Male	280 (54%)
Female	238 (46%)
Karnofsky Performance Status	
Mean	Range
61.2	10-100
Age (Years)	
Mean	Range
68	31-93
Other Metastatic Sites	
Lung	111 (21%)
Liver	90 (17%)
Brain	17 (3%)
Primary Cancer Sites	
Lung	130 (25%)
Breast	127 (25%)
Prostate	117 (23%)
GI	39 (8%)
Unknown Primary	34 (7%)
Others	71 (14%)
Radiation Prescription (cGy/fraction)	
2000/5	219 (42%)
800/1	209 (40%)
3000/10	26 (5%)
1000/1	10 (2%)
Others	54 (11%)
Site of Radiation	
Hip/Pelvis	30%
Spine	29%
Femur	12%
Rib Cage	9%
Humerus	8%
Clavicle	5%
Others	7%

Our findings

518 patients between January 1999 and January 2002 with bone metastases completed the ESAS at baseline prior to radiation treatment. This population contained approximately an even number of males and females with a median age of 68 years and a mean KPS of 60. The three most prevalent primary cancer sites were lung, breast and prostate, respectively. The majority of patients received either a single dose of 800cGy or 2000cGy in five fractions for their painful bone metastases. The two most common irradiated sites were the pelvis and spine. All other demographic information is included in table 1. The number of responders

and non-responders at month one, two and three along with their median and mean scores for all nine symptoms are included in table 2.

Table 2. ESAS mean and median scores for responders and non-responders

	Responder?	Month 1			Month 2			Month 3		
		N	Mean	Median	N	Mean	Median	N	Mean	Median
Tired	No	130	4.63	5.00	120	5.01	5.00	92	4.80	5.00
	Yes	130	4.68	5.00	105	4.36	5.00	97	4.13	5.00
Nausea	No	130	1.47	1.00	120	1.72	1.00	92	1.64	1.00
	Yes	130	1.42	0.00	105	1.10	0.00	97	1.05	0.00
Depressed	No	128	2.41	2.00	116	2.28	2.00	91	2.22	2.00
	Yes	128	2.42	2.00	103	2.42	2.00	93	2.29	2.00
Anxious	No	129	2.95	3.00	118	3.14	2.00	92	2.83	2.00
	Yes	129	3.30	3.00	104	3.30	3.00	95	3.35	3.00
Drowsy	No	129	3.38	3.00	120	3.37	3.00	92	3.07	2.00
	Yes	129	3.46	3.00	104	3.19	2.50	96	2.97	2.00
Appetite loss	No	130	4.28	5.00	120	4.00	4.00	92	3.84	4.00
	Yes	130	3.68	4.00	105	3.72	4.00	97	3.39	2.00
Sense of Well Being	No	129	4.18	4.00	119	4.13	4.00	88	4.05	4.00
	Yes	126	3.94	4.00	102	4.01	4.00	94	3.73	4.00
Short of Breath	No	129	1.93	1.00	119	2.44	1.00	91	2.48	2.00
	Yes	130	2.50	1.00	104	1.99	1.00	97	1.77	1.00

Of the 518 patients that completed ESAS at baseline, 256 patients completed the one month follow-up, 223 completed month two follow-up and 189 completed month three follow-up. Table 3 shows the results of the Wilcoxon rank-sum and One-way ANOVA statistical analyses at month one, two and three. These results are however, with the exception of the Wilcoxon rank-sum analysis at month three for nausea, not significant when applying the Bonferroni statistical correction for multiple comparisons (11).

Discussion

There has been very limited research done investigating the relationship between pre-treatment symptoms and response to radiation treatment. A fairly comprehensive analysis done at our centre which analyzed pre-treatment pain scores for 1,053 advanced cancer patients treated with radiotherapy for bone metastases was compared to response following radiation treatment. Patients with mild, moderate or severe pain at the beginning of treatment showed no significant difference in response up to three months post radiation treatment. Therefore the initial severity of pain was not shown to predict a response to radiation treatment (12). Our study also has yielded similar results when analyzing all other ESAS symptoms (with the exception of pain) in comparison with response. All baseline ESAS symptoms were not significantly related to either responders or non-responders at month one, two and three. Even though Wilcoxon rank-sum test at month three showed that the level of nausea predicted response to radiation, the lack of correlation between other commonly associated symptoms like anxiety and depression make it unlikely that nausea alone could predict for response at month three (13). Also the difference in median and mean nausea levels at baseline is so low between responders and non-responders that this finding would not be of any clinical significance.

Table 3. Wilcoxon rank-sum and One-way ANOVA analysis on ESAS symptoms

	Relationship with response rate (responders vs. non-responders)	
Baseline ESAS	Wilcoxon rank-sum p-value	One-way ANOVA p-value*
Month 1		
Tired	0.8711	0.9106
Nausea	0.1462	0.1833
Depressed	0.9739	0.9744
Anxious	0.5849	0.6720
Drowsy	0.9664	0.5974
Appetite loss	0.1511	0.1118
Well being	0.4407	0.2961
Shortness of breath	0.2789	0.2074
Month 2		
Tired	0.0960	0.0886
Nausea	0.0222	0.0268
Depressed	0.8288	0.6713
Anxious	0.7838	0.7481
Drowsy	0.6618	0.6005
Appetite loss	0.6220	0.5112
Well being	0.7402	0.3567
Shortness of breath	0.4320	0.5672
Month 3		
Tired	0.0988	0.0314
Nausea	**0.0038**	0.0110
Depressed	0.9864	0.8490
Anxious	0.3159	0.2411
Drowsy	0.7967	0.7444
Appetite loss	0.2891	0.2175
Well being	0.4362	0.2381
Shortness of breath	0.1220	0.1591

* log (baseline ESAS + 1) transformation was used for normalization
P< 0.005 considered significant

Kovner et al (8) determined based on their analysis of 42 metastastic cancer patients treated with palliative radiotherapy that had high levels of anxiety and depression prior to treatment had decreased pain and an increase in QOL following radiotherapy. However the analysis done by this study on a significantly greater number of patients refutes the effects of high anxiety and depression on response to radiation. Anxiety and depression are significantly associated with impairment of physical and psychosocial aspects of QOL, even after controlling for pain and illness severity (13). Therefore depression and anxiety have aspects that are independent from pain and levels are not always predictive for reductions in pain and increases in QOL (14).

Overall, a patient's presenting symptomology prior to palliative radiation for bone metastases has no predictive value in determining how a patient will respond. Therefore, it is recommended that patients be referred for palliative radiation to their painful bone metastases irrespective of the level of other ESAS symptoms. It is important that patients presenting even with moderate pain be referred for treatment, in order to avoid symptom progression (12).

Acknowledgments

The studentship was funded by the Michael and Karyn Goldstein Cancer Research Fund. We thank Stacy Lue for secretarial assistance.

References

[1] Falkmer U, Jarhult J, Wersall P, Cavallin-Stahl E. A systematic overview of radiation therapy effects in skeletal metastases. Acta Oncol 2003;42(5-6):620-33.

[2] Chow E, Harris K, Fan G, Tsao M, Sze W. Palliative radiotherapy trials for bone metastases: A systematic review. J Clin Oncol 2007;25(11):1423-36.

[3] Hoegler D. Radiotherapy for palliation of symptoms in incurable cancer. Curr Probl Cancer 1997;21(3):129-83.

[4] Wu J, Wong R, Johnston M, Bezjak A, Whelan T. Meta-analysis of dose-fractionation radiotherapy trials for the palliation of painful bone metastases. Int J Radiat Oncol Biol Phys 2003;55(3):594-605.

[5] Wong R, Wiffen PJ. Bisphosphonates for the relief of pain secondary to bone metastases. Cochrane Database Syst Rev 2002(2):002068.

[6] McQuay HJ, Collins SL, Carroll D, Moore RA. Radiotherapy for the palliation of painful bone metastases. Cochrane Database Syst Rev 2000(2):001793.

[7] Walsh D, Donnelly S, Rybicki L. The symptoms of advanced cancer: Relationship to age, gender, and performance status in 1,000 patients. Support Care Cancer 2000 May;8(3):175-9.

[8] Niv D, Shulamith K. Pain and quality of life. Pain Medicine 2001;1(2):150-61.

[9] Bruera E, Kuehn N, Miller MJ, Selmser P, Macmillan K. The edmonton symptom assessment system (ESAS): A simple method for the assessment of palliative care patients. J Palliat Care 1991;7(2):6-9.

[10] Chow E, Wu JS, Hoskin P, Coia LR, Bentzen SM, Blitzer PH. International consensus on palliative radiotherapy endpoints for future clinical trials in bone metastases. Radiother Oncol 2002;64(3):275-80.

[11] Shaffer JP. Multiple hypothesis testing. Ann Rev Psych 1995;46:561-84.

[12] Kirou-Mauro A, Hird A, Wong J, Sinclair E, Barnes EA, Tsao M, Danjoux C, Chow E. Is response to radiotherapy in patients related to the severity of pretreatment pain? Int J Radiat Oncol Biol Phys 2008;71(4):1208-12.
[13] Smith EM, Gomm SA, Dickens CM. Assessing the independent contribution to quality of life from anxiety and depression in patients with advanced cancer. Palliat Med 2003;17(6):509-13.
[14] Cordova MJ, Andrykowski, MA. Responses to cancer diagnosis and treatment: Posttraumatic stress and posttraumatic growth. Semin Clin Neuropsychiatry 2003;8(4):286-96.

In: Advanced Cancer. Pain and Quality of Life
Editors: E. Chow, J. Merrick, pp. 77-86
ISBN: 978-1-61668-207-1
© 2010 Nova Science Publishers, Inc.

Chapter VII

Improvement of Symptoms Following Palliative Radiation for Bone Metastases

Shaelyn Culleton, BSc(C), Liying Zhang, PhD, Emily Sinclair, MRT(T), Elizabeth Barnes, MD, May Tsao, MD, Cyril Danjoux, MD, Sarah Campos, BSc(C), Philiz Goh, BSc and Edward Chow, MBBS *

Rapid Response Radiotherapy Program, Department of Radiation Oncology, Odette cancer Centre, Sunnybrook Health Sciences Centre, University of Toronto, Toronto, Ontario, Canada

The purpose of this chapter was to assess pain and other common symptoms using the Edmonton System Assessment scale (ESAS) in patients with bone metastases following palliative radiotherapy. Methods: All patients with bone metastases treated with palliative radiotherapy were followed at baseline, then 1, 2, 4, 8 and 12 weeks after radiotherapy with ESAS. This scale includes pain, tiredness, nausea, depression, anxiety, drowsiness, appetite, sense of well being and shortness of breath. A Chi-squared test was used to search for the association between response effect and ESAS change at different weeks. To evaluate the response effect on the ESAS symptoms over time, a general linear mixed model was performed. Results: For the entire cohort of 518 patients, pain, anxiety, appetite, drowsiness and overall sense of well being significantly improved from baseline to last follow-up. Tiredness was the only symptom which showed worsening following palliative radiation in all patients. When looking at responders and non-responders with respect to pain, the greatest number of symptoms with a significant difference between the two groups occurred at week 12. Also when comparing the significant differences between responder and non-responders from week 1 to 12 inclusive, all ESAS symptoms were significantly better in responders with the exception of shortness of breath.

* Correspondence: Edward Chow, MBBS, PhD, FRCPC, Department of Radiation Oncology, Odette Cancer Centre, Sunnybrook Health Sciences Centre, 2075 Bayview Avenue, Toronto, ON M4N 3M5, Canada. Tel: 416-480-4998; Fax: 416-480-6002; E-mail: Edward.Chow@sunnybrook.ca

Conclusions: Palliative radiotherapy not only decreased pain at the radiated site in patients with bone metastases, but also improved many other symptoms in ESAS in conjunction with other systemic therapies.

Introduction

Skeletal metastases are a common occurrence and are seen in at least 50% of all cancer patients. Breast, prostate and lung cancers are the most frequently reported primaries that metastasize to bone and account for approximately 80% of all cases of bone metastases (1,2). Pain is the most commonly reported distressing symptom in 75% of patients with bone metastases. Palliative radiation has been proven to be an effective treatment for symptomatic bone metastases, with 24% of all patients experiencing complete pain relief and up to 59% reporting some pain relief (3).

Improving pain is the main goal in palliative radiation for bone metastases, however many advanced cancer patients experience other symptoms such as shortness of breath, depression and tiredness. It is therefore important to not only monitor the effects of radiation treatment on pain but to also see how the severities of other associated symptoms respond post-radiotherapy (4).

The Edmonton symptom assessment scale (ESAS) is an effective tool for monitoring pain and other symptoms in patients receiving palliative care. Its nine items include six symptoms related to physical well being (tiredness, drowsiness, appetite, pain, shortness of breath, and nausea) and three relating to psychological symptoms (depression, anxiety and overall well being) (5). Though the effects of radiation on depression and tiredness have been documented, analyzing all ESAS symptoms post radiation as well as comparing the results between responders and non-responders has not been reported (6-8). Therefore it is of interest to assess how response to radiation can affect the most common palliative cancer symptoms as well as a patient's overall sense of well being.

The primary objective of this study was to assess the overall change in ESAS symptoms in all patients following palliative radiation treatment for bone metastases. The secondary objective was to analyze the differences in ESAS symptoms between responders and non-responders to radiation treatment from week 1 to 12.

Our study

The Odette Cancer Centre (OCC) is one of two regional cancer centres providing radiotherapy in the Greater Toronto Area. The Rapid Response Radiotherapy Program (RRRP) at the OCC provides timely palliative radiation for symptomatic metastases. On initial consultation, patients with bone metastases were asked to rate the severity of symptoms they were experiencing using ESAS. This 11-point visual analogue scale asks patients to rate their symptoms from 0 (absence of symptom) to 10 (worst possible feeling of that symptom). The symptoms that ESAS assesses are pain, tiredness, nausea, depression, anxiety, drowsiness, appetite, overall sense of well being and shortness of breath. This tool has been proven to be very indicative of a patient's current status and is noted for its ease of administration as well as its brevity (5).

Patient demographics such as primary cancer site, age, Karnofsky Performance Status (KPS), analgesic intake and other sites of metastases were also recorded at the time of initial consultation. Radiation and site of radiation were also recorded. The initial baseline assessment was completed before radiation treatment and follow-up interviews were conducted by telephone or in person at weeks 1, 2, 4, 8, and 12 after the delivery of radiation treatment. We obtained ethics approval from the hospital for this study.

Statistical analysis

Response to radiation was determined by employing the International Consensus endpoints. A complete response to radiation is defined as a pain score of zero with no analgesic increase. Partial response is defined as a pain reduction of 2 or more without increased analgesic intake or a reduction of analgesic intake of 25% or more with no increase in pain score. Patients who responded to radiation treatment encompassed either one of the definitions for a complete and partial response (9).

To determine the percentage of patients who had an increase, decrease or no change in the severity of their symptoms comparing to the baseline score, an individual linear regression of ESAS symptom was applied for estimation of slope. It was considered as an increase, decrease or no change in the severity of symptom when an individual slope was positive, negative or zero. Chi-squared test was performed to evaluate the relationship between response effect and percentage change of ESAS symptoms at weeks 4, 8, and 12. Mean and median values were calculated for ESAS symptoms from baseline to week 12. General linear mixed model was used to determine the response effect on the ESAS symptoms over time. Results were considered significant at the 5% critical level ($p < 0.05$). All calculations were performed using SAS (version 9.1, SAS institute, Cary, NC) statistical software.

Our findings

Between January 1999 and January 2002, 518 patients with bone metastases completed baseline ESAS at the time of consultation. Demographic information is included in table 1. There were 280 males (54%) and 238 females (46%) in this study. Median and mean age of the study population was 68 years with an average KPS of 60. The most common primary cancer sites were lung (25%), breast (25%) and prostate (23%). The most frequently prescribed doses of radiation were 2000cGy/5 (42%) and 800cGy/1 (40%). The most common radiated sites were the pelvis (30%) and the spine (29%). Table 2 shows the median and mean scores for all 9 ESAS symptoms from baseline to week 12. At baseline pain, tiredness and lack of appetite were the most distressful symptoms reported by all patients with a median score of 5 for all three symptoms. Nausea and shortness of breath were shown to be the least severe symptoms at baseline with median scores of 0 and 1 respectively.

Table 1. Patient demographics

Sex	
Male	280 (54%)
Female	238 (46%)
Karnofsky Performance Status	
Median	Range
60	10-100
Age (Years)	
Mean	Range
68	31-93
Other Metastatic Sites	
Lung	111 (21%)
Liver	90 (17%)
Brain	17 (3%)
Primary Cancer Sites	
Lung	130 (25%)
Breast	127 (25%)
Prostate	117 (23%)
GI	39 (8%)
Unknown Primary	34 (7%)
Others	71 (14%)
Radiation Prescription (cGy/fraction)	
2000/5	219 (42%)
800/1	209 (40%)
3000/10	26 (5%)
1000/1	10 (2%)
Others	54 (11%)
Site of Radiation	
Hip/Pelvis	30%
Spine	29%
Femur	12%
Rib Cage	9%
Humerus	8%
Clavicle	5%
Others	7%

Table 2. Mean (M) and Median (P50) of ESAS symptoms in all patients from baseline to week 12

ESAS symptom	Week 0		Week 1		Week 2		Week 4		Week 8		Week 12		p-value*
	M	P50	M	P50	M	P50	M	P50	M	P50	M	P50	
Pain	4.46	5	3.15	3	2.86	2	2.84	2	2.82	2	3.37	3	< 0.0001
Tiredness	4.96	5	5.46	6	5.24	6	4.98	5	4.90	5	4.83	5	0.0043
Nausea	1.50	0	1.64	0	1.44	0	1.28	0	1.52	0	1.19	0	0.65
Depression	2.49	2	2.40	1	2.55	2	2.38	1	2.24	1	2.56	1	0.36
Anxiety	3.24	3	2.46	2	2.44	2	2.33	1	2.25	1	2.38	1	< 0.0001
Drowsiness	3.57	3	3.76	4	3.28	3	2.89	2	2.85	2	2.72	2	0.0015
Appetite	4.12	5	4.23	5	4.06	4	3.94	4	3.44	3	3.09	2	0.0071
Well Being	4.33	3	3.74	2	3.54	2	3.23	1	3.49	1	3.63	1	< 0.0001
Shortness of Breath	2.24	1	1.82	0	2.00	0	1.97	0	2.17	1	1.78	0	0.07

* p-value of week was obtained by general linear mixed model and indicated significance of ESAS symptoms change over time in all patients.

Table 3. Percent change in all ESAS symptoms from baseline to last FU

ESAS Symptoms	Percentage Change (%)		
	Increase	Decrease	No Change
Pain	40.5	50.9	8.6
Tiredness	52.8	39.4	7.8
Nausea	27.2	40.3	32.5
Depression	38.9	41.2	19.9
Anxiety	32.6	49.3	18.2
Drowsiness	36.9	52.6	10.5
Appetite	46.7	41.4	11.9
Sense of Well-Being	47.7	40.9	11.4
Shortness of Breath	29.5	46.0	24.6

Table 4. Percentage change of ESAS symptoms in responders and non-responders at weeks 4, 8 and 12

ESAS symptom	Responder			Non-responder			
	Increase (%)	Decrease (%)	No Change (%)	Increase (%)	Decrease (%)	No Change (%)	p-value*
At week 4							
Pain	22.4	67.2	10.4	43.2	49.2	7.6	**0.0015**
Tiredness	44.4	45.9	9.8	49.2	38.6	12.1	0.47
Nausea	21.8	32.3	45.9	23.5	42.4	34.1	0.12
Depression	33.8	42.9	23.3	33.6	38.9	27.5	0.70
Anxiety	26.5	57.6	15.9	32.1	42.0	26.0	**0.029**
Drowsiness	32.6	54.5	12.9	35.6	50.0	14.4	0.76
Appetite	36.1	51.9	12.0	46.2	38.6	15.2	0.096
Sense of Well-Being	25.8	62.9	11.4	38.6	40.9	20.5	**0.0015**
Shortness of Breath	29.9	45.5	24.6	28.8	40.2	31.1	0.48
At week 8							
Pain	33.0	60.6	6.4	43.4	53.3	3.3	0.19
Tiredness	43.1	50.5	6.4	52.5	43.4	4.1	0.33
Nausea	24.8	34.9	40.4	27.9	45.9	26.2	0.066
Depression	28.4	49.5	22.0	40.8	38.3	20.8	0.12
Anxiety	20.4	63.9	15.7	39.2	46.7	14.2	**0.0074**
Drowsiness	25.9	57.4	16.7	41.8	51.6	6.6	**0.0077**
Appetite	30.3	57.8	11.9	43.4	49.2	7.4	0.094
Sense of Well-Being	33.9	58.7	7.3	41.0	49.2	9.8	0.34
Shortness of Breath	33.9	45.0	21.1	36.1	37.7	26.2	0.49
At week 12							
Pain	37.8	54.1	8.2	53.7	44.2	2.1	**0.029**
Tiredness	40.8	57.1	2.0	57.9	40.0	2.1	0.056
Nausea	22.4	35.7	41.8	31.6	49.5	18.9	**0.0026**
Depression	33.0	50.5	16.5	44.2	35.8	20.0	0.12
Anxiety	17.5	66.0	16.5	46.8	43.6	9.6	**0.0001**
Drowsiness	28.6	64.3	7.1	47.9	47.9	4.3	**0.021**
Appetite	22.4	62.2	15.3	50.5	44.2	5.3	**0.0001**
Sense of Well-Being	38.8	56.1	5.1	44.7	48.9	6.4	0.60
Shortness of Breath	34.7	41.8	23.5	24.2	53.7	22.1	0.20

* p-value was obtained by Chi-squared test to see the relationship between response effect and percentage change of ESAS symptom at week 4, 8, and 12.

Of the 518 patients, 349 had at least one completed follow-up and 119 patients had a full five completed follow-ups. Using linear regression to determine percentage change in each patient's score, pain, anxiety, drowsiness, appetite and overall sense of well being all were shown to significantly improve from baseline to last follow-up. Tiredness was the only symptom that significantly worsened from baseline to last follow-up. Nausea, depression and shortness of breath showed no significant correlation from baseline to last follow-up. Table 3 shows all 518 patients' percent changes from baseline to their last follow-up regardless of response to radiation.

When comparing responders and non-responders at weeks 4, 8 and 12 (see table 4), all symptoms which showed a significant difference between the two populations had a greater improvement in the responders. At week 4, pain, anxiety and sense of well being were significantly better in the responders than the non-responders. At week 8 both anxiety and drowsiness were significantly better in responders. The greatest number of symptoms with a significant difference between responders and non-responders occurred at week 12. Pain, nausea, anxiety, drowsiness and appetite were all significantly better in responders when compared with non-responders at week 12.

When comparing those patients who responded to radiation to those who did not from weeks 1 through 12, all symptoms showed a significant difference except for shortness of breath (see table 5). Pain, tiredness, nausea, depression, anxiety, drowsiness, appetite and overall sense of well being were all significantly better in responders when compared to the non-responders. The only symptom which showed no significant difference between the responder and non-responder populations was shortness of breath.

Table 5. Average of ESAS symptoms between responders (R) and non-responders (NR) from week 1 to 12

ESAS Symptom	Week 1		Week 2		Week 4		Week 8		Week 12		p-value
	R	NR	R	NR	R	NR	R	NR	R	NR	Response effect†
Pain	2.33	3.92	2.08	3.64	1.81	3.89	2.29	3.28	2.52	4.22	< 0.0001
Tired	4.84	6.05	4.53	5.94	4.61	5.36	4.28	5.45	3.97	5.75	< 0.0001
Nausea	1.42	1.84	1.09	1.79	1.02	1.55	1.32	1.71	1.02	1.36	0.049
Depression	2.11	2.68	2.06	3.08	2.32	2.44	1.73	2.73	2.09	3.05	0.0004
Anxiety	2.21	2.69	1.99	2.94	2.20	2.47	1.48	2.99	1.83	2.96	< 0.0001
Drowsiness	3.06	4.42	2.52	4.08	2.78	2.99	2.13	3.54	1.94	3.55	< 0.0001
Appetite	3.87	4.57	3.26	4.86	3.44	4.44	2.91	3.92	2.35	3.87	0.015
Well Being	3.23	4.20	2.99	4.09	2.76	3.74	3.03	3.95	3.10	4.25	0.0007
Shortness of Breath	1.66	1.97	1.66	2.34	2.14	1.80	2.06	2.27	1.88	1.67	0.32

† *p-value of response effect* indicates significance of comparing symptoms change from week 1 to week 12 between responders and non-responders, when adjusting for week variable. General linear mixed model was performed in the analysis.

Disscussion

The symptoms included in ESAS are very appropriate for analyzing an advanced cancer patient's overall response after their course of radiation treatment. In a recent study by Walsh et al (10) involving 1,000 advanced cancer patients, many of the symptoms included in ESAS were among the most prevalent in the overall population. The most distressing symptoms according to this study were pain (84%), tiredness (69%), lack of appetite (66%), drowsiness (61%) and shortness of breath (50%). Walsh et al (10) also noted that many advanced cancer patients are polysymptomatic and although one symptom be the most dominant, all symptoms contribute to a patient's overall QOL. They also showed that advanced cancer symptoms are, for the most part, independent of age, gender, performance status and primary cancer site (10).

Radiotherapy for palliation of bone metastases has been proven to be an effective treatment for reducing pain and increasing patients' overall QOL (1,2,6). For patients with bone metastases, severe pain is often the most prevalent symptom for over 70% of these individuals, which is why palliation of pain using radiation is a primary concern (2,6,11-13). Limited mobility, fracture, hypercalcemia, reduced KPS, impaired daily functioning and diminished QOL are all noted consequences of bone metastases (2,14). In our study, most ESAS symptoms were shown to improve after radiation in all patients and the majority of those who responded to radiotherapy achieved a significant improvement within the first week after the start of radiation. In an overview of pain and QOL (15), they suggested that as a patient is cognitively aware that their radiation treatment is providing pain relief, their anxiety, depression and overall sense of well being also improved. This finding was also noticed in our overall study population when analyzing the change in their symptom scores from baseline to last follow-up. The only symptom that was negatively affected in all patients was tiredness.

Radiation induced tiredness is experienced by 80-90% of all cancer patients. On average 69% of advanced cancer patients experience tiredness on a regular basis irrespective of radiation treatment (6,10).Tiredness has a significant impact on the QOL of cancer patients and it is caused primarily by cancer pathology and other systemic treatments (7). Even though the responders did not show a significant increase or decrease in tiredness following radiation, it was the only symptom which had the highest consistent mean and median score before and after radiation treatment. Tiredness was also the only negatively effected ESAS symptom reported by all patients after radiation treatment.

In a study by Strauss et al (16) data from a sample of 239 cancer patients receiving radiotherapy showed a high negative correlation between tiredness and QoL. They found tiredness to be the most dominant factor in cancer patient suffering. Other studies have shown that exercise such as walking can significantly reduce the effects of radiotherapy induced tiredness in cancer patients but only a very limited number of studies have focused on tiredness in the palliative population (17-19). In one such study by Brown et al., a multidisciplinary program which included physical therapy, stretching, cognitive behavioral strategies, discussion and support was shown to be unsuccessful in reducing tiredness in palliative cancer patients (6). Overall, psychosocial and physical intervention in the treatment of tiredness among all palliative cancer patients has been shown to be inconclusive and more research is needed to combat the very negative effects of tiredness on QOL (6).

For those who responded to radiation treatment, all symptoms with the exception of shortness of breath had a significantly lower ESAS scores when compared with those who did not respond to radiation treatment. Furthermore, the greatest number of significant differences in symptoms between responders and non-responders were noted at week 12. As a possible explanation for these results, Niv and Shulamith reported that patients who are able to either reduce or stabilize their opiate consumption in turn decrease the side effects of these drugs which can include nausea, respiratory depression and confusion (15). This could partially explain why responders do appreciably better from weeks 1 through 12 in all but one ESAS symptom when compared with non-responders. In a study by Kovner et al (15) of 42 metastatic patients who received palliative radiotherapy for pain, those who responded with pain reduction also had a decrease in depression, anxiety and had increased vigor, curiosity, and overall QOL. The results from our respondent cohort were also consistent with this finding but when considering all 518 patients, depression scores did not change after radiation treatment. Depression is not an inevitable response to cancer or radiation treatment, which explains the consistency in depression scores for all patients before and after radiation in our study (8).

Kovner et al (15) also stated that those patients who were more active, had more anxiety and depression prior to treatment and had greater spirituality were shown to have a better response to radiation treatment and a greater QOL. Though we did not analyze predetermining factors to radiation response in this study, this could possibly be an area of further research and analysis. We also found in our study that patients who did not respond to radiation treatment not only had poor pain response but also worsened or showed no improvement in all other ESAS symptoms as well, with the exception of shortness of breath. This implies that radiation not only effectively relieves pain in respondents, but also improves many other problematic symptoms that are commonly experienced by patients with advanced cancer in conjunction with other systemic therapies.

Our study was limited to only English speaking patients. Also only 67% of the patients interviewed at baseline could be reached to complete at least one follow-up. Another limitation to this study was that only the change in ESAS symptoms were assessed and other advanced cancer symptoms such as constipation and dry mouth were not followed throughout a patient's course of radiation treatment. Lastly any changes in other systemic therapies were not considered in this study.

Conclusions

Our study has shown that overall pain, anxiety, drowsiness, appetite and sense of well being all improved following palliative radiation for bone metastases. Tiredness was the only symptom which worsened after radiation. All other ESAS symptoms (nausea, depression and shortness of breath) showed no significant difference post radiation. The greatest number of ESAS symptoms which showed a significant difference between responders and non-responders occurred at week 12. When comparing those who responded to radiation to those who did not, all but one symptom showed a significant difference in favour of responders. Shortness of breath was the only symptom which showed no significant difference between responders and non-responders. Non-responders not only achieved lack of adequate pain relief from radiation but did poorly in almost all ESAS symptoms as well when compared to those who responded to palliative radiation. We strongly recommend palliative radiation treatment be offered to patients with bone metastases.

Acknowledgments

The studentship was funded by the Michael and Karyn Goldstein Cancer Research Fund. We thank Ms Stacy Lue for her secretarial assistance. Conflict of interest: none

References

[1] Jasmin C, Capanna R, Coia L, Coleman R, Saillant G. Textbook of bone metastases. Hoboken, NJ: Wiley, 2005.

[2] Falkmer U, Jarhult J, Wersall P, Cavallin-Stahl E. A systematic overview of radiation therapy effects in skeletal metastases. Acta Oncol 2003;42(5-6):620-33.

[3] Chow E, Harris K, Fan G, Tsao M, Sze W. Palliative radiotherapy trials for bone metastases: A systematic review. J Clin Oncol 2007; 25(11):1423-36.

[4] Riechelmann RP, Krzyzanowska MK, O'Carroll A, Zimmermann C. Symptom and medication profiles among cancer patients attending a palliative care clinic. Support Care Cancer 2007;15(12):1407-12.

[5] Bruera E, Kuehn N, Miller MJ, Selmser P, Macmillan K. The edmonton symptom assessment system (ESAS): A simple method for the assessment of palliative care patients. J Palliat Care 1991;7(2):6-9.

[6] Brown P, Clark MM, Atherton P, Huschka M, Sloan JA, Gamble G, Girardi J, Frost MH, Piderman K, Rummans TA. Will improvement in quality of life (QOL) impact fatigue in patients receiving radiation therapy for advanced cancer? Am J Clin Oncol 2006;29(1):52-8.

[7] Greenberg DB, Sawicka J, Eisenthal S, Ross D. Fatigue syndrome due to localized radiation. J Pain Symptom Manage 1992;7(1):38-45.

[8] Jenkins C, Carmody TJ, Rush AJ. Depression in radiation oncology patients: A preliminary evaluation. J Affect Disord 1998;50(1):17-21.

[9] Chow E, Wu JS, Hoskin P, Coia LR, Bentzen SM, Blitzer PH. International consensus on palliative radiotherapy endpoints for future clinical trials in bone metastases. Radiother Oncol 2002;64(3):275-80.

[10] Walsh D, Donnelly S, Rybicki L. The symptoms of advanced cancer: Relationship to age, gender, and performance status in 1,000 patients. Support Care Cancer 2000;8(3):175-9.

[11] Gaze MN, Kelly CG, Kerr GR, Cull A, Cowie VJ, Gregor A, Howard GC, Rodger A. Pain relief and quality of life following radiotherapy for bone metastases: A randomised trial of two fractionation schedules. Radiother Oncol 1997; 45(2):109-16.

[12] Hoegler D. Radiotherapy for palliation of symptoms in incurable cancer. Curr Probl Cancer 1997;21(3):129-83.

[13] Janjan NA, Payne R, Gillis T, Podoloff D, Libshitz HI, Lenzi R, Theriault R, Martin C, Yasko A. Presenting symptoms in patients referred to a multidisciplinary clinic for bone metastases. J Pain Symptom Manage 1998;16(3):171-8.

[14] Barton MB, Dawson R, Jacob S, Currow D, Stevens G, Morgan G. Palliative radiotherapy of bone metastases: An evaluation of outcome measures. J Eval Clin Pract 2001;7(1):47-64.

[15] Niv D, Shulamith K. Pain and quality of life. Pain Medicine 2001;1(2):150-61

[16] Strauss B, Brix C, Fischer S, Leppert K, Fuller J, Roehrig B, Schleussner C, Wendt TG. The influence of resilience on fatigue in cancer patients undergoing radiation therapy (RT). J Cancer Res Clin Oncol 2007;133(8):511-8.

[17] Winsor P, Potter J, Nicol K. A randomized, controlled trial of aerobic exercise for treatment-related fatigue in men receiving radical external beam radiotherapy for localized prostate carcinoma. Cancer 2004; 101 (3) 550-7

[18] Sarna L, Conde F. Physical activity and fatigue during radiation therapy: a pilot study using actigraph monitors. Oncology Nursing Forum 2001; 28 (6): 1043-6

[19] Mock V, Dow K, Meares L, Grimm P, Dienemann J, Haisfield-Wolde M, Quitasol W, Mitchile S, Chakravarthy A, Gage I. Effect of exercise on fatigue, physical functioning and emotional distress during radiation therapy for breast cancer. Oncology Nursing Forum 1997; 24(6): 991-1000.

In: Advanced Cancer. Pain and Quality of Life
Editors: E. Chow, J. Merrick, pp. 87-94
ISBN: 978-1-61668-207-1
© 2010 Nova Science Publishers, Inc.

Chapter VIII

Pain Flare Following Palliative Radiotherapy for Symptomatic Bone Metastases

Amanda Hird, BSc(C)[1], Rebecca Wong, MD[2], Candi Flynn, BSc[1], Stephanie Hadi, BSc(C)[1], Eric de Sa, BSc[1], Liying Zhang, PhD[1], Carlo DeAngelis, PharmD[3] and Edward Chow, MBBS*[1]

[1]Rapid Response Radiotherapy Program, Department of Radiation Oncology, Odette Cancer Centre, Sunnybrook Health Sciences Centre, University of Toronto, Toronto, Ontario
[2]Palliative Radiotherapy Oncology Program, Department of Radiation Oncology, Princess Margaret Hospital, University of Toronto, Toronto Ontario and
[3]Pharmacy Department, Odette Cancer Centre, Sunnybrook Health Sciences Centre, University of Toronto, Toronto, Ontario, Canada

Pain flare following palliative radiotherapy (RT) for painful bone metastases is well-recognized with incidence rates of 2-44% reported in the literature. Objective was to investigate the impact of pain flare on patients with bone metastases treated with external beam RT. Methods: A five-item 'Pain Flare Qualitative Questionnaire' was developed to assess the psychological and functional impacts of the pain flare phenomenon. Results: Thirteen patients with pain flare completed the interview. There were three males and 10 females. The median age was 59 years (range: 48-89). The majority of participants had primary breast (9/13) or prostate cancer (2/13). Pain flare severely impacted patients' functional activity and carried resulted in negative mood and isolation from family and friends due to unbearable pain. Breakthrough pain medications were not adequate to control the pain increase in more than three quarters of the interviewed patients. Prophylactic medication was preferred as opposed to management with breakthrough

* ***Correspondence:*** Edward Chow, MBBS, PhD, FRCPC, Department of Radiation Oncology, Odette Cancer Centre, Sunnybrook Health Sciences Centre, 2075 Bayview Avenue, Toronto, ON M4N 3M5, Canada. Tel: 416-480-4998; Fax: 416-480-6002; E-mail: Edward.Chow@sunnybrook.ca

analgesia. Although patients felt the RT was worthwhile, there was hesitation to repeat the treatment if necessary due to the previously experienced flare effect. Conclusions: Pain flare is a common side effect following palliative RT for painful bone metastases. Based on our patient interviews, this even was debilitating and worrisome. Patients should be informed of this potential side effect and health care professionals should ensure patients are equipped with sufficient analgesia to manage this increase in metastatic bone pain. However, prevention of the pain flare as opposed to management with breakthrough pain medications was preferable in this study.

Introduction

Pain is the most prevalent symptom associated with bone metastases and is experienced by 60-75% of patients. Palliative radiotherapy (RT) is a well-established and effective treatment option for symptomatic bone metastases with overall pain response rates approaching 80% (1-3).

'Pain flare' is a temporary worsening of pain in the treated bony metastatic site immediately following RT. Pain flare has been a well-recognized side effect following treatment of painful bone metastases, particularly following radionucleotide therapy (4-12). However, reported rates of pain flare following external beam RT range from 2-44% and suggest a higher risk for patients treated with a single fraction (13-17). Hird and colleagues recently reported an overall pain flare incidence rate of 38% across three Canadian outpatient radiation clinics (18). Dexamethasone, a corticosteroid and anti-inflammatory medication, has been employed as an effective prophylactic agent for prevention of the pain flare phenomenon in the first two days following a single 8 Gy when prescribed at baseline. Specifically, the incidence of pain flare in the two days immediately following RT decreased from 60% to 3% in a recent pilot study (19).

Seemingly, pain flare occurs in a significant portion of patients treated for symptomatic bone metastases. However, the impact of pain flare on these patients has not been investigated. The purpose of this qualitative study was to examine the impact of pain flare on bone metastases patients treated with external beam RT, and to investigate patients' preference for pain flare prophylaxis versus management with breakthrough pain medications.

Our study

In February 2006, an observational study across three Canadian cancer centres: Odette Cancer Centre (OCC, Toronto, Ontario); Princess Margaret Hospital (PMH, Toronto, Ontario); Tom Baker Cancer Centre (TBCC, Calgary, Alberta), was initiated to determine the incidence of pain flare following palliative RT for bone metastases (18). An interim analysis was completed in October 2007. It was found that 35 out of 93 evaluable patients (38%) experienced a pain flare.

Anecdotally, the study investigators noted a significant burden to several of the patients experiencing a pain flare, as expressed by the patients during the telephone follow-up assessments. Therefore, the investigators developed a qualitative questionnaire to assess the impact of the flare experience on these patients.

Brainstorming with palliative radiation oncologists produced the 5-item Pain Flare Qualitative Questionnaire (see table 1). Open-ended questions were employed in order to facilitate open and unbiased responses from patients. Patients were eligible if they had experienced a pain flare in the incidence study by Hird et al (18). Patients were interviewed (by telephone) by a trained research assistant. Patient responses were recorded verbatim and analyzed for common themes between responders. Ethics approval was obtained from the hospital research ethics board to conduct the retrospective interviews.

Table 1. Pain Flare Qualitative Questionnaire Interviewer Guideline

Introduction to the interview
In *(insert date here)*, you received radiation to *(site)*. In the 10 days following your treatment, you indicated that your pain got a little bit worse. Do you recall this event? Would you mind if we asked you a total of 5 easy questions about this experience? We want to find out how the pain flare affected each patient, so there are no right or wrong answers to any of these questions.
Interview Questions
1. What did the pain increase mean to you at the time of the flare? (For example, what went through your mind when you were experiencing the flare?)   *2. Did the increase in pain interfere with your daily functioning? (For example, general activity, mood, walking ability, normal work, relations with others, sleep, enjoyment of life?)*   *3. What did you do to manage the increase in pain? (For example: extra pain medications, sitting, lying down, etc.)*   *4. In retrospect, what does the pain flare mean to you now?*   *5. Overall, do you feel the radiation treatment was worthwhile?*

In the pain flare incidence trial (18), patients completed the Brief Pain Inventory (BPI) before RT. The patient also kept a daily diary during treatment (if receiving multiple fractions) and for 10 days after RT. The diary collected the patients worst pain score for the preceding 24 hour period on a scale of 0-10, where 0 was the absence of pain and 10 was the worst possible pain; the patient's total intake of analgesia for the previous 24 hours, which was converted into an oral morphine equivalent dose (OMED); and a description of the worst pain as "worse", "the same", or "better" when compared to the baseline level. It was made clear to the patient that each pain score was to be based solely on the site treated with the RT.

Pain flare was defined (a priori) as a two-point increase in the worst pain score when compared to baseline on an 11-point scale (0-10) with no decrease in analgesic intake; or a 25% increase in analgesic intake employing OMED with no decrease in worst pain score. If the baseline worst pain was 9/10, pain flare was identified if the follow up worst pain score was 10/10 accompanied with a description of the current worst pain as "worse" when compared to the baseline worst pain. If the baseline worst pain was 10/10, pain flare was identified if the follow-up worst pain score was 10/10 with a description of the current worst pain level as "worse" than baseline worst pain. To distinguish pain flare from progression of pain, the worst pain score and OMED value must have returned back to baseline after the increase/flare.

Table 2. Patient demographics of the enrolled patients in the pain flare incidence study from the Odette Cancer Centre and Princess Margaret Hospital (N=111).

Sex	
Male	55 (50%)
Female	56 (50%)
Age (years) – Median (Range)	64 (40-89)
Oral Morphine Equivalent at Baseline (mg/day) – Median (Range)	12 (0-880)
Worst Pain Score at Baseline – Median (Range)	7 (0-10)
Radiation Dose	
8Gy	81 (73%)
20Gy/5 or 30Gy/10	30 (27%)
Primary Cancer Site	
Breast	43 (39%)
Prostate	27 (24%)
Lung	19 (17%)
Gastrointestinal	10 (9%)
Others	12 (11%)

All patients enrolled in the ongoing pain flare incidence investigation by Hird et al across three Canadian cancer centres (18).

Table 3. Patient demographics of pain flare patients (n=35) versus those contacted for the interview (n=13).

	Contacted Pain Flare Patients (n=13)*	**Patients Experiencing Pain Flare (n=35) †**	**a*p-value***
Sex			
Male	3 (23%)	12 (34%)	0.73
Female	10 (77%)	23 (66%)	
Age (years) – Median (Range)	59 (48-89)	60 (40-89)	0.99
Oral Morphine Equivalent at Baseline (mg-day) – Median (Range)	0 (0-190)	3 (0-590)	0.85
Worst Pain Score at Baseline – Median (Range)	4 (0-9)	6 (0-10)	0.33
Radiation Dose			
8Gy	8 (62%)	23 (66%)	0.79
20Gy/5 or 30Gy/10	5 (38%)	12 (34%)	
Primary Cancer Site			
Breast	9 (69%)	19 (54%)	0.78
Prostate	2 (15%)	5 (14%)	
Lung	0 (0%)	4 (11%)	
Gastrointestinal	0 (0%)	1 (3%)	
Others	2 (15%)	6 (17%)	

* Patients from Hird et al.'s cohort who were interviewed in the current study.

† All patients experiencing a pain flare from the Odette Cancer Centre or Princess Margaret Hospital from Hird et al.'s cohort (18).

p-values were obtained by Wilcoxon rank-sum test or Fisher exact test for comparing two groups. There were no significant differences between the pain flare cohort from Hird et al.'s study (18) and the patients interviewed in the current study.

The Wilcoxon rank-sum test or Fisher exact test was applied to compare patients from Hird et al.'s study population who experienced pain flare versus patients who completed the qualitative interview. Results were considered significant at the 5% critical level ($p < 0.05$). All calculations were performed using SAS (version 8.2 for Windows; SAS Institute, Cary, NC).

Our Findings

From February 2006 to October 2007, 111 patients were enrolled in the pain flare incidence study (see table 2) (18). There were 93 evaluable patients. From this cohort, 35 patients (38%) experienced pain flare. A total of 13/35 (37%) patients completed the qualitative interview. Ten out of 35 (29%) were deceased/hospitalized, 8/35 (23%) were unreachable, and 4/35 (11%) were from TBCC and not included in the analysis. The demographics of the cohort contacted for this analysis is compared to all patients experiencing a pain flare from Hird et al.'s study in Table 3. There were no statistically significant differences between Hird et al cohort of pain flare patients (18) and those included in the current study ($p > 0.05$).

The following sections outline the patient responses for each item from the Pain Flare Qualitative Questionnaire.

- Question 1: What did the pain increase mean to you at the time of the flare? (For example, what went through your mind when you were experiencing the flare?). Patients indicated their fear that the "cancer was getting worse" and that their "cancer pain was never going to end". Some believed the RT was not effective. One patient mentioned feeling confused – the RT was meant to improve bone pain rather than make it worse. Specifically, one patient described the flare as "a thousand times worse" when compared to the pain he had experienced at initial consultation in the clinic. Another described her pain flare experience as "excruciating". Generally, patients who were well informed of the possibility of a flare up of pain were not concerned by the experience. In fact, one patient mentioned feeling a sense of optimism – she believed that the flare meant that the RT was working. Nevertheless, some patients who were informed of the possibility of experiencing a pain flare reported feeling as though they were caught off guard, which in turn resulted in a great deal of worry and stress. Despite having the research study and the pain flare phenomenon explained to her prior to enrolment in the original pain flare incidence trial, one patient in particular was unaware this was a potential side effect of the RT. She was not pre-medicated in anticipation of this event, and a lack of understanding on pain flare prevented her from being psychologically prepared to deal with this pain increase.
- Question 2: Did the increase in pain interfere with your daily functioning? (For example, general activity, mood, walking ability, normal work, relations with others, sleep, enjoyment of life?). Overall, 10 patients indicated some level of functional interference while experiencing the pain flare, with the majority indicating that the pain flare completely interfered with daily activities. One patient specifically

indicated that the pain interfered with his relationships and put him in a "down" mood. He described himself as a "hermit" in the sense that he did not interact with people because the pain was so severe. Additionally, his wife described him as lethargic and said she could hear him "moaning during the night because of his pain". Another indicated that she needed assistance from her family with basic daily tasks. A female patient indicated she had to lie completely still because the pain significantly increased with the slightest movement. In general, patients indicated that daily activities had to be modified considerably during the time of the flare so as not to aggravate the pain they were experiencing.

- Question 3: What did you do to manage the increase in pain? (For example: extra pain medications, sitting, lying down, etc). Over three quarters of patients indicated they increased their pain medications. However, nine patients failed to achieve adequate control of the RT-induced flare pain despite this increase in OMED. Furthermore, some patients stated that they were reluctant to take additional breakthrough pain medications to control the pain flare due to the unfavourable side effects that may result (i.e. constipation, dry mouth, and fatigue). Alternative methods of pain flare management included rest, limited movement, and/or use of a hot water bottle.
- Question 4: In retrospect, what does the pain flare mean to you now? Most patients had not thought about this aspect of their pain flare experience. One patient indicated that she now knows that any pain relief she will obtain from RT comes with a discomfort. Similarly, another explained that she is now aware of what to expect in terms of what a pain flare feels like and how long it will last. Beyond this, patients experiencing adequate management of the flare with breakthrough pain medications did not have a response to this item. A single patient who did not recall the flare stated, "I don't know what the pain flare means at all".
- Question 5: Overall, do you feel the radiation treatment was worthwhile? The majority of patients indicated that RT was worthwhile, despite experiencing that pain flare. One patient mentioned that although the pain flare was problematic, the RT improved her daily functioning. Yet another expressed that if she wanted to improve functioning, she would have no choice but to experience the pain flare since RT seemed to be the only effective method of sustained pain relief. One patient expressed that she would have delayed RT since she achieved adequate pain relief following hormone therapy. Another patient indicated that the pain flare caused a significant amount of stress and did not result in any subsequent pain relief. The remaining patients were unsure whether the pain relief was from RT or due to pain medications.

At the end of the interview patients were asked if they would prefer the prevention of the pain flare altogether as opposed to management with breakthrough pain medications. Eleven out of 13 patients explicitly stated that they would prefer the prevention of the pain flare.

Discussion

Pain flare is common following external beam RT for symptomatic bone metastases. Our qualitative interview with patients experiencing a pain flare revealed several important trends. Not only was the pain flare debilitating to this cohort of patients by interfering with daily activities and general functioning, but it also resulted in the need for many patients to remain bed-bound. Furthermore, patients expressed anxiety and stress over treatment success. Increases in analgesia were not adequate to control RT-induced pain in the majority of patients. Although our study was limited by a small sample size, there was an overwhelming consensus to prevent the flare as opposed to managing it with breakthrough pain medications (85%).

Pain flare prophylaxis is preferential for two additional reasons: in order for the pain flare to be managed with as-needed pain medications, the patient in question must first experience a pain increase. Moreover, increases in pain medications can lead to increased side effects; including constipation, dry mouth, and drowsiness. The aforementioned situations may cause a further impairment in patient quality of life. Studies to explore prophylactic strategies for the prevention of the pain flare phenomenon are needed. Only through pain flare prevention can we completely eliminate additional and unnecessary patient suffering. Until this goal is reached, we encourage physicians to adequately educate their patients of the potential flare effect, ensure their patients are equipped with adequate breakthrough analgesia, and be attentive to the potential adverse effects of high dose opioid therapy.

Acknowledgments

This study was generously supported by the Michael and Karyn Goldstein Cancer Research Fund.

References

[1] Nielsen OS. Palliative radiotherapy of bone metastases: there is now evidence for the use of single fractions. Radiother Oncol 1999;52:95.

[2] Berk L. Prospective trials for the radiotherapeutic treatment of bone metastases. Am J Hosp Palliat Care 1995;12:24.

[3] Arcangeli G, Giovinazzo G, Saracino B, et al. Radiation therapy in the management of symptomatic bone metastases: The effect of total dose and histology on pain relief and response duration. Int J Rat Onc Biol Phys 1998;42:1119.

[4] Silberstein EB. Teletherapy and radiopharmaceutical therapy of painful bone metastases. Semin Nucl Med 2005;35(2):152-8.

[5] Kraeber-Bodere F, Campion L, Rousseau C, et al. Treatment of bone metastases of prostate cancer with strontium-89 chloride: efficacy in relation to the degree of bone involvement. Eur J Nucl Med 2000;27(10):1487-93.

[6] Roka R, Sera T, Pajor L, et al. Clinical experience with rhenium-188 HEDP therapy for metastatic bone pain. Orv Hetil 2000;141(19):1019-23.
[7] Slovin SF, Scher HI, Divgi CR, et al. Interferon--gamma and monoclonal antibody 131I-labeled CC49: outcomes in patients with androgenindependent prostate cancer. Clin Cancer Res 1998;4(3):643-51.
[8] Schoeneich G, Palmedo H, Dierke-Dzierzon C, et al. Rhenium-186 HEDP: palliative radionuclide therapy of painful bone metastases. Preliminary results. Scand J Urol Nephrol 1997;31(5):445-8.
[9] Limouris GS, Shukla SK, Condi-Paphiti A, et al. Palliative therapy using rhenium-186-HEDP in painful breast osseous metastases. Anticancer Res 1997;17(3B):1767-72.
[10] de Klerk JM, van het Schip AD, Zonnenberg BA, et al. Phase 1 study of rhenium-186-HEDP in patients with bone metastases originating from breast cancer. J Nucl Med 1996;37(2):244-9.
[11] Dafermou A, Colamussi P, Giganti M, et al. A multicentre observational study of radionuclide therapy in patients with painful bone metastases of prostate cancer. Eur J Nucl Med 2001;28(7):788-98.
[12] Bubley GJ. Is the flare phenomenon clinically significant? Urology 2001;58(2Suppl1):5-9.
[13] Kirkbride P, Aslanidis J. Single fraction radiation therapy for bone metastases - a pilot study using a dose of 12 Gy. [Abstract 581]. Clin Invest Med1996;19(4):S87.
[14] Foro P, Algara M, Reig A, et al. Randomized prospective trial comparing three schedules of palliative radiotherapy. Preliminary results. [Spanish]. Oncologia 1998;21(11):55-60.
[15] Loblaw DA, Wu JSY, Warde P, et al. Pain flare in patients with bone metastases after palliative radiotherapy: a nested randomized controlled trial. Sup Care Canc 2007;15(4):451-5.
[16] Chow E, Ling A, Davis L, et al. Pain flare following external beam radiotherapy and meaningful change in pain scores in the treatment of bone metastases. Radiother Oncol 2005;75:64-9.
[17] Roos DE, Turner SL, O'Brien PC, et al. Randomized trial of 8 Gy in 1 versus 20 Gy in 5 fractions of radiotherapy for neuropathic pain due to bone metastases (Trans-Tasman Radiation Oncology Group, TROG 96.05). Radiother Oncol 2005;75:54-63.
[18] Hird A, Hadi S, Loblaw A, et al. Pain flare following radiotherapy for painful bone metastases: a joint effort of three cancer centres to determine the incidence. Int J Rad Onc Biol Phys 2007;69(3) S32-3.
[19] Chow E, Loblaw DA, Harris K, et al. Dexamethasone for the prophylaxis of radiation-induced pain flare after palliative radiotherapy for bone metastases - a pilot study. Supp Care Canc 2007;15:643-7.

In: Advanced Cancer. Pain and Quality of Life
Editors: E. Chow, J. Merrick, pp. 95-118
ISBN: 978-1-61668-207-1
© 2010 Nova Science Publishers, Inc.

Chapter IX

Exploring the Optimal Definitions of Partial Response and Pain Progression in Patients Receiving Radiation Treatment for Painful Bone Metastases

Roseanna Presutti, BSc(C), Liying Zhang, PhD, Amanda Hird, BSc(C), Melissa Deyell, BMSc and Edward Chow, MBBS*

Rapid Response Radiotherapy Program, Department of Radiation Oncology, Odette Cancer Centre, Sunnybrook Health Sciences Centre, University of Toronto, Toronto, Ontario, Canada

The purpose of this chapter was to explore optimal definitions for partial response and pain progression in patients receiving palliative radiotherapy (RT) for painful bone metastases. Methods: Patients referred to the Rapid Response Radiotherapy Program (RRRP) for palliative RT from May 2003 to November 2007 were evaluated. The Brief Pain Inventory (BPI) evaluates worst, current, and average pain, as well as seven items of functional interference on an 11-point (0-10) numeric scale. The BPI was administered at baseline, 1- and 2-months following RT for all patients. Analgesic intake was collected and converted into an oral morphine equivalent dose (OMED). The total sum score of the BPI items was calculated at baseline and at subsequent follow-ups. The follow-up sum score was subtracted from the baseline sum score to determine the difference in the BPI sum score. Various cut-points for difference in worst pain score and percent change in analgesic intake were determined using multivariate analysis of variance (MANOVA). Results: A total of 400 patients were evaluated, 235 males and 165 females, with a median age of 68 years (range: 30-91). The median Karnofsky Performance Status (KPS)

* ***Correspondence:*** Edward Chow, MBBS, PhD, FRCPC, Department of Radiation Oncology, Odette Cancer Centre, Sunnybrook Health Sciences Centre, 2075 Bayview Avenue, Toronto, ON M4N 3M5, Canada. Tel: 416-480-4998; Fax: 416-480-6002; E-mail: Edward.Chow@sunnybrook.ca

was 70 (range: 30-90). At baseline, the mean worst pain score and OMED were 7.4 and 102mg/day respectively. Worst pain scores significantly decreased at the 1- and 2-month follow-up. Thirteen statistically significant and clinically relevant cut-points were identified in patients with BPI improvement or deterioration at 1- and 2-month follow-up.

Conclusion: The present study was a preliminary analysis and further investigation is required to validate our initial findings.

Introduction

Bone metastases are a common manifestation in advanced cancer. Pain is the most frequent complication reported, and over two thirds of patients will experience severe pain as a result of their bone metastases (1). External beam radiotherapy (RT) is an effective modality for the palliation of such metastases. Various randomized control trials have attempted to determine the optimal dose fractionation for alleviating metastatic bone pain. Bone metastases trials conducted by the Radiation Therapy Oncology Group (RTOG7402) initially concluded that low-dose, short-course schedules were as effective as high-dose, protracted schedules (2). However, when the data was reanalyzed using both pain score and analgesic intake, with or without retreatment, it was suggested that protracted fractionation schedules led to an improved complete response rate (3).

Subsequently, the Canadian Bone Metastases Trial compared a single 8Gy to 20Gy in five daily fractions in the treatment of bone metastases and found that pain relief—defined as reduction in the pain score at the treated site with reduced analgesics, or a pain score of zero at the treated site without an increase in analgesics—was significantly higher in patients receiving multiple fractions. However, when analgesic consumption was not included in the definition, the response rate was the same for both the single and fractionated arms (4). As the RTOG and Canadian trials demonstrate, different conclusions can be reached depending on the endpoint definitions employed.

In light of this, an International Bone Metastases Consensus Working Party on endpoint measurements was established in April 2000. Two years later, the Working Party published an international consensus on RT endpoints for future bone metastases clinical trials. Pain score and analgesic consumption were both incorporated into the RT response definition. According to these endpoints, a complete response (CR) is defined as a pain score of zero at the treated site, with no concomitant increase in analgesic intake. Partial response (PR) is defined as either a pain reduction of two or more at the treated site on a scale of zero to ten, without an increase in analgesic intake; or an analgesic reduction of 25% or more from baseline, without a concurrent increase in pain score. Finally, pain progression (PP) is defined as an increase in pain score of two or more points above baseline at the treated site, with stable analgesic intake; or an increase of 25% or more in analgesics relative to baseline measures, with a stable pain score or pain score one point above baseline (5).

The aforementioned endpoints were reached through consensus from previous bone metastases trials investigators and others with a recognized interest in bone metastases. Although the definition of complete response seems very reasonable, the definitions of partial response and disease progression may require more concrete parameters. The purpose of the current study was to explore the optimal definitions of partial response and pain progression following palliative RT for bone metastases.

Our study

This study is a secondary analysis of data collected from a prospective database that examined the effectiveness of palliative RT on alleviating the severity of both pain and functional interference. From May 2003 to November 2007, all patients referred to the Rapid Response Radiotherapy Program (RRRP) with painful metastatic bone lesions for palliative RT were evaluated. Patients were eligible if they could speak and understand English, were competent to complete the survey, had radiographic evidence of bone metastases and provided verbal consent. Ethics approval was obtained from Sunnybrook Health Sciences Centre Research Ethics Board.

Prior to RT, basic demographic information was collected for each patient, including primary cancer site and Karnofsky Performance Status (KPS). Using the Brief Pain Inventory (BPI), patients rated their worst, average and current pain intensity on an 11-point scale of 0 (no pain) to 10 (pain as bad as you can imagine). Patients were also asked to rate the level of pain interference for seven functional items—general activity, mood, walking ability, normal work, relations with other people, sleep and enjoyment of life—on a scale of 0 (no interference) to 10 (complete interference). In the present study, only worst pain scores were used when calculating response to RT. Previous investigations have found that worst pain scores correlate most strongly with the seven items of interference on the BPI and recommend that an 11-point scale evaluating worst pain scores be used when evaluating response rates to RT (6). Thus, only worst pain scores as assessed by the BPI are included in the present study. Additionally, analgesic consumption was recorded for each patient and converted into a daily oral morphine equivalent (OMED). Follow-up telephone interviews were conducted by a research assistant at 1- and 2-month intervals following RT, in order to collect analgesic intake and administer the BPI.

Statistical analysis

Descriptive statistics and distributions were generated for patient demographics and disease-related characteristics. To determine the optimal definitions of partial response and pain progression, the total sum score of the BPI (i.e. the sum of the seven functional interference items) was calculated at baseline and at the 1- and 2-month follow-ups. The change in BPI sum score was determined by subtracting the follow up sum score from the baseline sum score. In the present study, patients were considered to have BPI improvement if the difference in sum score was > 0. On the contrary, if the change was < 0, patients were considered to have deterioration in the BPI.

The difference in the worst pain score and the percent change in OMED were calculated from baseline to follow-up. All possible combinations for the difference of the worst pain score and the percentage change of OMED were created and related to the set of seven functional interference items from the BPI using multivariate analysis of variance (MANOVA). A multivariate Wilk's Lambda, Pillai's trace and Hotelling-Lawley Trace F statistics were calculated based on the effect of variance/covariance matrix. Two-sided p-values less than 0.05 were considered statistically significant. All analyses were performed using the Statistical Analysis Software (SAS Institute, version 9.1 for Windows) package.

Table 1. Patient characteristics (n=400)

	Number of Patients (%)
Sex	
Male	235 (58.8%)
Female	165 (41.2%)
Age (years)	
Median (range)	68 (30 – 91)
Karnofsky Performance Status	
n	385
Mean ± SD	70.2 ± 13.4
Median (range)	70 (30 – 90)
Primary cancer sites	
Breast	102 (25.5%)
Lung	99 (24.8%)
Prostate	98 (24.5%)
Kidney and Bladder	37 (9.3%)
Gastrointestinal	31 (7.8%)
Unknown	19 (4.8%)
Others	14 (3.5%)
Site of radiation treatment	
Extremities	135 (33.8%)
Spine	129 (32.3%)
Pelvis	86 (21.5%)
Ribs	25 (6.3%)
Others	25 (6.3%)
Radiation Dose/fraction	
8Gy/1	243 (60.8%)
20Gy/5	133 (33.3%)
30Gy/10	11 (2.8%)
Others	13 (3.3%)

Our findings

Between May 2003 and November 2007, a total of 400 patients receiving palliative RT for painful bone metastases were evaluated. The median age was 68 years (range: 30-91) with more males (59%) than females (41%). The median KPS score was 70 (range: 30-90). Breast, lung and prostate were the most common primary cancer sites, each representing approximately a quarter of the study population (Table 1). The most common irradiated painful bony sites were the extremities (34%), followed by the spine (32%), pelvis (22%), ribs (6%) and others (6%). The majority of patients (61%) received a single dose of 8Gy.

Table 2. Worst pain scores, seven interference items and analgesic consumption at baseline

Symptom	Mean ± SD	Median
Worst pain	7.4 ± 2.4	8
General activity	6.6 ± 3.2	8
Mood	5.0 ± 3.4	5
Walking ability	5.8 ± 3.6	7
Normal work	6.8 ± 3.5	8
Relations with others	3.4 ± 3.5	2
Sleep	4.8 ± 3.5	5
Enjoyment of life	6.5 ± 3.3	7
Total Daily Oral Morphine Equivalent (mg/day)	102 ± 218	24

Table 3. Worst pain, seven interference items and analgesic consumption at 1-month or at 2-month follow-up

At 1-month		
	Mean ± SD	Median
Worst pain	4.11 ± 3.14	4
	3.14	
General activity	4.24 ± 3.77	4
	3.77	
Mood	3.05 ± 3.55	2
	3.55	
Walking ability	3.64 ± 3.69	3
	3.69	
Normal work	4.65 ± 4.17	5
	4.17	
Relations with others	2.05 ± 3.16	0
	3.16	
Sleep	2.64 ± 3.28	1
	3.28	
Enjoyment of life	4.14 ± 3.66	4
	3.66	
Total Daily Oral Morphine Equivalent (mg/day)	96.45 ± 172.9	20
At 2-month		
	Mean ± SD	Median
Worst pain	3.71 ± 3.15	3
General activity	3.65 ± 3.63	3
Mood	2.73 ± 3.21	1
Walking ability	3.22 ± 3.65	2
Normal work	3.80 ± 3.94	3
Relations with others	1.84 ± 2.94	0
Sleep	1.91 ± 2.76	0
Enjoyment of life	3.38 ± 3.46	2
Total Daily Oral Morphine Equivalent (mg/day)	76.10 ± 126.1	16

At baseline, the mean worst pain score with standard deviation (SD) was 7.4 ± 2.4, with a mean (±SD) analgesic intake of 102 (±218) mg/day (Table 2). The mean (±SD) and median values for the seven functional interference items at baseline are outlined in Table 2. Following palliative RT, the mean (±SD) worst pain score was reduced to 4.11±3.14 and 3.71±3.15 at the 1- and 2-month follow-up, respectively. Table 3 outlines the corresponding values for functional interference and analgesic intake at the 1- and 2-month follow-up.

Table 4a. All possible combinations between changes in worst pain score and oral morphine equivalent in patients with BPI improvement at month 1 (n=84).

	Cutpoint	No. of patients		Cutpoint	No. of patients
1	CP4,-100	1	42	CP10,-20	2
2	CP4,20	1	43	CP,100	1
3	CP4,50	1	44	CP-3,-100	1
4	CP4,60	2	45	CP-2,-100	2
5	CP4,90	1	46	CP-2,-40	1
6	CP4,100	15	47	CP-1,-100	2
7	CP4,-50	1	48	CP-1,70	1
8	CP4,-10	1	49	CP-1,100	1
9	CP5,-100	3	50	CP-1,-10	1
10	CP5,0	1	51	CP0,-100	7
11	CP5,50	1	52	CP0,0	1
12	CP5,90	1	53	CP0,30	1
13	CP5,100	5	54	CP0,50	1
14	CP5,-30	1	55	CP0,100	2
15	CP5,-10	2	56	CP0,-50	1
16	CP6,-100	3	57	CP0,-40	1
17	CP6,0	2	58	CP0,-30	1
18	CP6,10	1	59	CP0,-20	1
19	CP6,20	1	60	CP0,-10	1
20	CP6,50	1	61	CP1,-100	3
21	CP6,60	1	62	CP1,10	1
22	CP6,100	12	63	CP1,80	1
23	CP,30	1	64	CP1,100	6
24	CP7,-100	1	65	CP1,-50	1
25	CP7,10	1	66	CP1,-40	2
26	CP7,100	2	67	CP2,-100	5
27	CP7,-10	1	68	CP2,0	1
28	CP8,-100	2	69	CP2,20	2
29	CP8,0	1	70	CP2,40	1
30	CP8,30	1	71	CP2,50	1
31	CP8,70	1	72	CP2,70	1
32	CP8,100	5	73	CP2,100	8
33	CP9,0	1	74	CP2,-50	1
34	CP9,50	1	75	CP2,-30	1
35	CP9,60	1	76	CP3,-100	4
36	CP9,70	1	77	CP3,0	2
37	CP9,90	1	78	CP3,50	1
38	CP9,100	3	79	CP3,60	2
39	CP10,40	1	80	CP3,-80	1
40	CP10,80	1	81	CP3,100	11
41	CP10,100	5	82	CP3,-30	1

Table 4b. Multivariate analysis of variance (MANOVA) on all possible 66 combinations of cutpoints and the improvement of 7 interference items at month 1.

Cutpoint	Statistic	Value	F statistic*	p-value*
CP9,100	Wilks' Lambda	0.8412	4.02	**0.0005**
CP9,100	Pillai's Trace	0.1588		
CP9,100	Hotelling-Lawley Trace	0.1888		
CP10,100	Wilks' Lambda	0.8650	3.32	**0.0026**
CP10,100	Pillai's Trace	0.1350		
CP10,100	Hotelling-Lawley Trace	0.1561		
CP5,-30	Wilks' Lambda	0.8795	2.92	**0.0069**
CP5,-30	Pillai's Trace	0.1205		
CP5,-30	Hotelling-Lawley Trace	0.1370		
CP5,90	Wilks' Lambda	0.8961	2.47	**0.0200**
CP5,90	Pillai's Trace	0.1039		
CP5,90	Hotelling-Lawley Trace	0.1160		
CP-1,-100	Wilks' Lambda	0.8994	2.38	**0.0245**
CP-1,-100	Pillai's Trace	0.1006		
CP-1,-100	Hotelling-Lawley Trace	0.1119		
CP0,30	Wilks' Lambda	0.9021	2.31	**0.0290**
CP0,30	Pillai's Trace	0.0979		
CP0,30	Hotelling-Lawley Trace	0.1085		
CP0,-40	Wilks' Lambda	0.9036	2.27	**0.0317**
CP0,-40	Pillai's Trace	0.0964		
CP0,-40	Hotelling-Lawley Trace	0.1067		
CP-1,70	Wilks' Lambda	0.9126	2.04	0.0538
CP-1,70	Pillai's Trace	0.0874		
CP-1,70	Hotelling-Lawley Trace	0.0958		
CP2,-30	Wilks' Lambda	0.9162	1.95	0.0661
CP2,-30	Pillai's Trace	0.0838		
CP2,-30	Hotelling-Lawley Trace	0.0915		
CP10,-20	Wilks' Lambda	0.9184	1.89	0.0746
CP10,-20	Pillai's Trace	0.0816		
CP10,-20	Hotelling-Lawley Trace	0.0889		
CP2,20	Wilks' Lambda	0.9225	1.79	0.0936
CP2,20	Pillai's Trace	0.0775		
CP2,20	Hotelling-Lawley Trace	0.0840		
CP0,-20	Wilks' Lambda	0.9226	1.79	0.0942
CP0,-20	Pillai's Trace	0.0774		
CP0,-20	Hotelling-Lawley Trace	0.0839		
CP8,100	Wilks' Lambda	0.9268	1.68	0.1175
CP8,100	Pillai's Trace	0.0732		
CP8,100	Hotelling-Lawley Trace	0.0790		
CP5,100	Wilks' Lambda	0.9275	1.66	0.1219
CP5,100	Pillai's Trace	0.0725		
CP5,100	Hotelling-Lawley Trace	0.0782		
CP4,60	Wilks' Lambda	0.9305	1.59	0.1428
CP4,60	Pillai's Trace	0.0695		
CP4,60	Hotelling-Lawley Trace	0.0747		
CP2,50	Wilks' Lambda	0.9311	1.57	0.1471
CP2,50	Pillai's Trace	0.0689		
CP2,50	Hotelling-Lawley Trace	0.0740		
CP10,40	Wilks' Lambda	0.9315	1.57	0.1500
CP10,40	Pillai's Trace	0.0685		
CP10,40	Hotelling-Lawley Trace	0.0735		

Table 4b. (continued)

Cutpoint	Statistic	Value	F statistic*	p-value*
CP9,70	Wilks' Lambda	0.9317	1.56	0.1518
CP9,70	Pillai's Trace	0.0683		
CP9,70	Hotelling-Lawley Trace	0.0733		
CP2,70	Wilks' Lambda	0.9329	1.53	0.1611
CP2,70	Pillai's Trace	0.0671		
CP2,70	Hotelling-Lawley Trace	0.0719		
CP1,80	Wilks' Lambda	0.9337	1.51	0.1671
CP1,80	Pillai's Trace	0.0663		
CP1,80	Hotelling-Lawley Trace	0.0711		
CP2,100	Wilks' Lambda	0.9349	1.48	0.1777
CP2,100	Pillai's Trace	0.0651		
CP2,100	Hotelling-Lawley Trace	0.0696		
CP4,-100	Wilks' Lambda	0.9351	1.48	0.1791
CP4,-100	Pillai's Trace	0.0649		
CP4,-100	Hotelling-Lawley Trace	0.0695		
CP7,100	Wilks' Lambda	0.9353	1.47	0.1817
CP7,100	Pillai's Trace	0.0647		
CP7,100	Hotelling-Lawley Trace	0.0691		
CP2,-100	Wilks' Lambda	0.9364	1.44	0.1915
CP2,-100	Pillai's Trace	0.0636		
CP2,-100	Hotelling-Lawley Trace	0.0679		
CP4,-10	Wilks' Lambda	0.9369	1.43	0.1962
CP4,-10	Pillai's Trace	0.0631		
CP4,-10	Hotelling-Lawley Trace	0.0673		
CP-3,-100	Wilks' Lambda	0.9385	1.40	0.2110
CP-3,-100	Pillai's Trace	0.0615		
CP-3,-100	Hotelling-Lawley Trace	0.0656		
CP5,0	Wilks' Lambda	0.9427	1.29	0.2571
CP5,0	Pillai's Trace	0.0573		
CP5,0	Hotelling-Lawley Trace	0.0608		
CP-2,-100	Wilks' Lambda	0.9452	1.23	0.2877
CP-2,-100	Pillai's Trace	0.0548		
CP-2,-100	Hotelling-Lawley Trace	0.0580		
CP3,0	Wilks' Lambda	0.9463	1.21	0.3017
CP3,0	Pillai's Trace	0.0537		
CP3,0	Hotelling-Lawley Trace	0.0568		
CP9,50	Wilks' Lambda	0.9484	1.16	0.3301
CP9,50	Pillai's Trace	0.0516		
CP9,50	Hotelling-Lawley Trace	0.0544		
CP3,60	Wilks' Lambda	0.9496	1.13	0.3475
CP3,60	Pillai's Trace	0.0504		
CP3,60	Hotelling-Lawley Trace	0.0531		
CP3,-80	Wilks' Lambda	0.9513	1.09	0.3731
CP3,-80	Pillai's Trace	0.0487		
CP3,-80	Hotelling-Lawley Trace	0.0512		
CP4,100	Wilks' Lambda	0.9525	1.06	0.3918
CP4,100	Pillai's Trace	0.0475		
CP4,100	Hotelling-Lawley Trace	0.0498		
CP8,30	Wilks' Lambda	0.9529	1.05	0.3977
CP8,30	Pillai's Trace	0.0471		
CP8,30	Hotelling-Lawley Trace	0.0494		

Table 4. (continued)

Cutpoint	Statistic	Value	F statistic*	p-value*
CP1,-40	Wilks' Lambda	0.9529	1.05	0.3980
CP1,-40	Pillai's Trace	0.0471		
CP1,-40	Hotelling-Lawley Trace	0.0494		
CP-1,100	Wilks' Lambda	0.9531	1.05	0.4008
CP-1,100	Pillai's Trace	0.0469		
CP-1,100	Hotelling-Lawley Trace	0.0492		
CP0,-10	Wilks' Lambda	0.9585	0.92	0.4924
CP0,-10	Pillai's Trace	0.0415		
CP0,-10	Hotelling-Lawley Trace	0.0432		
CP5,-10	Wilks' Lambda	0.9616	0.85	0.5473
CP5,-10	Pillai's Trace	0.0384		
CP5,-10	Hotelling-Lawley Trace	0.0400		
CP6,0	Wilks' Lambda	0.9637	0.80	0.5871
CP6,0	Pillai's Trace	0.0363		
CP6,0	Hotelling-Lawley Trace	0.0377		
CP2,-50	Wilks' Lambda	0.9638	0.80	0.5886
CP2,-50	Pillai's Trace	0.0362		
CP2,-50	Hotelling-Lawley Trace	0.0376		
CP7,10	Wilks' Lambda	0.9647	0.78	0.6055
CP7,10	Pillai's Trace	0.0353		
CP7,10	Hotelling-Lawley Trace	0.0366		
CP1,-50	Wilks' Lambda	0.9652	0.77	0.6163
CP1,-50	Pillai's Trace	0.0348		
CP1,-50	Hotelling-Lawley Trace	0.0360		
CP4,50	Wilks' Lambda	0.9672	0.72	0.6543
CP4,50	Pillai's Trace	0.0328		
CP4,50	Hotelling-Lawley Trace	0.0339		
CP6,60	Wilks' Lambda	0.9679	0.70	0.6679
CP6,60	Pillai's Trace	0.0321		
CP6,60	Hotelling-Lawley Trace	0.0331		
CP3,50	Wilks' Lambda	0.9710	0.64	0.7250
CP3,50	Pillai's Trace	0.0290		
CP3,50	Hotelling-Lawley Trace	0.0299		
CP6,-100	Wilks' Lambda	0.9711	0.63	0.7274
CP6,-100	Pillai's Trace	0.0289		
CP6,-100	Hotelling-Lawley Trace	0.0298		
CP1,10	Wilks' Lambda	0.9729	0.59	0.7616
CP1,10	Pillai's Trace	0.0271		
CP1,10	Hotelling-Lawley Trace	0.0278		
CP0,0	Wilks' Lambda	0.9732	0.59	0.7664
CP0,0	Pillai's Trace	0.0268		
CP0,0	Hotelling-Lawley Trace	0.0275		
CP6,100	Wilks' Lambda	0.9736	0.58	0.7735
CP6,100	Pillai's Trace	0.0264		
CP6,100	Hotelling-Lawley Trace	0.0271		
CP,30	Wilks' Lambda	0.9768	0.51	0.8292
CP7,-100	Pillai's Trace	0.0232		
CP7,-100	Hotelling-Lawley Trace	0.0238		
CP0,-30	Wilks' Lambda	0.9781	0.48	0.8498
CP0,-30	Pillai's Trace	0.0219		
CP0,-30	Hotelling-Lawley Trace	0.0224		
CP8,70	Wilks' Lambda	0.9786	0.47	0.8584

Table 4b. (continued)

Cutpoint	Statistic	Value	F statistic*	p-value*
CP8,70	Pillai's Trace	0.0214		
CP8,70	Hotelling-Lawley Trace	0.0219		
CP1,100	Wilks' Lambda	0.9798	0.44	0.8763
CP1,100	Pillai's Trace	0.0202		
CP1,100	Hotelling-Lawley Trace	0.0206		
CP1,-100	Wilks' Lambda	0.9827	0.38	0.9156
CP1,-100	Pillai's Trace	0.0173		
CP1,-100	Hotelling-Lawley Trace	0.0176		
CP9,60	Wilks' Lambda	0.9829	0.37	0.9187
CP9,60	Pillai's Trace	0.0171		
CP9,60	Hotelling-Lawley Trace	0.0174		
CP0,-100	Wilks' Lambda	0.9848	0.33	0.9404
CP0,-100	Pillai's Trace	0.0152		
CP0,-100	Hotelling-Lawley Trace	0.0154		
CP5,50	Wilks' Lambda	0.9854	0.32	0.9458
CP5,50	Pillai's Trace	0.0146		
CP5,50	Hotelling-Lawley Trace	0.0148		
CP2,40	Wilks' Lambda	0.9854	0.31	0.9464
CP2,40	Pillai's Trace	0.0146		
CP2,40	Hotelling-Lawley Trace	0.0148		
CP5,-100	Wilks' Lambda	0.9874	0.27	0.9641
CP5,-100	Pillai's Trace	0.0126		
CP5,-100	Hotelling-Lawley Trace	0.0128		
CP8,-100	Wilks' Lambda	0.9893	0.23	0.9775
CP8,-100	Pillai's Trace	0.0107		
CP8,-100	Hotelling-Lawley Trace	0.0108		
CP-1,-10	Wilks' Lambda	0.9893	0.23	0.9775
CP-1,-10	Pillai's Trace	0.0107		
CP-1,-10	Hotelling-Lawley Trace	0.0108		
CP0,100	Wilks' Lambda	0.9893	0.23	0.9775
CP0,100	Pillai's Trace	0.0107		
CP0,100	Hotelling-Lawley Trace	0.0108		
CP7,-10	Wilks' Lambda	0.9906	0.20	0.9845
CP7,-10	Pillai's Trace	0.0094		
CP7,-10	Hotelling-Lawley Trace	0.0095		
CP3,100	Wilks' Lambda	0.9911	0.19	0.9867
CP3,100	Pillai's Trace	0.0089		
CP3,100	Hotelling-Lawley Trace	0.0090		
CP3,-100	Wilks' Lambda	0.9912	0.19	0.9872
CP3,-100	Pillai's Trace	0.0088		
CP3,-100	Hotelling-Lawley Trace	0.0089		
CP2,0	Wilks' Lambda	0.9917	0.18	0.9894
CP2,0	Pillai's Trace	0.0083		
CP2,0	Hotelling-Lawley Trace	0.0084		

* Wilk's lamba, Pillai's trace and Hotelling-Lawley trace have same values for F-statistic and exact p-value. P-value < 0.05 was considered as significant.

Tables 4a and 5a list the possible cut-points (CP) for the worst pain score and percent change in OMED at the 1- and 2-month follow-up, respectively, for patients with improvement in their BPI sum score. For instance, CP4, 20 identified in Table 4a indicates that at follow-up the worst pain score was reduced by four points on the 0 to 10 scale of the BPI and there was also a concurrent reduction of 20% in OMED. Tables 4b and 5b show the multivariate analysis of variance (MANOVA) and the possible cut-point combinations for patients with improvement on the BPI. Cut-points with statistically significant values imply a partial response.

Table 5a. All possible combinations between changes in worst pain score and oral morphine equivalent in patients with BPI improvement at month 2 (n=92).

	Cutpoint	No. of patients		Cutpoint	No. of patients
1	CP4,-100	1	35	CP9,100	3
2	CP4,0	2	36	CP10,-100	1
3	CP4,10	1	37	CP10,70	1
4	CP4,60	2	38	CP10,100	6
5	CP4,70	1	39	CP,100	1
6	CP4,100	5	40	CP-3,-50	1
7	CP4,-40	1	41	CP-2,-100	1
8	CP4,-30	1	42	CP-2,20	1
9	CP5,-100	4	43	CP-2,-70	1
10	CP5,0	1	44	CP-1,0	1
11	CP5,20	1	45	CP-1,100	1
12	CP5,80	1	46	CP0,-100	5
13	CP5,100	6	47	CP0,0	1
14	CP5,-20	2	48	CP0,20	1
15	CP6,-100	4	49	CP0,50	1
16	CP6,10	1	50	CP0,100	3
17	CP6,20	1	51	CP0,-50	1
18	CP6,40	1	52	CP1,-100	5
19	CP6,70	1	53	CP1,0	1
20	CP6,100	8	54	CP1,20	1
21	CP6,-30	1	55	CP1,40	1
22	CP7,-100	1	56	CP1,70	2
23	CP7,50	1	57	CP1,100	8
24	CP7,80	1	58	CP1,-50	1
25	CP7,90	1	59	CP2,-100	4
26	CP7,100	10	60	CP2,0	1
27	CP8,-100	1	61	CP2,20	1
28	CP8,10	1	62	CP2,100	2
29	CP8,40	1	63	CP2,-70	1
30	CP8,100	6	64	CP3,-100	5
31	CP9,0	1	65	CP3,0	1
32	CP9,60	1	66	CP3,60	1
33	CP9,70	1	67	CP3,100	9
34	CP9,90	1			

All possible cut-points in worst pain score and percent change in OMED at 1- and 2-month follow-up are outlined in Tables 6a and 7a, respectively, for patients with deterioration in BPI sum score. From Table 6a, CP-2,-30 indicates that at follow-up, the worst pain score increased by 2 and the OMED percent increased by 30%. Tables 6b and 7b show the

MANOVA of the possible cut off point combinations for patients showing deterioration on the BPI. Statistical significance demonstrated by MANOVA ($p<0.05$) implies pain progression.

Table 5b. Multivariate analysis of variance (MANOVA) on all possible 53 combinations of cut points and the improvement of 7 interference items at month 2.

Cutpoint	Statistic	Value	F statistic*	p-value*
CP10,100	Wilks' Lambda	0.8004	4.45	**0.0002**
CP10,100	Pillai's Trace	0.1996		
CP10,100	Hotelling-Lawley Trace	0.2493		
CP8,10	Wilks' Lambda	0.8558	3.01	**0.0059**
CP8,10	Pillai's Trace	0.1442		
CP8,10	Hotelling-Lawley Trace	0.1686		
CP7,90	Wilks' Lambda	0.8803	2.43	**0.0229**
CP7,90	Pillai's Trace	0.1197		
CP7,90	Hotelling-Lawley Trace	0.1360		
CP2,100	Wilks' Lambda	0.8842	2.34	**0.0282**
CP2,100	Pillai's Trace	0.1158		
CP2,100	Hotelling-Lawley Trace	0.1309		
CP8,-100	Wilks' Lambda	0.8861	2.29	**0.0311**
CP8,-100	Pillai's Trace	0.1139		
CP8,-100	Hotelling-Lawley Trace	0.1285		
CP9,100	Wilks' Lambda	0.8963	2.07	0.0519
CP9,100	Pillai's Trace	0.1037		
CP9,100	Hotelling-Lawley Trace	0.1157		
CP1,0	Wilks' Lambda	0.9021	1.94	0.0689
CP1,0	Pillai's Trace	0.0979		
CP1,0	Hotelling-Lawley Trace	0.1086		
CP-1,100	Wilks' Lambda	0.9030	1.92	0.0721
CP-1,100	Pillai's Trace	0.0970		
CP-1,100	Hotelling-Lawley Trace	0.1074		
CP-1,0	Wilks' Lambda	0.9137	1.69	0.1183
CP-1,0	Pillai's Trace	0.0863		
CP-1,0	Hotelling-Lawley Trace	0.0944		
CP5,20	Wilks' Lambda	0.9161	1.64	0.1314
CP5,20	Pillai's Trace	0.0839		
CP5,20	Hotelling-Lawley Trace	0.0916		
CP1,-100	Wilks' Lambda	0.9164	1.63	0.1331
CP1,-100	Pillai's Trace	0.0836		
CP1,-100	Hotelling-Lawley Trace	0.0912		
CP2,20	Wilks' Lambda	0.9178	1.60	0.1415
CP2,20	Pillai's Trace	0.0822		
CP2,20	Hotelling-Lawley Trace	0.0896		
CP3,100	Wilks' Lambda	0.9236	1.48	0.1813
CP3,100	Pillai's Trace	0.0764		
CP3,100	Hotelling-Lawley Trace	0.0827		
CP8,100	Wilks' Lambda	0.9258	1.43	0.1985
CP8,100	Pillai's Trace	0.0742		
CP8,100	Hotelling-Lawley Trace	0.0802		
CP2,-100	Wilks' Lambda	0.9275	1.39	0.2132

Table 5b. (continued)

Cutpoint	Statistic	Value	F statistic*	p-value*
CP2,-100	Pillai's Trace	0.0725		
CP2,-100	Hotelling-Lawley Trace	0.0781		
CP4,-40	Wilks' Lambda	0.9352	1.24	0.2869
CP4,-40	Pillai's Trace	0.0648		
CP4,-40	Hotelling-Lawley Trace	0.0693		
CP9,70	Wilks' Lambda	0.9374	1.19	0.3120
CP9,70	Pillai's Trace	0.0626		
CP9,70	Hotelling-Lawley Trace	0.0668		
CP0,50	Wilks' Lambda	0.9417	1.11	0.3636
CP0,50	Pillai's Trace	0.0583		
CP0,50	Hotelling-Lawley Trace	0.0619		
CP4,0	Wilks' Lambda	0.9430	1.08	0.3803
CP4,0	Pillai's Trace	0.0570		
CP4,0	Hotelling-Lawley Trace	0.0605		
CP0,100	Wilks' Lambda	0.9434	1.07	0.3858
CP0,100	Pillai's Trace	0.0566		
CP0,100	Hotelling-Lawley Trace	0.0600		
CP6,100	Wilks' Lambda	0.9437	1.07	0.3899
CP6,100	Pillai's Trace	0.0563		
CP6,100	Hotelling-Lawley Trace	0.0597		
CP2,0	Wilks' Lambda	0.9438	1.06	0.3905
CP2,0	Pillai's Trace	0.0562		
CP2,0	Hotelling-Lawley Trace	0.0596		
CP6,20	Wilks' Lambda	0.9449	1.04	0.4052
CP6,20	Pillai's Trace	0.0551		
CP6,20	Hotelling-Lawley Trace	0.0584		
CP4,100	Wilks' Lambda	0.9459	1.02	0.4201
CP4,100	Pillai's Trace	0.0541		
CP4,100	Hotelling-Lawley Trace	0.0572		
CP0,-100	Wilks' Lambda	0.9473	0.99	0.4396
CP0,-100	Pillai's Trace	0.0527		
CP0,-100	Hotelling-Lawley Trace	0.0556		
CP-3,-50	Wilks' Lambda	0.9474	0.99	0.4407
CP-3,-50	Pillai's Trace	0.0526		
CP-3,-50	Hotelling-Lawley Trace	0.0555		
CP7,100	Wilks' Lambda	0.9475	0.99	0.4415
CP7,100	Pillai's Trace	0.0525		
CP7,100	Hotelling-Lawley Trace	0.0555		
CP5,-20	Wilks' Lambda	0.9481	0.98	0.4511
CP5,-20	Pillai's Trace	0.0519		
CP5,-20	Hotelling-Lawley Trace	0.0547		
CP-2,-70	Wilks' Lambda	0.9496	0.95	0.4730
CP-2,-70	Pillai's Trace	0.0504		
CP-2,-70	Hotelling-Lawley Trace	0.0530		
CP7,80	Wilks' Lambda	0.9501	0.94	0.4794
CP7,80	Pillai's Trace	0.0499		
CP7,80	Hotelling-Lawley Trace	0.0526		

Table 5b. (continued)

Cutpoint	Statistic	Value	F statistic*	p-value*
CP4,60	Wilks' Lambda	0.9511	0.92	0.4943
CP4,60	Pillai's Trace	0.0489		
CP4,60	Hotelling-Lawley Trace	0.0515		
CP9,0	Wilks' Lambda	0.9511	0.92	0.4946
CP9,0	Pillai's Trace	0.0489		
CP9,0	Hotelling-Lawley Trace	0.0514		
CP3,-100	Wilks' Lambda	0.9514	0.91	0.5001
CP3,-100	Pillai's Trace	0.0486		
CP3,-100	Hotelling-Lawley Trace	0.0510		
CP6,40	Wilks' Lambda	0.9538	0.86	0.5363
CP6,40	Pillai's Trace	0.0462		
CP6,40	Hotelling-Lawley Trace	0.0484		
CP5,0	Wilks' Lambda	0.9539	0.86	0.5380
CP5,0	Pillai's Trace	0.0461		
CP5,0	Hotelling-Lawley Trace	0.0483		
CP9,60	Wilks' Lambda	0.9590	0.76	0.6192
CP9,60	Pillai's Trace	0.0410		
CP9,60	Hotelling-Lawley Trace	0.0427		
CP5,-100	Wilks' Lambda	0.9596	0.75	0.6290
CP5,-100	Pillai's Trace	0.0404		
CP5,-100	Hotelling-Lawley Trace	0.0421		
CP2,-70	Wilks' Lambda	0.9606	0.73	0.6440
CP2,-70	Pillai's Trace	0.0394		
CP2,-70	Hotelling-Lawley Trace	0.0411		
CP10,70	Wilks' Lambda	0.9609	0.73	0.6489
CP10,70	Pillai's Trace	0.0391		
CP10,70	Hotelling-Lawley Trace	0.0407		
CP0,-50	Wilks' Lambda	0.9636	0.68	0.6927
CP0,-50	Pillai's Trace	0.0364		
CP0,-50	Hotelling-Lawley Trace	0.0378		
CP1,100	Wilks' Lambda	0.9641	0.67	0.7006
CP1,100	Pillai's Trace	0.0359		
CP1,100	Hotelling-Lawley Trace	0.0373		
CP5,80	Wilks' Lambda	0.9652	0.64	0.7196
CP5,80	Pillai's Trace	0.0348		
CP5,80	Hotelling-Lawley Trace	0.0360		
CP0,0	Wilks' Lambda	0.9656	0.64	0.7256
CP0,0	Pillai's Trace	0.0344		
CP0,0	Hotelling-Lawley Trace	0.0356		
CP4,70	Wilks' Lambda	0.9667	0.62	0.7420
CP4,70	Pillai's Trace	0.0333		
CP4,70	Hotelling-Lawley Trace	0.0345		
CP1,20	Wilks' Lambda	0.9716	0.52	0.8166
CP1,20	Pillai's Trace	0.0284		
CP1,20	Hotelling-Lawley Trace	0.0292		
CP7,-100	Wilks' Lambda	0.9741	0.47	0.8514
CP7,-100	Pillai's Trace	0.0259		
CP7,-100	Hotelling-Lawley Trace	0.0266		

Table 5b. (continued)

Cutpoint	Statistic	Value	F statistic*	p-value*
CP1,70	Wilks' Lambda	0.9766	0.43	0.8831
CP1,70	Pillai's Trace	0.0234		
CP1,70	Hotelling-Lawley Trace	0.0240		
CP6,70	Wilks' Lambda	0.9774	0.41	0.8931
CP6,70	Pillai's Trace	0.0226		
CP6,70	Hotelling-Lawley Trace	0.0231		
CP1,-50	Wilks' Lambda	0.9789	0.38	0.9099
CP1,-50	Pillai's Trace	0.0211		
CP1,-50	Hotelling-Lawley Trace	0.0215		
CP4,10	Wilks' Lambda	0.9797	0.37	0.9178
CP4,10	Pillai's Trace	0.0203		
CP4,10	Hotelling-Lawley Trace	0.0208		
CP6,-100	Wilks' Lambda	0.9803	0.36	0.9247
CP6,-100	Pillai's Trace	0.0197		
CP6,-100	Hotelling-Lawley Trace	0.0201		
CP1,40	Wilks' Lambda	0.9835	0.30	0.9525
CP1,40	Pillai's Trace	0.0165		
CP1,40	Hotelling-Lawley Trace	0.0168		
CP5,100	Wilks' Lambda	0.9841	0.29	0.9576
CP5,100	Pillai's Trace	0.0159		
CP5,100	Hotelling-Lawley Trace	0.0161		

* Wilk's lamba, Pillai's trace and Hotelling-Lawley trace have same values for F-statistic and exact p-value. P-value < 0.05 was considered as significant.

Table 6a. Possible cut-off points in patients with BPI deterioration at month 1 (n=56)

	Cutpoint	No. of patients		Cutpoint	No. of patients
1	CP4,-100	1	22	CP-1,-80	1
2	CP4,40	1	23	CP-1,100	3
3	CP4,90	1	24	CP-1,-10	1
4	CP4,100	1	25	CP0,-100	4
5	CP,10	1	26	CP0,30	1
6	CP-5,0	1	27	CP0,100	4
7	CP5,100	1	28	CP0,-10	2
8	CP6,-100	1	29	CP1,-100	1
9	CP-5,100	1	30	CP1,0	1
10	CP6,100	1	31	CP1,100	1
11	CP6,-30	1	32	CP1,-30	1
12	CP7,-100	2	33	CP2,-100	1
13	CP7,-40	1	34	CP2,0	1
14	CP,100	1	35	CP2,20	1
15	CP-4,90	1	36	CP2,80	1
16	CP-4,100	1	37	CP2,-60	1
17	CP-3,-100	1	38	CP2,-20	1
18	CP-3,-10	1	39	CP3,-100	3
19	CP-2,-100	2	40	CP3,20	1
20	CP-2,-30	1	41	CP3,-80	1
21	CP-1,30	1	42	CP3,100	2

Table 6b. Multivariate analysis of variance (MANOVA) on all possible 32 combinations of cut points and the deterioration of 7 interference items at month 1.

Cutpoint	Statistic	Value	F statistic*	p-value*
CP7,-100	Wilks' Lambda	0.3236	11.05	**<.0001**
CP7,-100	Pillai's Trace	0.6764		
CP7,-100	Hotelling-Lawley Trace	2.0901		
CP-4,100	Wilks' Lambda	0.6067	3.43	**0.0063**
CP-4,100	Pillai's Trace	0.3933		
CP-4,100	Hotelling-Lawley Trace	0.6484		
CP3,20	Wilks' Lambda	0.6839	2.44	**0.0365**
CP3,20	Pillai's Trace	0.3161		
CP3,20	Hotelling-Lawley Trace	0.4622		
CP0,100	Wilks' Lambda	0.6945	2.32	**0.0452**
CP0,100	Pillai's Trace	0.3055		
CP0,100	Hotelling-Lawley Trace	0.4399		
CP0,30	Wilks' Lambda	0.7248	2.01	0.0804
CP0,30	Pillai's Trace	0.2752		
CP0,30	Hotelling-Lawley Trace	0.3797		
CP4,-100	Wilks' Lambda	0.7377	1.88	0.1012
CP4,-100	Pillai's Trace	0.2623		
CP4,-100	Hotelling-Lawley Trace	0.3555		
CP-3,-10	Wilks' Lambda	0.7491	1.77	0.1230
CP-3,-10	Pillai's Trace	0.2509		
CP-3,-10	Hotelling-Lawley Trace	0.3349		
CP3,-80	Wilks' Lambda	0.7574	1.69	0.1409
CP3,-80	Pillai's Trace	0.2426		
CP3,-80	Hotelling-Lawley Trace	0.3204		
CP4,40	Wilks' Lambda	0.7709	1.57	0.1747
CP4,40	Pillai's Trace	0.2291		
CP4,40	Hotelling-Lawley Trace	0.2972		
CP1,100	Wilks' Lambda	0.7784	1.50	0.1961
CP1,100	Pillai's Trace	0.2216		
CP1,100	Hotelling-Lawley Trace	0.2847		
CP0,-10	Wilks' Lambda	0.7865	1.43	0.2212
CP0,-10	Pillai's Trace	0.2135		
CP0,-10	Hotelling-Lawley Trace	0.2714		
CP1,-100	Wilks' Lambda	0.8063	1.27	0.2919
CP1,-100	Pillai's Trace	0.1937		
CP1,-100	Hotelling-Lawley Trace	0.2402		
CP-1,-80	Wilks' Lambda	0.8311	1.07	0.3993
CP-1,-80	Pillai's Trace	0.1689		
CP-1,-80	Hotelling-Lawley Trace	0.2032		
CP-2,-30	Wilks' Lambda	0.8381	1.02	0.4329
CP-2,-30	Pillai's Trace	0.1619		
CP-2,-30	Hotelling-Lawley Trace	0.1932		
CP6,100	Wilks' Lambda	0.8438	0.98	0.4611
CP6,100	Pillai's Trace	0.1562		
CP6,100	Hotelling-Lawley Trace	0.1852		
CP-5,100	Wilks' Lambda	0.8577	0.88	0.5339
CP-5,100	Pillai's Trace	0.1423		
CP-5,100	Hotelling-Lawley Trace	0.1659		
CP-1,100	Wilks' Lambda	0.8636	0.84	0.5653
CP-1,100	Pillai's Trace	0.1364		
CP-1,100	Hotelling-Lawley Trace	0.1580		

Table 6. (continued)

Cutpoint	Statistic	Value	F statistic*	p-value*
CP2,-60	Wilks' Lambda	0.8672	0.81	0.5850
CP2,-60	Pillai's Trace	0.1328		
CP2,-60	Hotelling-Lawley Trace	0.1532		
CP0,-100	Wilks' Lambda	0.8730	0.77	0.6165
CP0,-100	Pillai's Trace	0.1270		
CP0,-100	Hotelling-Lawley Trace	0.1455		
CP2,-20	Wilks' Lambda	0.8799	0.72	0.6545
CP2,-20	Pillai's Trace	0.1201		
CP2,-20	Hotelling-Lawley Trace	0.1365		
CP2,-100	Wilks' Lambda	0.8807	0.72	0.6589
CP2,-100	Pillai's Trace	0.1193		
CP2,-100	Hotelling-Lawley Trace	0.1355		
CP2,80	Wilks' Lambda	0.8855	0.68	0.6849
CP2,80	Pillai's Trace	0.1145		
CP2,80	Hotelling-Lawley Trace	0.1293		
CP5,100	Wilks' Lambda	0.9089	0.53	0.8064
CP5,100	Pillai's Trace	0.0911		
CP5,100	Hotelling-Lawley Trace	0.1002		
CP1,-30	Wilks' Lambda	0.9166	0.48	0.8421
CP1,-30	Pillai's Trace	0.0834		
CP1,-30	Hotelling-Lawley Trace	0.0910		
CP-2,-100	Wilks' Lambda	0.9269	0.42	0.8857
CP-2,-100	Pillai's Trace	0.0731		
CP-2,-100	Hotelling-Lawley Trace	0.0788		
CP7,-40	Wilks' Lambda	0.9329	0.38	0.9079
CP7,-40	Pillai's Trace	0.0671		
CP7,-40	Hotelling-Lawley Trace	0.0720		
CP2,0	Wilks' Lambda	0.9335	0.38	0.9102
CP2,0	Pillai's Trace	0.0665		
CP2,0	Hotelling-Lawley Trace	0.0712		
CP3,-100	Wilks' Lambda	0.9394	0.34	0.9296
CP3,-100	Pillai's Trace	0.0606		
CP3,-100	Hotelling-Lawley Trace	0.0645		
CP4,100	Wilks' Lambda	0.9427	0.32	0.9396
CP4,100	Pillai's Trace	0.0573		
CP4,100	Hotelling-Lawley Trace	0.0608		
CP2,20	Wilks' Lambda	0.9438	0.31	0.9427
CP2,20	Pillai's Trace	0.0562		
CP2,20	Hotelling-Lawley Trace	0.0595		
CP6,-100	Wilks' Lambda	0.9589	0.23	0.9765
CP6,-100	Pillai's Trace	0.0411		
CP6,-100	Hotelling-Lawley Trace	0.0429		
CP6,-30	Wilks' Lambda	0.9759	0.13	0.9954
CP6,-30	Pillai's Trace	0.0241		
CP6,-30	Hotelling-Lawley Trace	0.0247		

* Wilk's lamba, Pillai's trace and Hotelling-Lawley trace have same values for F-statistic and exact p-value. P-value < 0.05 was considered as significance.

Table 7a. Possible cut-off points in patients with BPI deterioration at month 2 (n=35)

	Cutpoint	No. of patients
1	CP-6,-100	1
2	CP4,50	1
3	CP5,90	1
4	CP6,100	1
5	CP7,-100	1
6	CP7,80	1
7	CP-5,-50	1
8	CP9,60	1
9	CP-4,0	1
10	CP-4,100	1
11	CP-3,-100	2
12	CP-3,60	1
13	CP-2,100	1
14	CP-1,-100	2
15	CP-1,-90	1
16	CP0,-100	3
17	CP0,10	1
18	CP0,100	1
19	CP1,-100	2
20	CP1,-90	1
21	CP1,-40	1
22	CP2,40	1
23	CP2,100	2
24	CP3,-100	2
25	CP3,10	1
26	CP3,-80	1
27	CP3,100	2

All statistically significant cut-points are summarized in Table 8. One month following RT, CP9, 100 showed the most statistical significance (p=0.0005), followed by CP10, 100 (p=0.0026), CP5,-30 (p=0.0069), CP5, 90 (p=0.0200) and CP0, 30 (p=0.0290), respectively, in patients experiencing improvement in the BPI. For patients experiencing deterioration in the BPI deterioration at 1-month follow-up, two cut-points, CP7,-100 (p=<0.0001) and CP-4,100 (p=0.0063), were found to be statistically significant. Two months following RT, five statistically significant cut-points were identified in patients with BPI improvement, and one statistically significant cut-point, CP7, 80 (p=0.0157), was identified in patients with BPI deterioration.

Table 7b. Multivariate analysis of variance (MANOVA) on all possible 19 combinations of cut points and the deterioration of 7 interference items at month 2.

Cutpoint	Statistic	Value	F statistic*	p-value*
CP7,80	Wilks' Lambda	0.4758	3.30	**0.0157**
CP7,80	Pillai's Trace	0.5242		
CP7,80	Hotelling-Lawley Trace	1.1016		
CP0,100	Wilks' Lambda	0.5796	2.18	0.0794
CP0,100	Pillai's Trace	0.4204		
CP0,100	Hotelling-Lawley Trace	0.7254		
CP2,100	Wilks' Lambda	0.6061	1.95	0.1117
CP2,100	Pillai's Trace	0.3939		
CP2,100	Hotelling-Lawley Trace	0.6500		
CP9,60	Wilks' Lambda	0.6219	1.82	0.1352
CP9,60	Pillai's Trace	0.3781		
CP9,60	Hotelling-Lawley Trace	0.6081		
CP4,50	Wilks' Lambda	0.6490	1.62	0.1837
CP4,50	Pillai's Trace	0.3510		
CP4,50	Hotelling-Lawley Trace	0.5409		
CP3,-100	Wilks' Lambda	0.6496	1.62	0.1850
CP3,-100	Pillai's Trace	0.3504		
CP3,-100	Hotelling-Lawley Trace	0.5394		
CP2,40	Wilks' Lambda	0.6569	1.57	0.2000
CP2,40	Pillai's Trace	0.3431		
CP2,40	Hotelling-Lawley Trace	0.5222		
CP3,100	Wilks' Lambda	0.6845	1.38	0.2638
CP3,100	Pillai's Trace	0.3155		
CP3,100	Hotelling-Lawley Trace	0.4609		
CP7,-100	Wilks' Lambda	0.6933	1.33	0.2866
CP7,-100	Pillai's Trace	0.3067		
CP7,-100	Hotelling-Lawley Trace	0.4423		
CP-3,-100	Wilks' Lambda	0.7134	1.21	0.3428
CP-3,-100	Pillai's Trace	0.2866		
CP-3,-100	Hotelling-Lawley Trace	0.4018		
CP0,-100	Wilks' Lambda	0.7404	1.05	0.4267
CP0,-100	Pillai's Trace	0.2596		
CP0,-100	Hotelling-Lawley Trace	0.3507		
CP6,100	Wilks' Lambda	0.7510	0.99	0.4619
CP6,100	Hotelling-Lawley Trace	0.3316		
CP6,100	Pillai's Trace	0.2490		
CP3,-80	Wilks' Lambda	0.8360	0.59	0.7577
CP3,-80	Pillai's Trace	0.1640		
CP3,-80	Hotelling-Lawley Trace	0.1962		
CP5,90	Wilks' Lambda	0.8370	0.58	0.7611
CP5,90	Pillai's Trace	0.1630		
CP5,90	Hotelling-Lawley Trace	0.1948		
CP-1,-100	Wilks' Lambda	0.8669	0.46	0.8517
CP-1,-100	Pillai's Trace	0.1331		
CP-1,-100	Hotelling-Lawley Trace	0.1536		
CP-2,100	Wilks' Lambda	0.9041	0.32	0.9374

Table 7b. (continued)

Cutpoint	Statistic	Value	F statistic*	p-value*
CP-2,100	Pillai's Trace	0.0959		
CP-2,100	Hotelling-Lawley Trace	0.1060		
CP1,-40	Wilks' Lambda	0.9274	0.23	0.9718
CP1,-40	Pillai's Trace	0.0726		
CP1,-40	Hotelling-Lawley Trace	0.0783		
CP-4,100	Wilks' Lambda	0.9399	0.19	0.9839
CP-4,100	Pillai's Trace	0.0601		
CP-4,100	Hotelling-Lawley Trace	0.0640		
CP-4,0	Wilks' Lambda	0.9805	0.06	0.9996
CP-4,0	Pillai's Trace	0.0195		
CP-4,0	Hotelling-Lawley Trace	0.0199		

* Wilk's lamba, Pillai's trace and Hotelling-Lawley trace have same values for F-statistic and exact p-value. P-value < 0.05 was considered as significant.

Table 8. Summary of all possible cut-points

	Cut-points			
	Worst Pain	Analgesic intake	F statistic*	p-value*
Patients with BPI improvement at 1-Month follow-up (FU)				
CP9,100	Reduce 9 scores	100% reduction or 0 at FU	4.02	0.0005
CP10,100	Reduce 10 scores or 0 at FU	100% reduction or 0 at FU	3.32	0.0026
CP5,-30	Reduce 5 scores	30% increase	2.92	0.0069
CP5,90	Reduce 5 scores	90% reduction	2.47	0.0200
CP0,30	No change	30% reduction	2.31	0.0290
Patients with BPI improvement at 2-Month FU				
CP10,100	Reduce 10 scores or 0 at FU	100% reduction or 0 at FU	4.45	0.0002
CP8,10	Reduce 8 scores	10% reduction	3.01	0.0059
CP7,90	Reduce 7 scores	90% reduction	2.43	0.0229
CP2,100	Reduce 2 scores	100% reduction or 0 at FU	2.34	0.0282
CP8,-100	Reduce 8 scores	100% increase	2.29	0.0311
Patients with BPI deterioration at 1-Month FU				
CP7,-100	Reduce 7 scores	100% increase	11.05	<0.0001
CP-4,100	Increase 4 scores	100% reduction or 0 at FU	3.43	0.0063
Patients with BPI deterioration at 2-Month FU				
CP7,80	Reduce 7 scores	80% reduction	3.30	0.0157

* F-statistic and exact p-value was found by MANOVA Wilk's lambda or Pillai's trace or Hotelling-Lawley trace. P-value < 0.05 was considered as significance.

Discussion

The purpose of the present study was to explore optimal definitions for partial response and pain progression in patients receiving palliative RT for bone metastases. Numerous palliative RT trials for bone metastases have been conducted, in which a wide range of end-points were employed, especially in terms of partial response and pain progression. For instance, Steenland et al. defined partial response as a decrease in pain by two or more points and pain progression as an increase in pain, returning to initial pain score or higher when evaluated on an 11-point numeric scale in their 1999 trial (7). In contrast, Nielsen et al. used a visual analog scale (VAS), which used the descriptors none, mild, moderate and excruciating to evaluate pain and factored analgesic intake into their definition of pain progression. According to their study, partial response was a reduction of >50% on the VAS (8). Several trials did not provide a definition for partial response (4, 9-11) and others had no description for pain progression (4, 12). With such varying response definitions, it was recognized that the direct comparison of trial outcomes was invalid, and the unified definitions were necessary (13).

In 2002, the International Bone Metastases Consensus Group established definitions for complete response, partial response and pain progression. These endpoints were reached via the clinical experience of bone metastases experts and were not based on quantitative data. Individuals experiencing both a reduced worst pain score and increase in analgesic intake were not included in the response definitions, leading to a discrepancy in how to classify these patients. As a result, it has been recommended that the consensus response definitions be reassessed (14).

Based on our preliminary results, five clinically relevant and statistically significant cut-points were observed for partial response at both one and two months following RT. Although CP9, 100 (p=0.0005) and CP10, 100 (p=0.0026) had the greatest statistical significance at 1-month follow-up, these cut-points are closely related to the consensus definition for complete response. Cut-point 5,-30 (p=0.0069) represents a reduction in worst pain score by five points and a 30% increase in analgesic intake. This cut-point may be more relevant to defining partial response and also addresses the issue of calculating response in patients with decreased pain and increased analgesia. Furthermore, at the one month follow-up, CP0, 30 indicating no change in worst pain score and an analgesic reduction of 30%, was found to be statistically significant (p=0.029). This cut-point is similar to the International Consensus definition for partial response—analgesic reduction of 25% or more from baseline without an increase in worst pain score—and provides some degree of objectivity to the consensus definition.

Regarding patients with improvement in the BPI two months following RT, CP2, 100 (p=0.0282) represents a reduced worst pain by 2 scores with 100% reduction in analgesic intake or no analgesic intake at follow-up. This is also similar to the consensus definition of partial response (worst pain reduction of 2 or more at the treated site, without analgesic increase) in terms of worst pain score, however, differs in terms of analgesic consumption.

In an attempt to define pain progression, three cut-points were identified after the one and two-month follow-ups. However, CP7,80 (p=0.0157), which indicates a reduction of seven points in worst pain score and an 80% reduction in analgesic intake, is clinically irrelevant, and should be disregarded when considering pain progression. Only CP7,-100 (p=<0.0001) and CP-4,100 (p=0.0063) demonstrate both statistical significance and clinical relevance in the definition of progressive pain.

Although the primary objective of the present study is to explore the definition of partial response and pain progression using objective statistical analyses, it is also important to consider patient perspectives when defining response to palliative RT. We previously evaluated the meaningful change in pain scores as perceived by patients with bone metastases receiving palliative RT. It was found that when there was a decline in pain score of two or more on an 11-point numeric scale, patients perceived their current pain to be less than their baseline pain (15). In a similar investigation, the expectations of patients being treated with palliative RT for painful bone metastases were assessed in order to obtain a patient-derived definition for partial response. It was suggested that a pain score reduction of two-thirds from baseline as measured on an 11-point numeric scale may be indicative of partial response (16). A reduction of two-thirds is similar to the CP5,-30 identified in the present series which indicates a pain score reduction of approximately half on the 0-10 scale of the BPI. This cut-point demonstrates consistency with both statistical analyses and patient expectations when attempting to reach a more optimal definition for partial response. However, it is noted that patients were asked to consider pain scores only and not analgesic consumption in their expectation of partial response.

The present study was limited to only English speaking patients. Improvement and deterioration in the BPI were evaluated at 1- and 2-months post-RT. However, the International Bone Metastases Consensus Group recommends that pain response be assessed at 1-, 2- and 3-months post-RT (5). In order to maintain consistency, BPI sum scores may require evaluation 3-months following RT since we are attempting to reach a more optimal definition based on the International Consensus end-point definitions. On the other hand, one of our previous studies concluded that evaluating pain response 2-months post-RT may be more appropriate due to attrition rates and also because patients may require more than four weeks to achieve maximum pain relief (14). Therefore, the time intervals used in this study to measure BPI improvement and deterioration are supported.

Furthermore, cut-points that were statistically significant, but were not clinically relevant were removed from the analysis. Specifically, in patients found to have BPI improvement at 1-month follow-up, CP-1,-100 and CP0,-40 were eliminated. Also at 1-month follow up, CP 3, 20 and CP0, 100 were removed from the analysis for patients with deterioration in the BPI. Another possible limitation of this study lies in the method used to determine patient improvement or deterioration. Functional interference items were summed in order for such determination, which may not necessarily result in a linear relationship. Functional items of the BPI can be grouped into subscales of pain interference coupled with physical functions (general activity, walking ability and normal work) and psychological functions (mood, relations with other people, and enjoyment of life, sleep) (17, 18).

Response rates to RT are a function of the endpoint definition. The present study did not attempt to calculate response rate, rather it aimed to relate worst pain scores and percent change in analgesic intake to deterioration or improvement in the BPI. This would allow us to quantitatively define partial response and pain progression in patients with bone metastases. However, due to a small sample size, the present study was a preliminary analysis and the use of a larger sample size may result in more representative findings. Until our initial findings can be validated, the International Consensus end-points should continue to be used in order to maintain consistency when reporting RT response rates in bone metastases trials.

survival, we recommend the referral of patients after the orthopedic stabilization for a radiation oncology consult.

Kyphoplasty, vertebroplasty and cementoplasty have gained popularity as minimally invasive surgical procedures in patients with bone metastases. Some patients have been treated with these procedures alone. There have been few comparative studies addressing the benefits of adjuvant post procedure radiation therapy. Gerszten et al (3) did report using a combined kyphoplasty and spinal radiosurgery treatment in 26 patients with histologically confirmed pathological fractures, and an improvement in pain was seen in 24 patients. We encourage more prospective or retrospective research in this expanding area. Until then, extrapolating the evidence of benefits of adjuvant postoperative radiation therapy from the one retrospective study following the open orthopedic stabilization, we recommend patients likewise be treated with post procedure radiation therapy after kyphoplasty, vertebroplasty, or cementoplasty, unless they have received prior radiation to that site.

References

[1] Townsend P, Rosenthal H, Smalley S, et al. Impact of postoperative radiation therapy and other perioperative factors on outcome after orthopedic stabilization of impending or pathologic fractures due to metastatic disease. J Clin Oncol. 1994;12(11):2345-50.

[2] Townsend P, Smalley S, Cozad S, et al. Role of postoperative radiation therapy after stabilization of fractures caused by metastatic disease. Int J Radiat Oncol Biol Phys 1995;31(1):43-9.

[3] Gerszten P, Germanwala A, Burton S et al. Combination kyphoplasty and spinal radiosurgery: a new treatment paradigm for pathological fractures. Neurosurg Focus 2005;18(3):E8.

Acknowledgments

This study was supported by Michael and Karyn Goldstein Cancer Research Fund. We thank Stacy Lue for secretarial assistance. Conflict of Interest: None.

References

[1] von Moos R, Strasser F, Gillessen S, Zaugg K. Metastatic bone pain: treatment options with an emphasis on bisphosphonates. Support.Care Cancer 2008;16(10):1105-15.

[2] Tong D, Gillick L, Hendrickson FR. The palliation of symptomatic osseous metastases: final results of the Study by the Radiation Therapy Oncology Group. Cancer 1982;50(5):893-9.

[3] Blitzer PH: Reanalysis of the RTOG study of the palliation of symptomatic osseous metastasis. Cancer 1985;55:1468-72.

[4] Kirkbride P, Warde P, Panzarella A, et al: A randomized trial comparing the efficacy of single fraction radiation therapy plus ondansetron with fractionated radiation therapy in the palliation of skeletal metastases. Int J Radiat Oncol Biol Phys 2000;48(Suppl 3):185.

[5] Chow E, Wu JS, Hoskin P, Coia LR, Bentzen SM, Blitzer PH. International consensus on palliative radiotherapy endpoints for future clinical trials in bone metastases. Radiother Oncol. 2002;64(3):275-80.

[6] Harris K, Li K, Flynn C, Chow E. Worst, Average or Current Pain in the Brief Pain Inventory: Which Should be Used to Calculate the Response to Palliative Radiotherapy in Patients with Bone Metastases? Clin Oncol 2007;19:523-7.

[7] Steenland E, Leer JW, van Houwelingen H, Post WJ, van den Hout WB, Kievit J, et al. The effect of a single fraction compared to multiple fractions on painful bone metastases: a global analysis of the Dutch Bone Metastasis Study. Radiother Oncol 1999;52(2):101-9.

[8] Nielsen OS, Bentzen SM, Sandberg E, Gadeberg CC, Timothy AR. Randomized trial of single dose versus fractionated palliative radiotherapy of bone metastases. Radiother Oncol 1998;47(3):233-40.

[9] Koswig S, Budach V: Recalcification and pain relief following radiotherapy for bone metastases: A randomized trial of 2 different fractionation schedules (10 X 3 Gy vs. 1 X 8 Gy). Strahlenther Onkol 1999;175:500-8. [German]

[10] Kaasa S, Brenne E, Lund J, et al: Prospective randomized multicentre trial on single fraction radiotherapy (8 Gy X 1) versus multiple fractions (3 Gy X10) in the treatment of painful bone metastases: Phase III randomized trial. Radiother Oncol 2006;79:278-84.

[11] Haddad P, Behrouzi H, Amouzegar-Hashemi F, et al: Single versus multiple fractions of palliative radiotherapy for bone metastases: A randomized clinical trial in Iranian patients. Radiother Oncol 2006; 80:S65.

[12] Niewald M, Tkocz HJ, Abel U, Scheib T, Walter K, Nieder C, et al. Rapid course radiation therapy vs. more standard treatment: a randomized trial for bone metastases. Int J Radiat Oncol Biol Phys 1996;36(5):1085-9.

[13] Wu JS, Bezjak A, Chow E, Kirkbride P. Primary treatment endpoint following palliative radiotherapy for painful bone metastases: need for a consensus definition? Clin.Oncol (R Coll Radiol) 2002;14(1):70-7.

[14] Li KK, Hadi S, Kirou-Mauro A, Chow E. When should we define the response rates in the treatment of bone metastases by palliative radiotherapy? Clin Oncol 2008;20:83-9.

[15] Chow E, Chiu H, Doyle M, Hruby G, Holden L, et al. Patient expectation of the partial response and response shift in pain score. Support Cancer Ther 2007;4(2):110-8.

[16] Chow E, Ling A, Davis L, Panzarella T, Danjoux C. Pain flare following external beam radiotherapy and meaningful change in pain scores in the treatment of bone metastases. Radiother Oncol 2005; 75:64-9.

[17] Klepstad P, Loge JH, Borchgrevink PC, Mendoza TR, Cleeland CS, Kaasa S. The Norwegian brief pain inventory questionnaire: translation and validation in cancer pain patients. J Pain Symptom Manage 2002;24(5):517-25.

[18] Holen JC, Lydersen S, Klepstad P, Loge JH, Kaasa S. The Brief Pain Inventory: pain's interference with functions is different in cancer pain compared with noncancer chronic pain. Clin J Pain 2008; 24(3):219-25.

Section Three: Advanced Cancer

In: Advanced Cancer. Pain and Quality of Life
Editors: E. Chow, J. Merrick, pp. 123-127

ISBN: 978-1-61668-207-1
© 2010 Nova Science Publishers, Inc.

Chapter XI

Skeletal Related Events in Patients with Metastatic Bone Disease

Amanda E. Hird, BSc(C), Mark Clemons, MD, Liying Zhang, PhD and Edward Chow, MBBS*

Department of Radiation Oncology, Odette Cancer Centre,
Sunnybrook Health Sciences Centre, University of Toronto, Toronto, Ontario, Canada

Recent advances in effective systemic treatment and supportive care have resulted in an improved prognosis for patients with bone metastases. As patients are living with their metastatic bone disease for longer, skeletal related events (SREs) are of increasing concern. An SRE is defined as one of the following: the need for palliative surgery or radiation therapy (RT) for pain relief or stabilization of an osseous lesion, pathological fracture, spinal cord compression (SCC), or hypercalcaemia. Given that the occurrence of an SRE is associated with a worsening patient mortality, successful management of bone metastases is essential for not only reducing skeletal complications and maximizing patient quality of life (QOL), but also for improved survival.

Introduction

An estimated 166,400 new cases of cancer and 73,800 deaths from cancer will occur in Canada in 2008 (1). Bone metastases unfortunately remain a common site of recurrence, presenting in 5-73% of cancer patients (2), with breast and prostate cancer patients representing upwards of 80% of this population (3).

Metastatic bone disease is associated with significant morbidity and mortality. In terms of morbidity, pain is experienced by up to two thirds of patients (4-7). In terms of mortality, the prognosis for patients with bone metastases is highly influenced by tumor type,

* Correspondence: Edward Chow MBBS, PhD, FRCPC, Department of Radiation Oncology, Odette Cancer Centre, Sunnybrook Health Sciences Centre, 2075 Bayview Ave, Toronto, Ontario, Canada M4N 3M5. E-mail: Edward.Chow@sunnybrook.ca

performance status, and the presence of extraosseous disease (2,8-10). In a recent analysis, median survival was significantly longer in breast cancer patients with a first relapse in the axial skeleton (24 months) versus patients with initial relapse in the liver (3 months) (2). It has also been determined that survival after diagnosis of bone metastases is influenced by the subsequent development of extraosseous metastatic sites: 1.6 years versus 2.1 years in patients with bone-only disease (2).

Recent advances in effective systemic treatment and supportive care have resulted in an improved prognosis for patients with bone metastases (11-13). As patients are living with their metastatic bone disease for longer, skeletal related events (SREs) are of increasing concern. An SRE is defined as one of the following: the need for palliative surgery or radiation therapy (RT) for pain relief or stabilization of an osseous lesion, pathological fracture, spinal cord compression (SCC), or hypercalcaemia. Given that the occurrence of an SRE is associated with a worsening patient mortality (11,14-18), successful management of bone metastases is essential for not only reducing skeletal complications and maximizing patient quality of life (QOL), but also for improved survival.

However, reported incidences of SREs in the literature are often cited in clinical trial data from bisphosphonate studies (11). We therefore decided to explore SRE data in a large population of patients with bone metastases enrolled in an international study evaluating relevant quality of life (QOL) issues (19). Patients with radiologically documented bone metastases undergoing a variety of treatments (chemotherapy, bisphosphonates, hormone therapy, symptom management, and irradiation) were approached.

Skeletal related events

Our analysis of the prevalence of SREs was conducted in 365 Canadian and Australian patients with bone metastases. Patients were accrued from medical oncology clinics (61%), radiation oncology clinics (32%), inpatient units (5%), or in a pain/symptom management clinic (2%). Median patient age was 63 years (range 29 to 92) with a median time since bone metastases diagnosis of 1.5 years (range 0 to 26). The cohort was composed of slightly more females (58%) than males (42%). Most common primary cancer sites were breast (43%), prostate (19%), and lung (15%). Sixty one percent of patients had bone only metastases, while 16, 15, and 13% of patients also had lung, liver, and lymph node involvement, respectively. Fifty-five, 69, and 56% of patients were currently receiving or had previously received bisphosphonates, chemotherapy, and hormonal therapy, respectively.

Of the 365 patients the overall incidence of SREs was 244/365 (67%). At the time of interview, 52% of patients reported one, 10% reported two, and 4% reported three SREs. In this cohort of patients, the types of SRE were palliative RT (71%), pathological fracture (8%), nerve root/SCC (6%), need for surgery (5%), and hypercalcaemia (5%). The occurrence of an SRE was significantly related to Karnofsky performance status (KPS), with a lower performance status more indicative of a current SRE ($p<0.0001$). Age, duration of bone metastases diagnosis, primary cancer site, and use of bisphosphonates were not significantly related to the presence of an SRE. Patients previously or currently on systemic chemotherapy were more likely to experience an SRE ($p=0.0473$). Although the current or previous use of bisphosphonates did not significantly reduce the occurrence of SREs in this cohort, information on the duration or type of bisphosphonate therapy was not collected.

Given the predominance of SREs in this study, a number of management questions still remain pertaining to optimal time of initiation, duration, and type of bisphosphonate therapy. In the breast cancer setting, the American Society for Clinical Oncology (ASCO) practice guidelines (20) advises the initiation of bisphosphonates in women with obvious lytic disease on plain radiographs; or with an abnormal bone scan, normal radiographs but a CT or MRI scan showing bone destruction. Similarly in multiple myeloma, bisphosphonate therapy is introduced following radiographic evidence of lytic destruction to the bone cortex. In prostate cancer patients with significant bone loss, bisphosphonate therapy should be strongly considered regardless of hormonal status or systemic disease (15). Indications for bisphosphonate use in lung cancer remain controversial with respect to presentation of a clinically meaningful benefit when prognosis is generally limited (21).

Unanswered questions

Despite these recommendations, questions remain unanswered: a) what bisphosphonate regimen (agent, dose, frequency, and duration) is best; b) can integration of bisphosphonates in patients without documented bone metastases prevent future osseous involvement; c) how can their use be integrated with other bone-metastases specific treatments; d) and what is the cost-benefit evaluation in the palliative literature in terms of patient transportation to and from the cancer centre, toxicity, compliance, and cost-effectiveness. What is clear is that despite widespread use of BPs SREs remain common and we therefore need new strategies to optimize patient management (22-25)

As bone metastases and SREs are common even in the era of modern cancer therapies, there is an immediate need to continue to improve these therapies. Skeletal related events can severely influence QOL and, as suggested in our analysis, are correlated with a significantly lower KPS. Effective prevention of SREs in patients with bone metastases is essential to preservation of functioning and maintenance of QOL. While RT is effective for localized pain relief and remineralization of osseous lesions, systemic bisphosphonate therapy may inhibit tumor cell adhesion to bone, tumor growth, angiogenesis (26), and provide pain relief (27). Integration of bisphosphonate and RT may have a synergistic effect on metastatic bone lesions and potentially reduce the risk of SREs when used in combination (26). Moreover, investigation of targeted therapies may have more pronounced effect on management of metastatic bone disease. As prognosis for metastatic cancer patients improve, further research in-vivo will be useful for optimizing the management of this group.

References

[1] Canadian Cancer Society. Canadian Cancer Statistics 2008. 17 August 2008. Retrieved 12 October 2008 from <http://www.cancer.ca/Canada-wide/About%20cancer/Cancer%20statistics/Canadian%20Cancer%20Statistics.aspx?sc_lang=en>.

[2] Coleman RE. Clinical features of metastatic bone disease and risk of skeletal morbidity. Clin Cancer Res 2006;12(20 Suppl):6243-49.
[3] Coleman RE. Skeletal complications of malignancy. Cancer 1997;80(8 Suppl):1588-94.
[4] Mercadante S. Malignant bone pain: pathophysiology and treatment. Pain 1997;69(12):1-18.
[5] Janjan N. Bone metastases: approaches to management. Semin Oncol 2001;28(4 Suppl 11):28-34.
[6] Serafini AN. Therapy of metastatic bone pain. J Nucl Med 2001;42:895-906.
[7] Gralow J, Tripathy D. Managing metastatic bone pain: The role of bisphosphonates. J Pain Symp Manag 2007;33(4)462-72.
[8] Hansen BH, Keller J, Laitinen M, et al. Scandinavian Sarcoma Group Skeletal Metastasis Register. Survival after surgery for bone metastases in the pelvis and extremities. Acta Orthop Scand 2004;75:11-5.
[9] Katagiri H, Takahashi M, Wakai K, et al. Prognostic factors and a scoring system for patients with skeletal metastasis. J Bone Joint Surg Br 2005;87:698-703.
[10] van der Linden YM, Dijkstra SP, Vonk EJ, et al. Dutch Bone Metastasis Study Group. Prediction of survival in patients with metastases in the spinal column: results based on a randomized trial of radiotherapy. Cancer 2005;103:320-8.
[11] Lipton A. Treatment of bone metastases and bone pain with bisphosphonates. Supp Canc Ther 2007;4(2):92-100.
[12] Lipton A, Cook RJ, Major P, et al. Zoledronic acid and survival in breast cancer patients with bone metastases and elevated markers of osteoclast activity. Oncologist 2007;12:1035-43.
[13] Coleman RE. Metastatic bone disease: Clinical features, pathophysiology and treatment strategies. Cancer Treat Rev 2001;27:165-76.
[14] Hei YJ, Saad F, Coleman RE et al. Fractures negatively affect survival in patients with bone metastases from breast cancer [Abstract 6036]. 28th Annual San Antonio Breast Cancer Symposium; December 8-11, 2005.
[15] Saad F, Gleason D, Murray R, et al. Zoledronic acid provides long term reductions in skeletal morbidity for men with prostate cancer and bone metastases [Abstract 149]. American Society for Clinical Oncology Prostate Cancer Symposium; February 24-26, 2006.
[16] Theriault RL, Lipton A, Hortobagyi GN, et al. Pamidronate reduces skeletal morbidity in women with advanced breast cancer and lytic bone lesions: a randomized, placebo-controlled trial. Protocol 18 Aredia Breast Cancer Study Group. J Clin Oncol 1999;17:846–54.
[17] Oefelein MG, Ricchuti V, Conrad W, et al. Skeletal fractures negatively correlate with overall survival in men with prostate cancer. J Urol 2002;168:1005-7.
[18] Sugiura H, Yamada K, Sugiura T, Hida T, Mitsudomi T. Predictors of survival in patients with bone metastasis of lung cancer. Clin Orthop Relat Res 2008;466:729-36.
[19] Chow E, Hird A, Velikova G, et al. on behalf of the EORTC Quality of Life Group. Development of an EORTC disease-specific quality of life questionnaire module for patients with bone metastases. Eur J Cancer 2008 [e-pub ahead of print].

[20] Hillner BE, Ingle JN, Chlebowski RT, et al. American Society of Clinical Oncology 2003 update on the role of bisphosphonates and bone health issues in women with breast cancer. J Clin Oncol 2003;21(21):4042-57.

[21] Saba N, Khuri F. The role of bisphosphonates in the management of advanced cancer with a focus on non-small-cell lung cancer. Oncology 2005;68:18-22.

[22] Valdivielso JM, Fernandez E. Vitamin D receptor polymorphisms and diseases. Clinica Chimica Acta 2006;371(1-2):1-12.

[23] Simmons C, Ooi W, Dranitsaris G, et al. Phase II study of Vitamin D (10, 000 IU daily) supplementation in bisphosphonate-treated breast cancer patients with bone metastases [Abstract 176]. Breast Cancer Symposium; September 5-7, 2008.

[24] Masuda S, Jones G. Promise of vitamin D analogues in the treatment of hyperproliferative conditions. Mol Cancer Ther 2006;5(4):797–808.

[25] Lipton A, de Boer RH, Figueroa J, et al. Phase II study of denosumab in breast cancer patients with bone metastases naïve to intravenous bisphosphonate therapy: Extended efficacy and safety analysis [Abstract 266]. Breast Cancer Symposium; September 7-8, 2007.

[26] Ural AU, Avcu F, Baran Y. Bisphosphonate treatment and radiotherapy in metastatic breast cancer. Med Oncol 2008;25:350-5.

[27] Wong RKS, Wiffen PJ. Bisphosphonates for the relief of pain secondary to bone metastases. Cochrane Database Syst Rev 2002(2):002068.

In: Advanced Cancer. Pain and Quality of Life
Editors: E. Chow, J. Merrick, pp. 129-143
ISBN: 978-1-61668-207-1
© 2010 Nova Science Publishers, Inc.

Chapter XII

A Critical Discussion of Symptom Clusters in Metastatic Cancer

Harleen Bedi, BSc(C), Amanda Hird, BSc(C), Sarah Campos, BSc(C) and Edward Chow, MBBS, PhD, FRCPC*

Rapid Response Radiotherapy Program, Department of Radiation Oncology,
Odette Cancer Centre, Sunnybrook Health Sciences Centre,
University of Toronto, Toronto, Ontario, Canada

Advanced cancer patients often present with multiple concurrent symptoms that may have synergistic effect on patient morbidity. Previous research in oncology has suggested that certain symptoms tend to occur together, stay relatively stable over time, and remain relatively independent of other symptoms, with or without a shared etiology. Research on the co-management of symptoms through the analysis of symptom clusters can improve palliative care in oncology. This literature review analyzes symptom cluster studies in metastatic cancer. Common advanced cancer symptoms are discussed to explore their relationship within a cluster. Methods: A literature search was conducted to identify studies on symptom clusters in advanced cancer. Additionally, studies analyzing conceptual issues, statistical modelling and physiological mechanisms of symptoms common to advance cancer were examined. Results: The literature review identified 11 relevant studies published between 1997 and 2008. Eight studies focussed on metastatic cancer while three studies investigated symptom clusters in oncology patients representing various disease stages. Discussion: Investigation of symptom clusters is complicated and is influenced by several conceptual, methodological and patient related factors. Studies reviewed differed in their definitions of symptom clusters, types of assessment questionnaires and statistical analyses. Further research to explore the mechanisms underlying symptom clusters and the stability of clusters over time will validate research on this concept.

Introduction

Oncology patients often present with multiple symptoms that co-occur and may be caused by the cancer itself, its treatment, or a combination of the two (1). A symptom is defined as a "subjective experience reflecting the biopyschosocial functioning, sensations, or cognition of an individual" (2, pg 669). Symptoms are multidimensional and can include a patient's perceptions of prevalence, intensity and distress (3).

Past research in cancer symptom management has followed a reductionist approach by investigating a few clinically significant symptoms individually (4). Though this approach reveals extensive information about certain symptoms, it does not determine particular groups of symptoms commonly observed in cancer patients co-occur and correlate. Dodd et al (5) pioneered the concept of "symptom clusters" to research on the concurrence and co-management of symptoms commonly observed in cancer. A symptom cluster was proposed to be constructed of symptoms that were related without necessarily sharing a common etiology (5).

Exploration of symptom clusters has revealed new avenues in symptom management and palliative care of cancer patients. Research on the influence of groups of symptoms on patient outcomes has led to increased awareness of symptom clusters, and was recently supported by the National Institutes of Health (NIH) at the State-of-the-Science Conference on "Symptom Management in Cancer: Pain, Depression and Fatigue" (6).

Successive studies of symptom clusters have refined the definition of what should qualify as a symptom cluster. Kim et al (7) defined a symptom cluster as a group of two or more related symptoms that co-occur and form a stable group independent of other clusters. Additionally, Miaskowski et al (4) suggested symptoms should share a common etiology, have common variance and produce outcomes different from individual symptoms to be considered related. Nevertheless considerable debate exists around determining a common, working definition of symptom clusters (4,8-10).

Contemporary research in symptom clusters has either followed the deterministic model or the heuristic model. The deterministic model investigates the validity and reliability of pre-defined symptom clusters (10). In contrast, the heuristic model statistically examines relationship between a list of symptoms to derive clusters (10). Generally symptom clusters studies have employed a cross-sectional design to examine the concurrence of symptoms at any given time (10). Nonetheless, analysis of symptom clusters in chronic diseases such as cancer can benefit from longitudinal studies that investigate symptom profiles over time.

Common statistical approaches employed for derivation of symptom clusters include correlation and related measures of association, graphical modelling, factor analysis and cluster analysis. Correlation and related measures of association provide concrete mathematical evidence for the concurrence of two or more symptoms (10). On the other hand, graphical modelling is an effective tool for visual representation of conditional relationships in multivariate random observations (10). Alternatively, factor analysis can

* *Correspondence:* Edward Chow MBBS, PhD, FRCPC, Department of Radiation Oncology, Odette Cancer Centre, Sunnybrook Health Sciences Centre, 2075 Bayview Avenue, Toronto, ON, Canada M4N 3M5. Tel: 416-480-4998; Fax: 416-480-6002; E-mail: Edward.Chow@sunnybrook.ca

identify groups of symptoms which share an underlying mechanism (10). Furthermore, cluster analysis can identify clinical subgroups that present common symptom patterns (10).

Despite the variance among previous studies in terms of definition, methodological approaches to derivation and statistical analyses, symptom clusters are a major issue in metastatic cancer. The investigation of symptom clusters has the potential to greatly contribute to the symptom management and palliative care of this population. The present study delved into the origin of symptom cluster research in metastatic cancer populations. An exhaustive review of literature on symptom clusters in advanced cancer was conducted to understand the current state of knowledge on this concept. Additionally, symptoms commonly observed in advanced cancer are summarized and the physiological or psychological mechanisms underlying a cluster of symptoms are explored. Moreover, limitations in concept definition, methodology and application of research findings are critically analyzed. Recommendations for future research on symptom clusters in advanced cancer population are proposed.

Our Study

A literature search was conducted in the following databases to identify studies investigating symptom clusters in advanced cancer patients: Medline (1950 to October 2008), PubMed, Embase (1980 to 2008), Embase reviews (including Cochrane Central Register of Controlled Trials (CCTR), National Health Service Economic Evaluation, Cochrane Database of Systematic Reviews (COCH), Cochrane Methodology Register Database (CMR), Database of Abstracts of Reviews of Effects (DARE), Health Technology Assessment Database (DTA) and ACP Journal Club. The search was restricted to publications in English and studies conducted on humans. The keywords used for search included "symptom cluster", "symptom constellation", "co-occurrence of symptoms". The results were combined with "metastases" and "advanced cancer". Studies on conceptual issues in symptom clusters and statistical modelling were analyzed. Additionally, studies examining physiological mechanisms underlying symptoms common to advanced cancer were reviewed to investigate the reasons for occurrence of symptom clusters.

Findings

The literature review identified 11 relevant studies published between 1997 and 2008. Eight studies focussed on metastatic cancer while three studies investigated symptom clusters in oncology patients representing various disease stages. A summary of cancer site investigated, sample size, symptoms clusters derived, statistical analysis method employed and assessment tool used by each study is presented in tables 1 and 2.

Table 1. Review of symptom clusters in advanced cancer patients

Reference	Cancer site	Sample Size	Symptom cluster	Statistical Analysis	Assessment Tools
Chow et al (11)	Bone metastases	518	Cluster 1: fatigue, pain, drowsiness, poor sense of well-being Cluster 2: anxiety, depression Cluster 3: shortness of breath, nausea, poor appetite	Principal component analysis with varimax rotation	Edmonton Symptom Assessment System
Hadi et al (12)	Bone metastases	348	Cluster 1: walking ability, general activity, normal work, enjoyment of life, worst pain Cluster 2 : relations with others, mood, sleep	Principal component analysis with varimax rotation	Brief Pain Inventory
Chow et al (13)	Brain metastases	170	Cluster 1: fatigue, pain, drowsiness, shortness of breath Cluster 2: anxiety, depression Cluster 3: shortness of breath, nausea, poor appetite	Principal component analysis with varimax rotation	Edmonton Symptom Assessment System
Sarna and Brecht (15)	Advanced lung cancer (women)	60	Cluster 1: Emotional/Physical Suffering- pain frequency, pain severity, bowel, appearance, outlook Cluster 2: Gastrointestinal- nausea frequency, nausea severity, appetite Cluster 3: Respiratory Distress- cough, breathing, insomnia, Cluster 4: Malaise- fatigue, concentration	Principal component analysis with varimax rotation	13-item Symptom Distress Scale
Chan et al (14)	Advanced lung cancer (undergoing radiation treatment)	27	Cluster 1: breathlessness, anxiety, fatigue	Multivariate analysis of variance	100 mm horizontal visual analog scale
Reference	Cancer site	Sample Size	Symptom cluster	Statistical Analysis	Assessment Tools
Fan et al (9)	Metastases to miscellaneous sites (common primary: lung, breast, prostrate)	1296	Cluster 1: Nausea, appetite loss, poor sense of well-being, pain Cluster 2: fatigue, drowsiness, shortness of breath Cluster 3: anxiety, depression	Principal component analysis with varimax rotation	Edmonton Symptom Assessment System
Teunissen et al (17)	Metastases to miscellaneous sites (common primary: GI, breast, gynaecological, head and neck)	181	Cluster 1: nausea, dysphagia, dyspnea, confusion, depressed mood	Multivariate analysis	49-symptom checklist (derived by the Dutch Centres for Development of Palliative Care)
Walsh and Rybicki (18)	Metastases to miscellaneous sites (common primary: lung, breast, colorectal, prostrate)	922	Cluster 1: Fatigue: anorexia-cachexia (fatigue, weakness, lack of energy, anorexia, early satiety, weight loss, taste change, dry mouth) Cluster 2: neuropsychological (sleep, depression, anxiety) Cluster 3: upper gastrointestinal (dizziness, dyspepsia, belching, bloating) Cluster 4: nausea-vomiting Cluster 5: aerodigestive (dyspnea, cough, hoarseness, dysphagia) Cluster 6: debility (edema, confusion) Cluster 7: pain (pain, constipation)	Cluster analysis (agglomerative hierarchical with average linkage)	38-item Eastern Cooperative Oncology Group performance status and severity checklist

Table 2. Review of symptom clusters in cancer patients combined across different stages

Reference	Cancer site	Sample Size	Symptom cluster	Statistical Analysis	Assessment Tools
Fox and Lyon (19)	Ovarian cancer survivors (mostly stage III advanced)	76	Cluster 1: depression, fatigue	Hierarchical multiple regression analysis	Short Form- 36 Health Status Survey subscales, Fox Simple Quality of Life Scale
Bender et al (20)	Breast cancer	154 (40 Early Sage, 88 Sage I/II/III, 26 Stage IV)	Cluster 1 : Fatigue- fatigue, weakness, lacking energy Cluster 2 : Cognitive impairment- memory problems, concentration loss Cluster 3 : mood problems- anxiety, depression	Hierarchical cluster analysis	Profile of Mood States, Symptom Checklist, Daily symptom diary, Kupperman Index, Menopausal Quality of Life Scale, Functional Assessment of Cancer Therapy: Anemia/ Fatigue Scale
Glaus et al (21)	Breast cancer (receiving hormone therapy)	373 (301 Early Stage, 72 Late Stage)	Cluster 1 : menopausal- hot flashes/sweats, weight tiredness/ fatigue, weight gain, vaginal dryness, decreased sexual interest	Cluster Analysis (agglomerative hierarchical method)	Checklist for Patients with Endocrine Therapy, International Breast Cancer Study Group Linear Snalogue Scale for patients with endocrine treatment

Dodd et al (5) pioneered symptom cluster research in 2001. The study attempted to validate a symptom cluster including pain, fatigue and sleep insufficiency in cancer patients receiving chemotherapy. Information on symptom distress was collected by the 33-item Quality of Life- Cancer (QoL-CA) questionnaire. The deterministic model was analyzed by two-stage hierarchical multiple regression. Inter-correlations among fatigue, pain and sleep insufficiency were observed to be small and the hierarchical regression model explained only 48.4% of the total variance in functional status (5). Thus, the study was unable to confirm the symptom cluster of pain, fatigue and sleep insufficiency in the cancer population. However, the initial work stimulated further research in symptom clusters to improve quality of life in cancer patients.

Symptom clusters in bone metastases

Two studies have investigated symptom clusters in bone metastases patients. Chow et al (11) examined if bone pain clustered with other advanced cancer symptoms in 518 patients. Principal component analysis (PCA) with varimax rotation on the symptoms assessed by the Edmonton Symptom Assessment System (ESAS) questionnaire yielded a three cluster solution that accounted for 66% of the total variance. Cluster 1 included fatigue, pain, drowsiness, poor sense of well-being while anxiety and depression comprised cluster 2. Lastly, cluster 3 consisted of shortness of breath, nausea, and poor appetite. Cronbach's alpha coefficient ranged from 0.61 to 0.81, demonstrating high internal reliability. The clusters were found to disintegrate during the follow-ups conducted 1, 2, 4, 8 and 12 weeks post radiation treatment in both responders and non-responders to radiotherapy (RT) (11). Nevertheless some symptoms often appeared in the same cluster, for instance fatigue and drowsiness, and anxiety and depression remained together at each assessment.

Following a similar design, Hadi et al (12) attempted to validate symptom clusters in bone metastases. The Brief Pain Inventory (BPI) was used to assess symptom distress in 348 patients with bone metastases. In contrast to Chow et al (11), PCA with varimax rotation yielded a two factor solution that accounted for 67% of the total variance. Cluster 1 included walking ability, general activity, normal work, enjoyment of life and worst pain while cluster 2 included relations with others, mood and sleep. The two symptom clusters disintegrated at 4, 8, and 12 weeks post RT in the responder group and followed an inconsistent pattern in the non-responders. The disintegration of symptom clusters in responders following RT alluded to the effectiveness of palliative RT in alleviating symptomatic bone pain and reducing functional interference over time (12).

Symptom clusters in brain metastases

Only one study investigating symptom clusters in brain metastases was identified in the literature search. Chow et al (13) utilized a design similar to their previous study on bone metastases (11) to explore symptom clusters in 170 brain metastases patients referred to an outpatient palliative RT clinic. The most common primary cancer sites were lung, breast and gastrointestinal. Principal component analysis with varimax rotation on the ESAS questionnaire revealed three clusters; cluster 1 contained fatigue, drowsiness, shortness of breath, and pain; cluster 2 consisted of anxiety and depression; and cluster 3 included poor appetite, nausea and poor sense of well-being. Similar to preceding longitudinal studies (11, 12), the symptom clusters were observed to change in follow-up weeks, alluding to their dynamic nature.

Symptom clusters in advanced lung cancer

Two studies focussed on symptom clusters in advanced lung cancer patients. Chan et al (14) investigated the existence of a symptom cluster consisting of breathlessness, fatigue, and anxiety in patients undergoing palliative RT. Data was collected from 27 patients at three time points: 1 day prior to RT (Baseline, T0), week 3 (T1) and week 6 (T2) after commencement of RT using 100 mm horizontal visual analog scales (VAS). The three symptoms shared moderate to strong relationships (Spearman coefficient= 0.49-0.66) and the cluster had a high internal consistency (Cronbach a = 0.69 to 0.82) at the three time points.

Another study by Sarna and Brecht (15) applied factor analysis with varimax orthogonal rotation to the 13-item Symptom Distress Scale. The study sampled 60 women with advanced lung cancer and generated four symptom clusters explaining 63.3% of the total variance. The four clusters identified were emotional or physical suffering, gastrointestinal distress, respiratory distress and malaise. Nevertheless, reliability and validity of these findings is questionable due to the small sample size and lack of male representation in the studied population (16).

Symptom clusters in patients with metastases to miscellaneous sites

Three studies investigated symptom clusters in patients with any site of metastases. Fan et al (9) analyzed 1296 metastatic patients, primarily with metastases to the bone (64%) from primary lung, breast, and prostate cancer. Principal component analysis with varimax rotation was employed on the 9-symptom ESAS scale. Based on Kim et al's (7) definition, three clusters were identified, which accounted for 62% of the total variance. Cluster 1 was composed of nausea, lack of appetite, poor sense of well-being and pain. Cluster 2 included fatigue, drowsiness and shortness of breath, while cluster 3 was comprised of anxiety and depression.

Teunissen et al (17) conducted a prospective analysis on 181 advanced metastases patients. Gastrointestinal, breast, gynaecological or head and neck were the most common primary cancer sites in this cohort, and bone, lymph node, liver, lung and viscera were the most common sites of metastasis. A 49-symptom checklist derived by the Dutch Centres for Development of Palliative Care was utilized. Multivariate analysis of 20 symptoms, which occurred in more than 10% of the patient sample, yielded a symptom cluster composed of nausea, dysphagia, dyspnea, confusion and depressed mood. The obtained symptom cluster was later validated to accurately predict survival in hospitalized cancer patients.

In contrast, Walsh and Rybicki (18) utilized the 38-item Eastern Cooperative Oncology Group (ECOG) performance status and symptom severity checklist to measure symptom distress in 922 patients with metastatic cancer. The ECOG checklist graded each symptom on a four point scale as present/absent, mild, moderate or severe. The most common primary cancer sites were lung, breast, colorectal and prostate. Twenty five symptoms with greater than 15% prevalence were statistically analyzed. Cluster analysis using agglomerative hierarchical method with average linkage yielded seven symptom clusters (fatigue, anorexia-cachexia, neuropsychological, upper gastrointestinal, nausea-vomiting, aerodigestive, debility, and pain) when a cut-off of correlation > 0.68 was employed. The symptoms within each cluster are listed in Table 1.

Symptom clusters in cancer patients combined across different stages

Fox and Lyon (19) explored symptom clusters in survivors of ovarian cancer. The multipurpose Short Form- 36 (SF-36) Health Status Survey subscales for general health status and the Fox Simple Quality of Life Scale (FSQOLS) for quality of life assessment were employed. Following Kim et al's (2005) definition, hierarchical multiple regression analysis identified a symptom cluster of depression and fatigue, which explained 41% of total variance.

Bender et al (20) analyzed symptom data from three independent studies to identify symptom clusters common across three phases of breast cancer. The study population consisted of 40 women in early stage (received primary surgery but not yet initiated adjuvant therapy); 88 in stage I, II, or III (completed surgery and adjuvant chemotherapy, may have been receiving hormonal therapy); and 26 in stage IV (metastatic cancer). Information on symptom distress was extracted from a variety of self-report questionnaires such as Profile of Mood States (POMS), symptom checklist, daily symptom diary, Kupperman Index, Menopausal Quality of Life Scale, and Functional Assessment of Cancer Therapy (FACT): Anaemia/Fatigue Scale. Hierarchical cluster analysis identified symptom clusters related to fatigue, cognitive impairment and mood problems common in each of the three different phases of breast cancer.

Glaus et al (21) explored a menopausal symptom cluster and its relationship with fatigue in 373 breast cancer patients undergoing hormonal treatment (301 with early stage cancer and 72 with late stage cancer). The Checklist for Patients with Endocrine Therapy (C-PET) and the International Breast Cancer Study Group (IBCSG) Linear Analogue Scale for patients with endocrine treatment were used for symptom assessment. Agglomerative hierarchical cluster analysis confirmed a menopausal symptom cluster, composed of hot flashes, weight tiredness, weight gain, vaginal dryness, and decreased sexual interest.

Discussion

The field of symptom clusters is complicated due to the presence of several confounding factors. The symptom cluster studies conducted in advanced cancer populations differed in the type of symptom assessment questionnaires employed and methods of statistical analyses.

Mularski et al (22) noted that the use of different assessment tools of uncertain quality had made it difficult to compare results across studies on symptom clusters. Additionally, the necessity of uniformity in assessment tools utilized by quality of life studies has been emphasized by the National Institutes of Health, State-of-the-Science Conference Statement on "Improving End-of-Life Care" (23). The differences in symptom clusters identified by two studies on bone metastases (11,12) (see table 1) can be attributed to the different assessment questionnaires employed. A lack of consensus on a symptom assessment tool and statistical methodology is a limitation in the extrapolation of findings and generalization of symptom clusters from various studies (9, 14, 15, 17, 18, 20, 21) (see table 1 and 2).

Most common assessment tools utilized in symptom cluster studies include the ESAS, M.D. Anderson Symptom Inventory, Symptom Distress Scale and BPI. These self-report, multi-symptom assessment questionnaires are widely used to measure the presence, severity and frequency of symptoms such as pain, fatigue, nausea, depression, lack of appetite, dyspnea in general cancer patients (24). Nevertheless, symptom clusters in advanced cancer may be specific to the type of cancer, treatment, or a combination of both factors (24). A comparison of symptom clusters identified by Chow et al (11) in bone metastases patients and brain metastases patients (13) exemplifies the disadvantage of using a general questionnaire. Both studies utilized the ESAS to assess symptom distress. Consequently, the symptom clusters derived included symptoms common to both cancer types and do not allow an effective diagnosis or clinical management of the particular cancer populations examined. Thus, assessment tools specifically designed and validated for a particular cancer population are preferred over a general questionnaire (22) to ensure the extraction of symptom clusters that are relevant to the specific symptomatology of that cancer.

Additionally, several symptom cluster studies were conducted in patients with different cancer types (9,17,18) and disease stages (19-21). It is necessary to recognize that patients with different stages and types of cancer have different symptom experiences. In their analysis of ovarian cancer survivors with different stages of the disease, Fox and Lyon (19) identified a cluster that correlated depression with fatigue. The study did not explore more specific quality of life items affecting ovarian cancer-specific disease and treatment-related symptoms. Moreover, symptom distress can be confounded by the use of symptom management strategies, such as opioids used to relieve pain, RT and chemotherapy (1). For instance, Sarna and Brecht (15) observed that symptom distress was significantly related to treatment (chemotherapy was associated with fewer serious problems with insomnia). Hence, symptom management efforts must be considered when assessing symptom distress.

There is much variability in how symptoms within a cluster may be correlated. The "partial mediation model" (25) alludes to the complexity in understanding dynamics of symptom concurrence in advanced cancer. The model explains how two symptoms can influence each other indirectly through effect on a common symptom, for instance, pain could affect sleep and indirectly influence subjective reports of fatigue (25). Thus, the validity of symptom clusters must be confirmed by investigating the underlying pathophysiology behind observed symptom groups, or by reviewing previous literature and conducting further research. Owing to the complications in statistical analysis of symptom clusters, Kim et al (10) have proposed the use of a multimodal strategy for further investigations. Their study suggested using a graphical modelling of multiple symptoms to gain insight into the type and direction of relationship between symptoms, followed by structural equation modelling to test the viability of the model.

Several studies have correlated psychological distress (anxiety, depression, psychological distress or sadness) with physical burden (fatigue, weakness or decreased physical activity) in advanced cancer patients (10, 15,19). For instance, Chen and Chang (26) observed an increased occurrence of insomnia, pain, anorexia, fatigue, and wound or pressure sores in depressed patients. Similarly, Lloyd-Williams et al (27) have affirmed a significant correlation between a patient's subjective feeling of physical symptoms, such as pain and fatigue, and psychological distress.

Subsequent research by Teunissen et al (28) investigated the effect of anxiety and depression on presence and severity of physical symptoms in hospitalized advanced cancer patients. Anxiety and depression were measured by the Hospital Anxiety and Depression Scale (HADS) and the ESAS. Conversely, this study did not find a relationship between anxiety or depressed mood and symptom presence or symptom intensity. In a review of research by Chen and Chang (26), Teunissen et al (28) noted that the relationship between depression and physical symptom distress could be confounded owing to a high Karnofsky score (KPS) (Table 3) (29) in the cancer population analyzed (mean KPS of study sample was 81%) and the chemotherapy treatment being administered. When Teunissen et al (28) applied the DSM-criteria (Diagnostic and Statistical Manual of Mental Disorders) to analyze depression in patients observed by Lloyd-Williams et al (27), no significant differences in symptom rating could be found between depressed and non-depressed patients. Therefore, contrary to the assumption made in palliative medicine, presence and intensity of physical symptom distress may not be a reliable predictor of anxiety or depression in the advanced cancer population or vice-versa (28).

Table 3. The Karnofsky Performance Status Scale (KPS) (29)

Score	Description
100	Normal, no complaints, no evidence of disease.
90	Able to carry on normal activity; minor signs or symptoms of disease.
80	Normal activity with effort; some signs or symptoms of disease.
70	Cares for self, unable to carry on normal activity or do active work.
60	Requires occasional assistance, but is able to care for most of his/her needs.
50	Requires considerable assistance and frequent medical care.
40	Disabled, requires special care and assistance.
30	Severely disabled, hospitalization indicated. Death not imminent.
20	Very sick, hospitalization indicated. Death not imminent.
10	Moribund, fatal processes progressing rapidly.
0	Dead

The KPS is used to measure the functional status, daily mobility and degree of dependence on medical care of cancer patients. The scale has intervals of 10% and measures performance on a range of 0% (dead) to 100% (normal, no complaints, no evidence of disease). Higher scores on the KPS indicate better physical mobility and functioning while lower scores signify greater symptom burden (40).

A significant volume of research has been conducted to advance knowledge on the occurrence of symptom clusters in advanced cancer. However, research on mechanisms underlying the manifestation of symptom clusters specific to advanced cancer has not been discussed extensively in the palliative literature. Several studies investigating symptom clusters in oncology populations have referred to the “sickness behaviour” described in animal models to explain symptom clusters observed. For instance, the sickness symptom cluster observed by Chen and Tseng (16) in the general cancer population was composed of fatigue, pain, sleep disturbance, lack of appetite and drowsiness. This cluster was found to be remarkably similar to the “sickness behaviour” described for animals (16). The sickness behaviour in animals is characterized by pyrexia, fatigue, somnolence, psychomotor retardation, anhedonia and impaired cognitive functioning (16,30). This behaviour is thought to be mediated by proinflammatory cytokines (such as interleukin-1, interleukin-6, interferon-a and tumour necrosis factor-a) and the study questioned the existence of a similar underlying mechanism in humans (31).

Analyses of causal factors underlying commonly observed symptoms in advanced cancer can provide the theoretical framework for correlations between symptoms in a cluster. Few symptoms commonly observed in advanced cancer include anorexia, cachexia, dyspnea, delirium, nausea, vomiting and fatigue. Anorexia and cachexia are major causes of morbidity and mortality in advanced cancer (32). While both anorexia and cachexia can result in weight loss and reduced tolerance to RT, chemotherapy and surgery, mechanisms underlying their expression are different (32,33). Anorexia occurs when appetite signals, normally derived from neuropeptide Y within the hypothalamus, are diminished while satiety signals generated by melacortins are amplified (32). In contrast, cachexia is a systemic inflammatory response caused by cytokines (tumour or host generated) such as leukemia-inhibiting factor and tumour necrosis factor, or specific cachexins that detrimentally alter carbohydrate, lipid and protein metabolism (32). Management of cachexia also depends upon correction of several secondary causes, such as emotional distress, pain, dyspnea, and several reversible gastrointestinal disorders (33).

Dyspnea is a subjective sense of difficulty in breathing which is associated with a multidimensional physical, social and emotional component (32,34). While the occurrence of dyspnea has been related to weakness of respiratory muscles (34,35), no tests exist yet to indicate its severity. Hence, reports on symptom distress due to dyspnea vary with a patient's subjective experience. Under metastatic conditions, dyspnea can result from complications of therapy or comorbidities (such as cachexia and anemia) (32). Additionally, Dudgeon et al (35) observed a significant correlation between intensity of dyspnea and the intensity of anxiety. The cluster composed of breathlessness, anxiety and fatigue, identified by Chan et al (14), exemplifies the need to investigate common mechanisms underlying the presentation of these symptoms in advanced lung cancer populations.

Advanced cancer patients that present with delirium can be challenging to manage under palliative settings (36). Delirium can be manifested as disturbance in consciousness, reduced concentration, impaired memory or language disturbance (32). It can be precipitated due to several factors such as medication, infection, central nervous system malignancies, pain, and surgery (32,36). Several patient related factors such as age, pre-existing cognitive dysfunction, nutritional deficits, hearing or visual dysfunction and unfamiliar surroundings may predispose the development of delirium (32). A few symptom cluster studies have correlated cognitive impairment with depression (17) and fatigue (15). Additionally, Bender et al (20) identified a cognitive impairment cluster that was common to breast cancer patients across different stages of the disease. Notably, above studies did not utilize validated tools, such as the Delirium Rating Scale, the Confusion Assessment Method, or the Mini-Mental Status Examination (32), to screen for delirium. Rather the assessments were made from single-item screening question or general symptom distress checklists (28). Thus the correlations observed must be confirmed by further investigations of the causal mechanisms.

Furthermore, nausea and vomiting are frequently observed in advanced cancer. While nausea is an unpleasant, subjective feeling of wanting to vomit, vomiting is the forceful expulsion of gastric contents (32, 37). Metabolic abnormalities, brain metastases, chemotherapy, RT, constipation and certain medications (opioids, antibiotics, non-steroidal anti-inflammatory drugs, and vitamin / mineral supplements) can dispose a patient to develop nausea and vomiting (32,37). Emotional distress (for instance, anxiety, and fear) and pain can also stimulate the development of nausea (32,37). Nausea and vomiting centres in the medulla have been hypothesized to share common afferent neural pathways (32), which may explain their concurrence in advanced cancer patients (18).

Advanced cancer patients often report fatigue as a distressing symptom. Cancer-related fatigue is defined "as an unusual, persistent, subjective sense of tiredness, related to cancer or cancer treatment that interferes with usual functioning" (38, pg 152). Though the exact pathways for fatigue are unknown, it is speculated that multiple factors such as cancer treatment (chemotherapy/radiotherapy), co-morbid illnesses, cachexia, anaemia, sleep disorders, psychological factors (anxiety/depression), pain, nausea, dyspnea, medications may predispose the development of fatigue (32). Therefore, the clustering of fatigue with symptoms such as anorexia (18), pain (11,13), anxiety (14) and depression (19) can be explained. Further investigations of pathophysiology of symptoms common in advanced cancer would validate the symptom clusters observed in this population.

Symptom clusters research in advanced cancer is complicated due to several variables that can confound the symptom experience. Subjective reports of symptom distress can be confounded by long-term experience with the disease, presence of multiple symptoms, duration of disease experience or any other perceptual disorders (3). Additionally, factors such as education level, language skills, and ethnicity can affect a patient's reports of symptom distress (3,9). In an investigation of symptom clusters in women with advanced lung cancer, Sarna and Brecht (15) confirmed that personal and subjective factors can affect the symptom experience. For instance, higher education levels were significantly associated with poorer outlook and associated distress, and lower income was correlated with serious disruptions in sleeping (15). Therefore, adoption of objective measures of symptom presence and severity, administered by trained nurses or physicians, could eliminate problems associated with a subjective, self-report questionnaire.

It is important to monitor how symptom clusters observed in advance cancer population change over time to establish a definite relationship between symptoms within a cluster. Longitudinal studies can provide information on the effectiveness of management strategies commonly employed to treat or contain the cancer. Only a few studies have delved into the longitudinal patterns in symptom clusters observed in advanced cancer patients (11-14). These studies confirmed the effectiveness of palliative RT in alleviating symptomatic bone pain and reducing symptom burden and functional interference over time. Additionally, Chan et al (14) confirmed the concurrence of breathlessness, fatigue, and anxiety in advanced lung cancer patients by observing a strong correlation between the three symptoms 3 weeks and 6 weeks after palliative radiotherapy. Further investigations on the stability of symptom clusters over time, would validate the concept of symptom clusters and improve quality of life in advanced cancer populations by allowing a co-management of various symptoms that form a cluster.

Importantly, prioritization of certain symptoms by patients can increase the possibility of those symptoms being relieved through clinical intervention (39). This hypothesis was confirmed for some physical symptoms, such as pain and constipation (39). However symptom prioritization had little influence over the alleviation of subjective symptoms such as nausea, fatigue, physical function, role function and activity (39). In view of the fact that patients who prioritize certain symptoms report higher initial scores for those symptoms and describe a significantly better treatment outcome than those who do not do so, palliative care could be focussed on relieving the most prioritized symptoms to optimize patient care and increase cost effectiveness in palliative oncology.

Acknowledgments

This study was supported by the Michael and Karyn Goldstein Cancer Research Fund. We would like to thank Rene E. Harrison, PhD, Department of Biological Sciences, University of Toronto for her comments.

References

[1] Barsevick AM, Whitmer K, Nail LM, Beck SL, Dudley WN. Symptom cluster research: Conceptual, design, measurement, and analysis issues. J Pain Symptom Manage 2006;31(1):85-95.

[2] Dodd M, Janson S, Facione N, Faucett J, Froelicher ES, Humphreys J, et al. Advancing the science of symptom management. J Adv Nurs 2001;33(5):668-76.

[3] Lenz ER, Pugh LC, Milligan RA, Gift A, Suppe F. The middle-range theory of unpleasant symptoms: An update.(middle-range nursing theory). Adv Nurs Sci 1997;19(3):14-27.

[4] Miaskowski C, Dodd M, Lee K. Symptom clusters: The new frontier in symptom management research. J Natl Cancer Inst Monogr 2004(32):17-21.

[5] Dodd MJ, Miaskowski C, Paul SM. Symptom clusters and their effect on the functional status of patients with cancer. Oncol Nurs Forum 2001;28(3):465-70.

[6] National Institutes of Health Consensus State-of-the-Science Statements. Symptom Management in cancer: pain, depression, and fatigue 2002;19(4):1-29. Accessed 2008 Nov 12. URL: http://consensus.nih.gov

[7] Kim HJ, McGuire DB, Tulman L, Barsevick AM. Symptom clusters - concept analysis and clinical implications for cancer nursing. Cancer Nurs 2005;28(4):270-82.

[8] Armstrong TS. Symptoms experience: A concept analysis. Oncol Nurs Forum 2003;30(4):601-6.

[9] Fan G, Hadi S, Chow E. Symptom clusters in patients with advanced-stage cancer referred for palliative radiation therapy in an outpatient setting. Support Cancer Ther 2007;4(3):157-62.

[10] Kim HJ, Abraham IL. Statistical approaches to modeling symptom clusters in cancer patients. Cancer Nurs 2008;31(5):E1-E10.

[11] Chow E, Fan G, Hadi S, Filipczak L. Symptom clusters in cancer patients with bone metastases. Support Care Cancer 2007;15(9):1035-43.

[12] Hadi S, Fan G, Hird AE, Kirou-Mauro A, Filipczak LA, Chow E. Symptom clusters in patients with cancer with metastatic bone pain. J Palliat Med 2008;11(4):591-600.

[13] Chow E, Fan G, Hadi S, Wong J, Kirou-Mauro A, Filipczak L. Symptom clusters in cancer patients with brain metastases. Clin Oncol (R Coll Radiol) 2008;20(1):76-82.
[14] Chan CW, Richardson A, Richardson J. A study to assess the existence of the symptom cluster of breathlessness, fatigue and anxiety in patients with advanced lung cancer. Eur J Oncol Nurs 2005;9(4):325-33.
[15] Sarna L, Brecht M. Dimensions of symptom distress in women with advanced lung cancer: A factor analysis, Heart and Lung: The Journal of Acute and Critical Care, 1997;26(1):23-30.
[16] Chen ML, Tseng HC. Symptom clusters in cancer patients. Support Care Cancer 2006;14(8):825-30.
[17] Teunissen SC, de Graeff A, de Haes HC, Voest EE. Prognostic significance of symptoms of hospitalised advanced cancer patients. Eur J Cancer 2006;42(15):2510-6.
[18] Walsh D, Rybicki L. Symptom clustering in advanced cancer. Support Care Cancer 2006;14(8):831-6.
[19] Fox SW, Lyon D. Symptom clusters and quality of life in survivors of ovarian cancer. Cancer Nurs 2007;30(5):354-61.
[20] Bender CM, Ergun FS, Rosenzweig MQ, Cohen SM, Sereika SM. Symptom clusters in breast cancer across 3 phases of the disease. Cancer Nurs 2005;28(3):219-25.
[21] Glaus A, Boehme C, Thurlimann B, Ruhstaller T, Hsu Schmitz SF, Morant R, et al. Fatigue and menopausal symptoms in women with breast cancer undergoing hormonal cancer treatment. Ann Oncol 2006;17(5):801-6.
[22] Mularski RA, Dy SM, Shugarman LR, Wilkinson AM, Lynn J, Shekelle PG et al. A systematic review of measures of end-of-life care and its outcomes. Health Serv Res 2007;42(5):1848-70.
[23] National Institutes of Health State-of-the-Science Conference Statement. "Improving End-of-Life Care and Outcomes" 2004 Dec 6-8;21(3):1-28. Accessed 2008 Oct 21. URL: http://consensus.nih.gov/2004/2004EndOfLifeCareSOS024PDF.pdf
[24] Lacasse C, Beck SL. Clinical assessment of symptom clusters. Seminars in Oncology Nursing 2007;23(2):106-12.
[25] Beck SL, Dudley WN, Barsevick A. Pain, sleep disturbance, and fatigue in patients with cancer: Using a mediation model to test a symptom cluster. Oncol Nurs Forum 2005;32(3):542.
[26] Chen ML, Chang HK. Physical symptom profiles of depressed and nondepressed patients with cancer. Palliat Med 2004;18(8):712-8.
[27] Lloyd-Williams M, Dennis M, Taylor F. A prospective study to determine the association between physical symptoms and depression in patients with advanced cancer. Palliat Med 2004;18(6):558-63.
[28] Teunissen SC, de Graeff A, Voest EE, de Haes JC. Are anxiety and depressed mood related to physical symptom burden? A study in hospitalized advanced cancer patients. Palliat Med 2007;21(4):341-6.
[29] Karnofsky DA, Abelmann WH, Craver LF, Burchenal JH. The use of the nitrogen mustards in the palliative treatment of carcinoma. With particular reference to bronchogenic carcinoma. Cancer 1948; 1(4):634-656.

[30] Kent S, Bluthe RM, Kelly KW, Dantzer R. Sickness behaviour as a new target for drug development. Trends Pharmacol Sci 1992;13:24-9.

[31] Cleeland CS, Bennett GJ, Dantzer R, Dougherty PM, Dunn AJ, Meyers CA, et al. Are the symptoms of cancer and cancer treatment due to a shared biologic mechanism? A cytokine-immunologic model of cancer symptoms. Cancer 2003;97(11):2919-25.

[32] Lagman RL, Davis MP, LeGrand SB, Walsh D. Common symptoms in advanced cancer. Surg Clin North Am 2005;85(2):237-55.

[33] MacDonald N. Cancer cachexia and targeting chronic inflammation: A unified approach to cancer treatment and palliative/supportive care. J Support Oncol 2007;5(4):157-62.

[34] Dudgeon DJ, Lertzman M. Dyspnea in the advanced cancer patient. J Pain Symptom Manage 1998;16(4):212-9.

[35] Dudgeon DJ, Lertzman M, Askew GR. Physiological changes and clinical correlations of dyspnea in cancer outpatients. J Pain Symptom Manage 2001;21(5):373-9.

[36] Lawlor PG, Gagnon B, Mancini IL, Pereira JL, Hanson J, Suarez-Almazor ME, et al. Occurrence, causes, and outcome of delirium in patients with advanced cancer: A prospective study. Arch Intern Med 2000;160(6):786-94.

[37] Twycross R, Back I. Nausea and vomiting in advanced cancer. Eur J Palliat Care 1998;5(2):39-45.

[38] Mock V, Atkinson A, Barsevick A, Cella D, Cimprich B, Cleeland C, et al. National Comprehensive Cancer N. NCCN practice guidelines for cancer-related fatigue. Oncology (Williston) 2000;14(11A):151-61.

[39] Stromgren AS, Goldschmidt D, Groenvold M, Petersen MA, Jensen PT, Pedersen L, et al. Self-assessment in cancer patients referred to palliative care: A study of feasibility and symptom epidemiology. Cancer 2002;94(2):512-7.

[40] Chen ML, Lin CC. Cancer symptom clusters: a validation study. J Pain Symptom Manage 2007;34(6):590-9.

In: Advanced Cancer. Pain and Quality of Life
Editors: E. Chow, J. Merrick, pp. 145-151
ISBN: 978-1-61668-207-1
© 2010 Nova Science Publishers, Inc.

Chapter XIII

Meaningful Change in Pain Scores in the Treatment of Bone Metastases

Edward Chow, MBBS*[*1], Amanda Hird, BSc(C)[2], Rebecca Wong, MD[2], Liying Zhang, PhD[1], Jackson Wu, MD[3], Lisa Barbera, MD[1], May Tsao, MD[1], Elizabeth Barnes, MD[1] and Cyril Danjoux, MD[1]

[1]Odette Cancer Centre, Sunnybrook Health Sciences Centre, University of Toronto, Toronto, Ontario
[2]Princess Margaret Hospital, University Health Network, University of Toronto, Toronto, Ontario and
[3]Tom Baker Cancer Centre, University of Calgary, Calgary, Alberta, Canada

The purpose was to validate the meaningful change in pain scores in the treatment of bone metastases. Methods: Patients with bone metastases treated with external beam radiotherapy were asked to score their 'worst' pain on a scale of 0-10 before treatment (baseline), daily during treatment and for 10 days after completion of external beam radiation. Patients were also asked to indicate if their pain at the time of follow up was "worse", "the same", or "better" when compared to the pre-treatment level. The change in pain score was accompanied with patient perception. Results: One hundred and seventy-eight patients were evaluated in this study. There were 82 male and 96 female patients with the median age of 65.5 years. A total of 1431 pain scorings were obtained. Patients perceived an improvement in pain when their self-reported pain score decreased by at least two points. Conclusion: Our current study validates the previous finding of meaningful change in pain score as reduction of patient self reported pain score by at least two points. This finding of the meaningful change in pain scores supports the investigation-defined partial response in clinical trials and the international consensus endpoints.

* ***Correspondence:*** Edward Chow, MBBS, PhD, FRCPC, Department of Radiation Oncology, Odette Cancer Centre, Sunnybrook Health Sciences Centre, 2075 Bayview Avenue, Toronto, Ontario, Canada M4N 3M5. Tel: 416-480-4998; Fax: 416-480-6002; E-mail: Edward.Chow@sunnybrook.ca

Introduction

The benefits of palliative radiotherapy (RT) for bone metastases are mainly assessed by the change in pain intensity often measured by pain scores. Previous studies have shown that clinicians and family members tend to overestimate the benefits of treatment interventions (1-8). Patient self-assessment should therefore be the preferred measure of the benefit or success of the treatment.

Patients are often not informed of what pain score they provided at baseline when they are asked to score their current pain. However we have noticed that patients may inform their pain score is increasing/worsening in numbers but at the same time state their pain is getting better or vice versa. It is therefore important to determine a meaningful improvement or decline in scores to assess the benefits of the treatment such as palliative RT. In our previous study of 797 pain scorings from 88 patients, patients were able to perceive their current pain to be less than the baseline pain when they reported a decline of their pain score of two or more from the baseline (9). The current study was to validate the above finding in a separate population.

Our Study

Patients with bone metastases treated with external beam RT were eligible. Patients were asked to score their 'worst' pain on a scale of 0 – 10 with the Brief Pain Inventory (zero means absence of pain and 10 is the worst possible pain) before treatment, daily during treatment and for 10 days after the completion of external beam RT. Patients either recorded the information in a diary or requested a telephone follow up by the research assistant.

At each follow up, they were asked to compare their current 'worst' pain with their pretreatment 'worst' pain using the following categories based on their own perception: worse, the same, or better. Changes in pain score with respect to the baseline pain score were compared with patient perception of changes in pain. When the change in pain score is a negative value, it means the patient's current 'worst' pain score was lower than the baseline pretreatment 'worst' pain score.

The analgesic intake was recorded at baseline and at each follow up and converted into daily oral morphine equivalent. Patients with pathological fractures, spinal cord compression, or language barrier were excluded. Ethics approval was obtained for the study.

Descriptive statistics were reported as percentages for proportions, and as medians and ranges for continuous variables. All statistical analyses were performed using version 9.1 of the Statistical Analysis System (SAS).

Findings

From February 2006 to March 2008, one hundred and seventy-eight patients were enrolled from three cancer centres in Canada (Odette Cancer Centre, 90; Princess Margaret Hospital,

80; Tom Baker Cancer Centre, 8). There were 82 male and 96 female patients. Their median age was 65.5 years. The median 'worst' pain score before treatment for all patients was 7 (range 0 – 10). The median analgesic intake in daily oral morphine equivalent was 6 mg (range 0 – 880). Breast, prostate and lung were the most common primary sites. Other patient characteristics are listed in table 1. The radiation dose fractionations employed are listed in table 2 and sites of irradiation in table 3.

Table 1. Patient characteristics (n=178)

Gender	
Male	82 (46%)
Female	96 (54%)
Age	
Median	65.5 years
Range	40-90 years
Primary Cancer Site	
Breast	64 (36%)
Prostate	42 (24%)
Lung	39 (22%)
Bladder + Kidney	12 (7%)
Gastrointestinal	10 (6%)
Others	11 (6%)
Worst Pain	
Mean ± SD	6.3 ± 2.7
Median (range)	7 (0-10)
Daily Total Oral Morphine Equivalent (mg)	
Mean ± SD	54.6 ± 115.3
Median (range)	6 (0-880)

Table 2. Radiation dose fractions (n=178)

Radiation Regimens	Number of Patients
8 Gy in 1 fraction	99 (56%)
20 Gy in 5 daily fractions	55 (31%)
30 Gy in 10 daily fractions	8 (4%)
Other multiple fractions	16 (9%)

Table 3. Sites of irradiation (n=178)

Site of Radiation	Number of Patients
Spine	73 (41%)
Extremities	54 (30%)
Pelvis	38 (21%)
Others	13 (7%)

Table 4. Pain perception in 1,431 scorings

Change in Pain Score	Patient Perception		
	Pain Level	Frequency	%
-10 (n=4)	W	0	0%
	S	0	0%
	B	4	100%
-9 (n=17)	W	0	0%
	S	1	6%
	B	16	94%
-8 (n=31)	W	0	0%
	S	10	32%
	B	21	68%
-7 (n=42)	W	0	0%
	S	5	12%
	B	37	88%
-6 (n=41)	W	1	2%
	S	6	15%
	B	34	83%
-5 (n=52)	W	1	2%
	S	14	27%
	B	37	71%
-4 (n=121)	W	6	5%
	S	44	36%
	B	71	59%
-3 (n=117)	W	9	8%
	S	18	15%
	B	90	77%
-2 (n=217)	W	18	8%
	S	68	31%
	B	131	60%
-1 (n=234)	W	46	20%
	S	92	39%
	B	96	41%
(n=289)	W	72	25%
	S	190	66%
	B	27	9%
+1 (n=117)	W	78	67%
	S	24	20%
	B	15	13%
+2 (n=63)	W	45	71%
	S	10	16%
	B	8	13%
+3 (n=44)	W	33	75%
	S	7	16%
	B	4	9%
+4 (n=19)	W	19	10%
	S	0	0%

Change in Pain Score	Patient Perception		
	B	0	0%
	Pain Level	Frequency	%
+5 (n=9)	W	9	100%
	S	0	0%
	B	0	0%
+6 (n=8)	W	8	100%
	S	0	0%
	B	0	0%
+7 (n=4)	W	4	100%
	S	0	0%
	B	0	0%
+8 (n=1)	W	1	100%
	S	0	0%
	B	0	0%
+9 (n=1)	W	1	100%
	S	0	0%
	B	0	0%

Change in pain score = current pain score – baseline pain score
Patient perception = current pain compared with baseline pain
W, worse; S, same; B, better

A total of 1,431 pain scorings were obtained in the study cohort. Table 4 lists the change in pain score and patient perception of pain. From our data, there was consistency of the change in pain score with the patient perception when the change in pain score was from -10 to -2. The majority of patients reported feeling better when compared with the baseline. However when the change in pain score was only -1, 39% of patients reported the same and 41% of patients reported better when compared with the baseline. When there was no change in pain score, 66% of patients reported same when compared with the baseline. For change in pain score from +1 to +9, the majority of patients gave the response of 'worse' when compared with the baseline.

Contributions of pain scorings varied from one patient to another depending on the dose fractionations they received. We were able to capture 65% of the anticipated pain score data. Thus, we randomly selected the same contributions from all patients and reanalyzed the data, but found no change in outcome (data not shown). We also removed the baseline pain scores near the ceiling (i.e. 9 or 10) to account and correct for the ceiling effect, but again our findings remained unchanged (data not shown). The change in pain score reflects a combined effect of RT and concurrent systemic therapies including analgesics.

Discussion

In our previous study, except when the change in pain score was -7, there was consistency of the change in score with the patient perception for change of pain score from -10 to -2. When the change in pain score was -2, 78% of the pain scorings were accompanied with a response of 'better' (9). Our current study showed consistency of the change in score with the patient perception from change in pain score from -10 to -2. When the change in pain score was -2, 60% of the pain scorings were accompanied with a response of 'better'.

For the previous study, when the change in pain score was -1, the responses for the 'same' and 'better' categories were similar in frequency (9). The current study had the same findings: 39% vs. 41%. In the previous study, for change in pain score from 0 to +5, there was no consistent pattern in patient perception. For the change in pain score of +6 or above, 67% of pain scorings were accompanied with a response of 'worse' (9). In our current study, when there was no change in pain score, 66% of pain scorings were accompanied with a response of 'same'. For change in pain score from +1 to +9, the majority of pain scorings were accompanied with a response of 'worse'.

In our study, we asked patients their pain score and pain perception over a period of 11 days (for patients who received a single treatment) to 22–24 days (for patients who received 10 daily treatments). It is unlikely that during this time frame, patients' internal frame of reference may have changed.

With our two studies, we are confident that patients perceived the current pain to be less than the baseline pain when they reported a decline of their pain score of two or more from the baseline. Recent bone metastases randomized trials (10,11) and international consensus in palliative RT endpoints for future clinical trials in bone metastases (12) defined partial response as a reduction of pain score by two or more points on a pain scale of 0-10. This definition appears to be supported by our data. Our current study however only focused on the pain score. The international consensus takes both pain score and analgesic consumption into consideration when defining partial response.

Our study suggests if the change in pain score was zero, the pain seemed to be stable. However for a positive change even from +1 onwards, patients in our study cohort reported worse pain, which should draw the attention of the health care professionals. This needs to be taken into account when trialists define pain progression.

Acknowledgments

We thank Ms. Stacy Lue for secretarial support. This study was generously supported by Michael and Karyn Goldstein Cancer Research Fund. We thank staff and research assistants at the three cancer centres for the accrual. Conflicts of interest notification: None

References

[1] Brunelli C, Constantini M, Di Giulio P, et al. Quality-of-life evaluation: when do terminal cancer patients and health-care providers agree? J Pain Symptom Manage 1998;15:151–8.

[2] Grossman SA, Sheidler VR, Swedeen K, Mucenski J, Piantadosi S. Correlation of patient and caregiver ratings of cancer pain. J Pain Symptom Manage 1991;6:53–7.

[3] Higginson IJ, McCarthy M. Validity of the support team assessment schedule: do staffs' ratings reflect those made by patients or their families? Palliat Med 1993;7:219–28.

[4] Higginson IJ. Can professionals improve their assessment? [commentary] J Pain Symptom Manage 1998;15:149–50.

[5] Nekolaichuk CL, Bruera E, Spachynski K, MacEachern T, Hanson J, Maguire TO. A comparison of patient and proxy symptom assessments in advanced cancer patients. Palliat Med 1999;13:311–23.

[6] Slevin ML, Plant H, Lynch D, Drinkwater J, Gregory WM. Who should measure quality of life, the doctor or the patient? Br J Cancer 1988;57:109–12.

[7] Sneeuw KCA, Aaronson NK, Sprangers MAG, Delmar SB, Wever LDV, Schornagel JH. Value of caregiver ratings in evaluating the quality of life of patients with cancer. J Clin Oncol 1997;15:1206–17.

[8] Sprangers MAG, Aaronson NK. The role of health care providers and significant others in evaluating the quality of life of patients with chronic disease: a review. J Clin Epidemiol 1992;45:743–60.

[9] Chow E, Ling A, Davis L, Panzarella T, Danjoux C. Pain flare following external beam radiotherapy and meaningful change in pain scores in the treatment of bone metastases. Radiat Oncol 2005;75:64-9.

[10] Hartsell WF, Scott C, Brunner DW, et al. Phase III randomized trial of 8 Gy in fraction vs. 30 Gy in 10 fractions for palliation of painful bone metastases: preliminary results of RTOG 97-14. Int J Radiat Oncol Biol Phys 2003;57:S124.

[11] Steenland E, Leer JW, van Houwelingen H, et al. The effect of a single fraction compared to multiple fractions on painful bone metastases: a global analysis of the Dutch bone metastasis study. Radiother Oncol 1999;52:101–9.

[12] Chow E, Wu J, Hoskin P, Coia L, Bentzen S, Blitzer P on behalf of the International Bone Metastases Consensus Working Party. International consensus on palliative radiotherapy endpoints for future clinical trials in bone metastases. Radiother Oncol 2002;64:275–80.

In: Advanced Cancer. Pain and Quality of Life
Editors: E. Chow, J. Merrick, pp. 153-164
ISBN: 978-1-61668-207-1
© 2010 Nova Science Publishers, Inc.

Chapter XIV

Multidisciplinary Approach to Metastatic Bone Disease

Janet Nguyen, BSc(C), Emily Sinclair, MRT (T), Albert Yee, MD, Joel Finkelstein, MD, Michael Ford, MD, Anita Chakraborty, MD, Macey Farhadian, RN, Robyn Pugash, MD, Gunita Mitera, MRT (T), Cyril Danjoux, MD, Elizabeth Barnes, MD, May Tsao, MD, Arjun Sahgal, MD and Edward Chow, MBBS*

Bone Metastases Site Group, Sunnybrook Health Sciences Centre,
University of Toronto, Toronto, Canada

The purpose of this chapter was to review the coordinated, multidisciplinary approach to the management and care of cancer patients with metastatic bone disease at the one-stop bone metastases clinic (BMC) at the Odette Cancer Centre. Patients with symptomatic bone metastases are referred to the BMC and assessed by a team consisting of specialists in various disciplines such as interventional radiology, orthopedic surgery, palliative medicine, and radiation oncology. At initial consultation, patient demographics, reasons for referral, and case disposition were recorded. From June 2006 to December 2008, a total of 254 patients with bone metastases were seen at the BMC. The median age was 64 years (range 29-94) and median KPS score was 70 (range 10-100). The majority of patients arrived from home (85%), while 5% of patients came from a hospital. Approximately 16% of patients had 2 or more reasons for referral, yielding a total of 295 reasons. Bone pain was the main reason for referral (69%), followed by a pathological fracture (10%) and impending fracture (8%). Out of 254 patients, only 240 case dispositions were recorded, with 3 patients receiving 2 treatment recommendations. Almost a third of patients (28%) received palliative radiation, 20% needed further investigation and/or imaging, 17% were referred to other support /specialist services such

* *Correspondence:* Edward Chow, MBBS, PhD, FRCPC, Department of Radiation Oncology, Odette Cancer Centre, Sunnybrook Health Sciences Centre, 2075 Bayview Avenue, Toronto, Ontario, Canada M4N 3M5. Tel: 416-480-4998; Fax: 416-480-6002; E-mail: Edward.Chow@sunnybrook.ca

as palliative care or physiotherapy, and 15% of patients were offered surgery. A co-ordinated multidisciplinary clinic is useful in managing symptomatic bone metastases in cancer patients.

Introduction

In 2008, it is estimated that there will be 166,400 new cases of cancer and 73,800 deaths will result from cancer in Canada (1). Skeletal metastases are a frequent complication of cancer, particularly in breast, lung, prostate, thyroid, and renal cancers (2,3). Due to advances in systemic treatments, survival in cancer patients is increasing, and as a result the prevalence of patients with bone metastases is also expected to increase (3,4). Patients with breast and prostate cancer with bone-only metastases can have a relatively long median survival, ranging from 2 to 5 years (2,5). It is important that appropriate management and prevention of skeletal complications are achieved in order to maintain quality of life in these patients (6,7). There is a need to reassess the management strategies in patients with bone metastases due to the following reasons (2,6,8-13):

- Pain from bone metastases is the most common cause of cancer-associated pain;
- Bone metastases typically cause severe symptoms and these develop earlier than symptoms due to liver or lung metastases;
- Complications resulting from bone metastases are common and can seriously impact patients' quality of life. Pain and impaired mobility occur in 65-75% of patients with bone metastases; pathological fractures occur in 10-30% ; hypercalcemia occurs in 10-15%; and spinal cord compression or nerve root compression is seen in 5% of patients;
- There has been a noticeable increase in the prevalence of bone metastases due to longer survival duration of patients and;
- Multidisciplinary care of this group is needed to address specific problems in the management of bone metastases.

Pain is the most common symptom resulting from bone metastases, however bone pain is often under-treated (6,7). Treatment for bone metastases involves a multidisciplinary approach, which includes surgery, radiotherapy, chemotherapy, and other treatments (13). There have been clinical trials and reviews in a variety of disciplines addressing the optimal management of bone metastases, some of which discuss the potential of newer generations of bisphosphonates (5,9,14), the efficacy of radiotherapy, as well as the expanding need for effective surgical treatment (13). When bone pain is mechanical in origin, it cannot be adequately treated with radiotherapy or systemic therapies, and therefore surgical stabilization is recommended (2, 15).

In Janjan and colleagues' review of their multidisciplinary bone metastases clinic, they note that lack of coordination of care among many specialties contributes to inadequately treating cancer-related pain (6). Their report describes an integrated clinic model for the management of bone metastases, with 108 patients (seen by physicians from diagnostic radiology, nuclear medicine, pain and symptom management, physical medicine and rehabilitation, orthopedic surgery, medical oncology, and radiation oncology), being retrospectively evaluated. Presenting symptoms, extent of disease, past therapies, and evaluation of current treatment options were reviewed, and they concluded that coordination of care could overcome many practical difficulties in the management of metastatic disease in symptomatic patients. Surgery and radiotherapy are often used in combination with other treatments, therefore a multidisciplinary approach is especially important in reaching the goals of treatment for patients, some of which are to relieve pain, restore and maintain function, and to prevent skeletal related events (SREs). SREs are classified as the need for radiotherapy or surgery for palliation of pain, hypercalcemia, pathological fracture, or spinal cord compression (SCC) (6,8).

The Division of Orthopedics at Sunnybrook Health Sciences Centre and the Rapid Response Radiotherapy Program at Sunnybrook Odette Cancer Centre initiated a first-of-its-kind clinic, the Bone Metastases Clinic, at Sunnybrook Odette Cancer Centre in January 1999. The clinic aims to provide a coordinated multidisciplinary approach to the management of symptomatic bone metastases patients. This multidisciplinary service will also save the time and effort that a patient would otherwise expend during separate, sequential visits to various specialists for consultation.

A review of the BMC from 1999 to 2005 has previously been reported with a total of 272 patients seen at the BMC during that period 4. From 1999 to 2005, at initial consultation patient demographics, cancer history, disease status, and symptom profiles were collected, as well as patient Edmonton Symptom Assessment Scale (ESAS) scores. The purpose of this paper was to update our experience at the BMC from 2006 to 2008.

Our study

The BMC is managed by a team in various specialties: interventional radiology, nursing, orthopedic surgery, pain and palliative medicine, radiation oncology, and radiation therapy. The clinic is held on every second and fourth Friday of every month.

A prospective database has been set up for patients referred for assessment at BMC since January 1999. Pathological diagnosis of cancer and documentation of bone metastases either by pathological confirmation, clinical examination, or imaging, are required for referral to the BMC. Patients were entered into the database if they were able to speak English, give verbal consent, and respond to questions that assessed their symptoms. Patients were excluded from the database if they were confused, refused, or were unable to complete the symptom assessment.

At initial consultation, patient demographics, cancer history, disease status, and symptom profiles were collected. Patients were asked to complete the Brief Pain Inventory (BPI) from June 2006 to May 2008. Then from May 2008 to December 2008, patients completed the EORTC Bone Metastases Module (EORTC QLQ-BM22). The BPI evaluates current, average, and worst pain on a scale of 0-10, as well as 7 questions evaluating the interference of pain in their daily life. The EORTC QLQ-BM22 consists of 22 questions assessing pain site(s), pain characteristics, functional interference, and psychosocial aspects, and rates on a scale of 1-4. Analgesic consumption, total pain relief, site(s) of bone metastases, and the risk of fractures at the initial visit were assessed and also recorded along with either the BPI or the EORTC QLQ-BM22. The functional status of the patient was scored as follows: normal with pain-free use of the extremity and spine; normal use with pain; significant limited use (i.e. use of prosthesis, walker, cane, crutches, and sling); and nonfunctional extremity/spine (wheelchair-bound, bedridden).

Patients were assessed by an orthopedic surgeon, a radiation oncologist, and a pain specialist at initial consultation. The team then made a joint recommendation based on their assessments, along with nursing and radiation therapy support. An interventional radiologist was consulted if the patient was considered a candidate for percutaneous vertebroplasty or cementoplasty.

Our findings

From June 2006 to December 2008, a total of 254 patients with bone metastases were referred to the BMC. One hundred and thirty-two patients were male (52%) and 122 were female (48%). Their median age was 64 years (range 29-94). The three most common primary sites were breast (22%), lung (17%), and renal cell (17%). The median KPS score at initial consultation was 70 (range 10-100). The majority of patients arrived from home (85%) while only 5% came from a hospital. Patients identified the spine (43%), pelvis and hips (21%), and lower limbs (17%) to be the most painful bony sites (see table 1). There were a total of 295 reasons for referral, where nearly one-fifth of patients (21%) had two or more reasons for referral. The top three reasons for referral were bone pain (69%), pathological fracture (10%), and impending fracture (8%) (see table 2).

Brief pain inventory scores are summarized in table 3. The median worst, average, and current pain score were 7, 4, and 3 respectively. Pain interfering with normal work was the most severe problem expressed by patients, with a median score of 8. Pain interfering with general activity, walking ability, and enjoyment of life came next at a median score of 7. There were only 91 patients who had analgesic intake recorded, measured by total daily oral morphine equivalent (OME) in milligrams. Sixteen of those patients had zero OME; therefore they may have been taking non-opioids or no pain medication(s) at all, however the names of the pain medication(s) were not recorded. The mean OME was 109.12 ± 144.21 mg, with a median of 36 mg (range 0 – 640 mg). Out of 91 patients with analgesic intake recorded, pain relief data was collected from 77 patients – with 0 being no relief and 100 being complete relief. The mean score was 69.31 ± 67.26, and median pain relief experienced by patients was 70 (range 0 – 100).

Scores from the EORTC QLQ-BM22 are summarized in table 4. A number of patients noted that they experience pain in the back, constant pain, pain not relieved by pain medication, and pain when walking quite a bit (median score of 3).

Table 1. Patient characteristics (n=254)

Sex	
Male	132 (52%)
Female	122 (48%)
Age (Years)	
Median (Range)	64 (29-94)
Mean ± SD	63.11 ± 12.72
Source of Referral	
SPEC: Previous patients reviewed in BMC for new reason	179 (70%)
FU: Previous Patients Followed-Up	62 (24%)
NP: New Patients	13 (5%)
Locations where cases arrived from	
Home	216 (85%)
Hospital	12 (5%)
Unknown	14 (6%)
Primary cancer site	
Breast	55 (22%)
Lung	53 (21%)
Renal Cell	43 (17%)
Prostate	37 (15%)
Gastrointestinal	23 (9%)
Unknown	10 (4%)
Bladder	7 (3%)
Gynecological	6 (2%)
Others	19 (7 %)
Painful bony sites	
Spine	109 (43%)
Pelvis/Hips	53 (21%)
Lower limbs	42 (17%)
Upper limbs	21 (8%)
Trunk (Ribs, Clavicle, Scapula)	7 (3%)
Karnofsky performance status	
Median (range)	70 (10-100)

Table 2. Reason(s) for referral*

Bone Pain	175 (69%)
Pathological Fracture	25 (10%)
Impending Fracture	20 (8%)
Review Recent Imaging	18 (7%)
Assess need for more treatment	15 (6%)
Lesion Seen in Diagnostic Imaging	13 (5%)
Neuropathic Pain	8 (3%)
Assess Progression of disease	8 (3%)
Post Surgery	6 (2%)
Cord Compression	2 (1%)
Others	13 (5%)

Note: *295 reasons in total for n = 254. Eighteen patients' reason(s) for referral were not listed.

Table 3. Pain scores and Analgesic intake according to the Brief Pain Inventory

	N	Mean	Standard Deviation	Median	Range
Worst pain in past day	92	6.47	3.00	7	0 – 10
Average pain in past day	90	4.39	2.47	4	0 – 10
Current Pain	92	3.40	2.87	3	0 – 10
General activity‡	88	5.77	3.59	7	0 – 10
Mood ‡	87	4.25	3.56	4	0 – 10
Walking ability‡	85	5.81	3.66	7	0 – 10
Normal work‡	82	7.12	3.34	8	0 – 10
Relations with other people‡	85	2.81	3.50	0	0 – 10
Sleeping‡	86	4.34	3.89	4	0 – 10
Enjoyment of life‡	87	6.23	3.57	7	0 – 10
Total Morphine Equivalent (mg)	91*	109.12	144.21	36	0 – 640
Pain relief experienced**	77	69.31	67.26	70	0-100

Notes: 0, no pain; 10, worst pain

‡How much pain interferes with this issue. 0, no interference; 10, completely interferes

*Out of 91 responses, 16 patients had 0 morphine equivalent

**0, no relief; 100, complete relief

Table 4. Pain scores according to the Bone Metastases Module (EORTC QLQ-BM22)*

	N	Mean	Standard Deviation	Median	Range
Pain in back	42	3	1.17	3	1 – 4
Pain in leg(s) or hip(s)	41	3	1.16	2	1 – 4
Pain in arm(s) or shoulder(s)	42	2	1.15	1	1 – 4
Pain in chest or rib(s)	42	1	3.59	1	1 – 4
Pain in buttock(s)	40	2	0.74	1	1 – 4
Constant pain	41	2	1.15	3	1 – 4
Intermittent pain	40	3	1.14	2	1 – 4
Pain not relieved by pain medication	36	2	1.15	3	1 – 4
Pain when sitting	42	2	3.89	4	1 – 4
Pain when lying down	42	2	1.14	2	1 – 4
Pain when trying to stand up	39	3	1.21	2	1 – 4
Pain when walking	38	3	1.17	3	1 – 4
Pain when bending/climbing stairs	32	2	1.14	2	1 – 4
Pain with strenuous activity	27	3	1.25	3	1 – 4
Trouble sleeping	42	2	1.18	2	1 – 4
Need to modify daily activities	39	2	1.16	2	1 – 4
Feel isolated from family/friends	38	2	1.22	1	1 – 4
Worried about loss of mobility	38	2	1.16	2	
Worried about being dependent on others	39	2	1.15	2	1 – 4
Worried about health in the future	38	2	1.26	2	1 – 4
Felt hopeful the pain will get better	37	4	0.90	4	1 – 4
Felt positive about health	38	3	1.01	3	1 – 4

Notes: *Refers to issues in the past week
1, not at all; 2, a little; 3, quite a bit; 4, very much.

Orthopedic assessment

The orthopedic surgeon's assessment was recorded at initial consultation with the patient. The functional status of the affected extremity/spine, the presence or risk of fractures, and the severity of the risk was recorded. The report was completed 79% of the time (n=201). The majority of patients had normal use with pain (37%), followed by significant limited use (25%) and normal, pain-free use of extremity/spine (13%). Only 7% of patients were reported to have nonfunctional use of the extremity/spine (see table 5).

At the orthopedic surgeon's assessment for presence or risk of fractures, 17% of patients had a high risk of fractures, 7% had low risk, and 25% had a present fracture at initial consultation (see table 6). Out of the 34 patients presenting with a high risk, 22 (65%) had a high risk of fractures at the extremities, with 41% (9/22) involving a lytic lesions = 2.5 cm in size, and 45% (10/22) having = 50% of the cortex involved. Seventeen patients were reported to have a high risk of fracture at the spine, with 47% (8/17) due to mechanical instability, 29% (5/17) because of spinal cord compression, and 24% (4/17) for cauda equine syndrome or = 2 nerve root deficits.

Table 5. Functional status of extremity/spine (n=201 orthopedic assessments filled out)

Status	
Normal use with pain	75 (37%)
Significant limited use	51 (25%)
Normal, pain free use of extremity/spine	26 (13%)
Nonfunctional extremity/spine	14 (7%)
Unknown	35 (17%)

Table 6. Presence of bone metastasis fractures/risk of fracture (n=201)

Presence of fracture	
Pathological fracture	44 (22%)
Wedge	7 (3%)
Fracture risk assessment	
High risk	34 (17%)
Low risk	14 (7%)
Medium risk	2 (1%)
Extremities risks	
Lytic lesion 2.5 to 5 cm in size	6 (3%)
50-74% cortex involved	5 (2%)
≥ 75% cortex involved	5 (2%)
Lytic lesions ≥ 5 cm in size	3 (1%)
Subtrochanteric region of femur	3 (1%)
Spinal risks	
Mechanical instability	8 (4%)
Spinal cord compression	5 (2%)
Cauda equine syndrome OR ≥ 2 nerve root deficits	4 (2%)

Case dispositions and recommendations

Following thorough examination of a patient's symptoms, the BMC physicians consulted to decide the best course of action to take. Out of 254 patients who were examined, only 240 case dispositions were recorded. Sixty-seven patients (28%) received palliative radiation, 20% required further investigation, 17% were referred to other support services such as physiotherapy, and 15% were offered surgery (see table 7).

Table 7. Case disposition and treatment recommendation(s) (n=240*)

Palliative radiation	67 (28%)
Further investigation required	48 (20%)
Referred to other support services	41 (17%)
Offered surgery	37 (15%)
No action	34 (14%)
Inappropriate referral	3 (1%)
Others	10 (4%)

Notes: *20 patient's case dispositions are unknown out of 254 patients. 3 patients received 2 treatment recommendations.

Discussion

As many as two-thirds of patients with bone metastases experience severe pain, thus this is usually the reason for the significantly decreased quality of life in patients (10,11). Over 80% of bone metastases are located in the axial skeleton, with the spine, ribs, and hips being the most frequently involved sites (9). This concurs with the top three painful bony sites recorded for the 254 patients seen at the BMC. Patients with bone metastases are at risk for SREs (12). Radiotherapy remains the standard choice of treatment for bone pain, and is also used where there is a risk for pathological fracture, or neurological complications arising from SCC or cauda equine syndrome (7, 9,16). Surgery tends to be indicated where there is intractable pain, high risk of fractures, acute spinal cord injury, or in cases where the pain is mechanical and cannot be treated by radiotherapy or systemic therapies (2,13,15,17). Prophylactic surgery can allow for stabilization of significantly destructive lytic lesions, whereas support frames or surgical fusion can be used to prevent SCC (7). However, due to the risks that come with surgery, particularly in elderly patients, a thorough assessment of all the available treatment options will allow the physicians and the patient to make the best choice (7,10). Oetiker and colleagues did a review of palliative surgery for bone metastases patients. They state that it is important to plan early and effective treatment to maximize the quality of life for these patients, and surgery can be very effective in relieving pain and for stabilization. However, they do note that an orthopedic surgeon must recognize that there is a need to manage this group of patients from a multidisciplinary perspective to ensure the best possible care for the bone metastases patient (16).

Bisphosphonates are known to give impressive results for treating hypercalcemia, as well as possibly reducing symptoms from bone metastases and the incidence and severity of SREs

(5,7,17,18). In Brown and Coleman's review (5) of using bisphosphonates to manage bone metastases in breast cancer patients, they note that radiotherapy is the first-choice treatment for treating local pain in many bone metastases patients, and excellent results are frequently achieved. However, since many patients also have widespread, poorly localised and non-mechanical pain, bisphosphonates may be a valuable alternative (5). They have found several studies showing that using intravenous clodronate, ibandronate, pamidronate, and zoledronic acid showed pain relief in bone metastases patients, with reductions in analgesic intake and an improvement in quality of life (5).

Pain from bone metastases typically develop slowly, and become progressively more severe (4). In the early stages, pain can be managed with analgesics or anti-inflammatory agents, however patients may still experience intermittent pain, such as a flare of pain upon movement (19) – a common complaint among patients with bone metastases (20). This type of pain then interferes with patients' ability to function, as well as restricting them from normal activities. This is seen in the BPI scores recorded at the BMC, where a median score of 8 was seen for pain interfering with normal work.

Once pain from bone metastases progress, other treatments must be considered. External beam radiotherapy achieves good results in most situations where patients have well-localized bone pain (5), and generally used in conjunction with either systemic treatment or supportive care (ie. analgesic therapy or bisphosphonates) (10). One-fifth of all radiotherapy treatments are given for pain due to bone metastases, and more than 40% of patients achieve at least 50% pain relief at 1 month. However, patients may also experience episodes of pain flare shortly after receiving radiotherapy. Approximately 14% of patients receiving a single dose of radiation have pain flare on day one as well as day two. Thus it is important to provide symptom control when alternative treatments are considered. Since pain relief from radiotherapy is also not permanent, pain progression generally happens at a median 5 to 6 months after treatment (21).

In Mercadante and colleagues' review of management of painful bone metastases, they state that 20-30% of patients treated with radiotherapy and analgesic may not have optimal pain relief, and therefore this may be where minimally invasive procedures, such as percutaneous vertebroplasty (PV), can play an important role (10). A prospective study was done by Cheung et al. investigating the efficacy of PV on pain relief and improvement of quality of life on patients with metastatic bone fractures (22). They used the ESAS for common cancer symptoms, the Townsend Functional Assessment Scale (TFAS) to assess mobility, site-specific pain score, as well as recording analgesic intake to assess changes in quality of life and pain before and after the intervention. A significant improvement was found in TFAS scores, all nine symptoms on the ESAS, site-specific pain, and there was a general trend of reduced analgesic intake post-PVP.

There is a real need for reducing complications due to bone metastases, as well as to improve the quality of life in these patients (5). Efficient management of bone metastases in patients requires a multidisciplinary approach due to the associated symptoms, clinical presentations, and complex underlying medical conditions (6,9). Closer collaboration between different disciplines would lead to quantifying clinical strategies and targeting them efficiently to those patients who have the most to gain (2). It is generally agreed that treatment should be individualized according to each patient's life expectancy, performance status, and quality of life (8,10).

From the inception of the BMC in 1999 until 2005, a total of 272 patients were seen (4). The median age was 65 years (range 28-95) and median KPS score at initial consultation was 60 (range 30-90), and this is fairly similar to the numbers seen in this review. Approximately a third (28%) of patients seen had two or more reasons for referral, which is nearly double the 16% of patients who had two or more reasons for referral to the BMC in 2006 – 2008. The most common reasons for referral in Li and colleague's review of the BMC were bone pain (42%), bone metastases (21%), high risk for pathological fracture (12%), and pathological fracture (10%). Bone pain continues to be the prevalent reason for referral to the BMC from 2006 – 2008 (69%). Out of the 272 patients, 40% of patients received palliative radiotherapy, 19% received interventional surgery, 7% were referred to other support services, and 7% needed further investigation or imaging. Although radiotherapy continues to be the most common case disposition seen (28%), there was an increase seen for patients who required further investigation or imaging (20%) and/or other support services (17%) in the past 3 years. During the initial six years at the BMC, the ESAS was used to record patient's symptoms; therefore there was no information on analgesic intake at that time.

When the total of 272 patients seen from 1999 – 2005 is compared with the 254 patients seen at the BMC from 2006 – 2008, it is evident that the BMC did approximately the same amount of work in 3 years as it did in its first six years. This is indicative of the increased awareness and need for multidisciplinary care in this group of patients. It is likely that the number of referrals to the BMC will continue to rise, which means there will be also be a need for increased funding as well as human resources. The ultimate goal of the BMC is to improve the overall quality of life for patients with bone metastases by maintaining and expanding this one-stop clinic approach for more patients who require this care. This is important given that as the population ages, the burden of cancer and bone metastases may also increase.

The Odette Cancer Centre Bone Metastases Clinic's integrated approach to the care of bone metastases patients allows for more streamlined care, in addition to eliminating the inconvenience of separate visits to a variety of specialists for consultation. Patients referred to the BMC receive a multidisciplinary assessment to decide the best course of action in order to maximize the benefits and palliate present symptoms. In order to further improve patient care at the BMC, there should be one quality of life instrument tool employed in order to keep results consistent, (ie. the EORTC QLQ-BM22). Analgesic information should be carefully recorded as well. Methods should also improve to collect orthopedic assessments and patient-rated quality of life questionnaires, as there were a number of patients and orthopedic surgeons who did not complete the assessments. Patient satisfaction of and cost-effectiveness of the clinic may need to be investigated in order to ensure the BMC continues to give efficient multidisciplinary care to patients with bone metastases.

Acknowledgments

This study was supported by the Michael and Karyn Goldstein Cancer Research Fund and Novartis Oncology. We thank Stacy Lue for secretarial assistance.

References

[1] [CCS/NCIC] Canadian Cancer Society/National Cancer Institute of Canada. 2008. Canada Cancer Statistics 2008. Toronto, Canada: Canadian Cancer Society/National Institute of Canada.

[2] Coleman RE. Skeletal complications of malignancy. Cancer 1997;80(8 Suppl):1588-94.

[3] Andersson L, Chow E, Finkelstein J, Connolly R, Danjoux C, Szumacher E, Wong R, Stephen D, Axelrod T. The ultimate one-stop for cancer patients with bone metastases: New combined bone metastases clinic. Can Oncol Nurs J 1999;9(2):103-4.

[4] Li KK, Sinclair E, Pope J, Farhadian M, Harris K, Napolskikh J, Yee A, Librach L, Wynnychuk L, Danjoux C, Chow E. A multidisciplinary bone metastases clinic at Toronto Sunnybrook Regional Cancer Centre – A review of the experience from 1999 to 2005. J Pain Res 2008:1;43-8.

[5] Brown JE, Coleman RE. The present and future role of bisphosphonates in the management of patients with breast cancer. Breast Cancer Res 2002;4(1):24-9.

[6] Janjan NA, Payne R, Gillis T, Podoloff D, Libshitz HI, Lenzi R, Theriault R, Martin C, Yasko A. Presenting symptoms in patients referred to a multidisciplinary clinic for bone metastases. J Pain Sympt Manage 1998;16(3):171-8.

[7] Mystakidou K, Katsouda E, Stathopoulou E, Vlahos L. Approaches to managing bone metastases from breast cancer: The role of bisphosphonates. Cancer Treat Rev 2005;31(4):303-11.

[8] Schachar NS. An update on the nonoperative treatment of patients with metastatic bone disease. Clin Orthop 2001;382:75-81.

[9] Selvaggi G, Scagliotti GV. Management of bone metastases in cancer: A review. Crit Rev Oncol Hematol 2005;56(3):365-78.

[10] Mercadante S, Fulfaro F. Management of painful bone metastases. Curr Opin Oncol 2007;19(4):308-14.

[11] Carlin BI, Andriole GL. The natural history, skeletal complications, and management of bone metastases in patients with prostate carcinoma. Cancer 2000;88(12 Suppl):2989-94.

[12] Lipton A. Future treatment of bone metastases. Clin Cancer Res 2006;12(20 Pt 2):6305s-8s.

[13] Manabe J, Kawaguchi N, Matsumoto S, Tanizawa T. Surgical treatment of bone metastasis: Indications and outcomes. Int J Clin Oncol 2005;10(2):103-11.

[14] Kohno N. Treatment of breast cancer with bone metastasis: Bisphosphonate treatment - current and future. Int J Clin Oncol 2008;13(1):18-23.

[15] Coleman RE. Clinical features of metastatic bone disease and risk of skeletal morbidity. Clin Cancer Res 2006;12(20 Pt 2):6243s-9s.

[16] Oetiker RF, Meier G, Hefti F, Bereiter H. [Palliative surgery for bone metastases]. Ther Umsch 2001;58(12):738-45.

[17] Talbot M, Turcotte RE, Isler M, Normandin D, Iannuzzi D, Downer P. Function and health status in surgically treated bone metastases. Clin Orthop 2005;438:215-20.

[18] Chow E, Ling A, Davis L, Panzarella T, Danjoux C. Pain flare following external beam radiotherapy and meaningful change in pain scores in the treatment of bone metastases. Radiother Oncol 2005;75(1):64-9.

[19] Coleman RE. Future directions in the treatment and prevention of bone metastases. Am J Clin Oncol 2002;25(6 Suppl 1):S32-8.

[20] Portenoy RK, Hagen NA. Breakthrough pain: Definition, prevalence and characteristics. Pain 1990;41(3):273-81.

[21] Steenland E, Leer JW, van Houwelingen H, Post WJ, van den Hout WB, Kievit J, et al. The effect of a single fraction compared to multiple fractions on painful bone metastases: A global analysis of the dutch bone metastasis study. Radiother Oncol 1999;52(2):101-9.

[22] Cheung G, Chow E, Holden L, Vidmar M, Danjoux C, Yee AJ, Connolly R, Finkelstein J. Percutaneous vertebroplasty in patients with intractable pain from osteoporotic or metastatic fractures: A prospective study using quality-of-life assessment. Can Assoc Radiol J 2006;57(1):13-21.

In: Advanced Cancer. Pain and Quality of Life
Editors: E. Chow, J. Merrick, pp. 165-175
ISBN: 978-1-61668-207-1
© 2010 Nova Science Publishers, Inc.

Chapter XV

Gender Difference in Patients with Advanced Cancer

Harleen Bedi, BSc (C), Roseanna Presutti, BSc (C), Amanda Hird, BSc (C), Sarah Campos, BSc (C), Liying Zhang, PhD, Gunita Mitera, MRT (T), Emily Sinclair, MRT (T), Elizabeth Barnes, MD, May Tsao, MD, Arjun Sahgal, MD, Cyril Danjoux, MD, Carlo DeAngelis, PhD and Edward Chow, MBBS, PhD, FRCPC*

Rapid Response Radiotherapy Program, Department of Radiation Oncology,
Odette Cancer Centre, Sunnybrook Health Sciences Centre,
University of Toronto, Toronto, Ontario, Canada

To examine if there is a gender difference in Edmonton Symptom Assessment System (ESAS) symptoms in patients with advanced cancer. Methods: Consecutive advanced cancer patients referred for outpatient palliative radiotherapy at the Rapid Response Radiotherapy Program (RRRP) completed the ESAS prior to radiation treatment. Baseline demographics were obtained for each patient. Correlation between gender, demographics, and the ESAS items was calculated using univariate logistic regression analysis. Results: A total of 1,107 patients were referred to RRRP from January 1999 to January 2002 and July 2007 to October 2008. There were 601 (54%) male and 506 (46%) female patients. The median age was 69 years (range 21 – 95). Males were older (male median age=70 years; female median age=66 years; $p<0.0001$). The most common primary cancer sites were lung (32%), breast (22%), and prostate (21%). Females reported significantly higher mean scores ($\pm$ SD) for tiredness (5.1 ± 3.0 versus 4.7 ± 3.0, $p=0.027$), nausea (1.6 ± 2.6 versus 1.1 ± 2.1, $p=0.0004$) and anxiety (3.4 ± 3.2 versus 2.7 ± 3.0, $p=0.0017$). Conclusions: There is a gender difference in certain symptom distress

* Correspondence: Edward Chow, MBBS, PhD, FRCPC, Department of Radiation Oncology, Odette Cancer Centre, Sunnybrook Health Sciences Centre, 2075 Bayview Avenue, Toronto, ON M4N 3M5, Canada. Tel: 416-480-4998; Fax: 416-480-6002; E-mail: Edward.Chow@sunnybrook.ca

scores in patients with advanced cancer. Our findings should be validated in future studies.

Introduction

It has been suggested that males and females differ in their approach to life, values and life roles (1). The reports of symptom intensity and response to treatment may also differ between the sexes. In a survey of the general US population, Mirowsky and Ross (2) found that women experienced distress (measured using six indexes representing sadness, happiness, anger, anxiety, malaise and aches) about 30 percent more often than men. Additionally, in a cross-national epidemiological survey of major depression and bipolar disorder, Weissman et al (3) found that women were twice as likely to develop depressive disorders as compared to men. Insomnia and fatigue, which were the most common symptoms associated with major depression, also affected women more than men. The literature on gender differences in palliative oncology patients is limited. While some studies have observed that women report greater intensity and prevalence of symptoms, others have failed to observe any significant gender differences. Given the contradictory findings, it is of interest to investigate if the genders differ in their responses to symptom questionnaires. In this study the Edmonton Symptom Assessment Scale (ESAS) was utilized to examine symptom experience in advanced cancer patients. The ESAS questionnaire is an effective tool for measuring symptoms in patients receiving palliative care and has been widely used in oncology populations. It consists of a nine item visual analog scale of which six symptoms relate to physical well-being (pain, tiredness, nausea, drowsiness, lack of appetite and shortness of breath) while three measure psychological symptoms (depression, anxiety and overall well-being). The ESAS distress score is a sum of the nine symptoms (4) and tends to reflect physical well-being (5).

Advanced cancer patients often present with multiple symptoms that co-occur and may be caused by the cancer itself, its treatment, or a combination of the two (6). Investigation of gender differences in symptom experience could help facilitate effective management of these symptoms by providing comprehensive, individualized care. Thus, the primary objective of the present study was to examine if there were any gender differences in symptom distress assessed using the ESAS questionnaire in patients with advanced cancer prior to palliative radiation therapy (RT).

Our study

Patients referred for outpatient palliative radiotherapy at the Rapid Response Radiotherapy Program (RRRP) at the Odette Cancer Centre with a pathological diagnosis of cancer were evaluated in this study. Patients completed the ESAS questionnaire using a touch-screen kiosk located at the clinic or with a trained research assistant prior to RT (baseline). The patients were asked to rate these symptoms on the ESAS on a scale of 0 to 10. A score of 0 indicated no symptom distress while a score of 10 represented worst symptom distress. This questionnaire has been validated in cancer outpatients and is noted for its ease of administration and brevity (5).

Baseline demographics, including the reason for referral and primary cancer site were obtained for each patient as part of routine clinical practice. Patients were evaluated on their performance status using the Karnofsky Performance Scale (KPS) (Figure 1). Ethics approval for this study was obtained from the hospital research ethics board.

Score	Description
100	Normal, no complaints, no evidence of disease.
90	Able to carry on normal activity; minor signs or symptoms of disease.
80	Normal activity with effort; some signs or symptoms of disease.
70	Cares for self, unable to carry on normal activity or do active work.
60	Requires occasional assistance, but is able to care for most of his/her needs.
50	Requires considerable assistance and frequent medical care.
40	Disabled, requires special care and assistance.
30	Severely disabled, hospitalization indicated. Death not imminent.
20	Very sick, hospitalization indicated. Death not imminent.
10	Moribund, fatal processes progressing rapidly.
0	Dead

Figure 1. The Karnofsky Performance Status Scale (KPS) (25)

The mean, standard deviation (SD) and median scores of nine ESAS symptoms were calculated for the total population and for males and females separately. Demographics and ESAS scores were compared for males and females using Student t-test (for continuous variables) and chi-squared test (for categorical variables). Demographics that were found to be significantly different between the sexes were considered as possible confounding variables and were controlled in the statistical analysis that examined gender differences in the ESAS symptoms. As a secondary analysis, prostate and breast primary cancer sites were excluded from the analysis to avoid a gender bias. Univariate logistic regression analysis of gender (females vs. males) was performed to search for the association with demographics and the ESAS symptoms. The same analysis was conducted to adjust for the confounding factors as well. Log-transform was used for nine ESAS items to account for a non-normal distribution. A two-sided p-value of less than 0.05 was considered statistically significant. All calculations were performed using SAS (version 9.1, SAS institute, Cary, NC) statistical software.

Findings

From January 1999 to January 2002 and July 2007 to October 2008, 1107 patients were seen at the RRRP. During the interval from 2002 to 2007, the Brief Pain Inventory (BPI) was substituted for the ESAS. The ESAS was reinstituted at the RRRP in 2007 after a Cancer Care Ontario (CCO) initiative to standardize patient assessment tools in order to coordinate patient care and symptom management across the province in September 2006 (7).

Our study evaluated 601 (54%) male and 506 (46%) female patients. The median age was 69 years (range: 21 to 95) and the median KPS was 60 (range: 10 to 100) (see figure 1). Males were significantly older than females in this study (median age of males 70 years, females 66 years, p<0.0001). Breast and prostate were the most common primary cancer sites in females and males respectively. Lung was the second most common primary cancer site in both groups. The KPS score of males was significantly higher than that of females (mean KPS of males 63 ± 16, females 61 ± 16, p= 0.029). However, there were no clinically significant differences between male and female performance status (median KPS 60 for both genders). Most patients were referred for bone metastases and brain metastases (see table 1).

Table 1. Demographics in total population at baseline (n = 1107)

Demographics	Males	Females	p-value[1]
Age (years)			
n	601	506	
Mean ± SD	70 ± 11	66 ± 13	
Median (Range)	71 (21 - 95)	66 (30 – 95)	**<0.0001**
KPS			
n	587	496	
Mean ± SD	63 ± 16	61 ± 16	
Median (Range)	60 (10 -100)	60 (20 – 100)	**0.029**
Primary cancer site			**<0.0001**[2]
Lung	203 (34%)	152 (30%)	0.18
Breast	2 (>1%)	236 (47%)	**<0.0001**
Prostate	228 (38%)	0 (0%)	**<0.0001**
Gastrointestinal	58 (61%)	37 (7%)	0.17
Other Genitourinary	49 (8%)	29 (6%)	0.12
Others	44 (7%)	36 (7%)	
Unknown	17 (3%)	16 (3%)	
Reason of referral			
Bone Pain	230 (38%)	160 (32%)	**0.020**[2]
Bone metastases	198 (33%)	180 (36%)	0.36
Brain metastases	64 (11%)	79 (16%)	**0.014**
Mass	23 (4%)	28 (5%)	0.18
Cord Compression	17 (3%)	11 (2%)	0.49
Others	69 (11%)	48 (9%)	-

[1] Student t-test was used for continuous variables; chi-squared test was used for categorical variables (significance level <0.05)

[2] p-value was obtained from the cross-table of gender and a) all primary cancer sites (excluding answers with "Others" and "Unknown"); b) all reasons of referral (excluding answers with "Others")

The ESAS symptoms scored as the most distressing in the total population were (mean ± SD) tiredness (4.9 ± 3.0), pain (4.8 ± 3.3), well-being (4.5 ± 2.7), and appetite loss (4.0 ± 3.3) (Table 2). Mean and median distress scores of males and females for the 9 ESAS items are listed in Table 2. Of all the 9 ESAS items, females reported significantly higher mean scores for tiredness (5.1 ± 3.0 versus 4.7 ± 3.0, p=0.027), nausea (1.6 ± 2.6 versus 1.1 ± 2.1, p=0.0004) and anxiety (3.4 ± 3.2 versus 2.7 ± 3.0, p=0.0017). The results did not change after controlling for age in both genders.

Table 2. Mean and median severity of 9 ESAS items

	Population	n	Mean	Standard deviation	Median	p-value[2]
Pain	Total	1106	4.8	3.3	5.0	
	Female	505	4.9	3.4	5.0	
	Male	601	4.6	3.3	5.0	0.43
Tired	Total	1079	4.9	3.0	5.0	
	Female	492	5.1	3.0	5.0	
	Male	321	4.7	3.0	5.0	0.027
Nausea	Total	1081	1.3	2.4	0.0	
	Female	492	1.6	2.6	0.0	
	Male	589	1.1	2.1	0.0	0.0004
Depression	Total	1059	2.3	2.8	1.0	
	Female	483	2.5	3.0	1.0	
	Male	576	2.2	2.7	1.0	0.11
Anxious	Total	1064	3.0	3.1	2.0	
	Female	484	3.4	3.2	3.0	
	Male	580	2.7	3.0	2.0	0.0017
Drowsy	Total	1068	3.3	3.1	3.0	
	Female	487	3.6	3.2	3.0	
	Male	581	3.1	3.0	3.0	0.056
Appetite	Total	1080	4.0	3.3	4.0	
	Female	491	4.1	3.3	4.0	
	Male	589	4.0	3.3	4.0	0.61
Wellbeing	Total	1045	4.5	2.7	5.0	
	Female	476	4.5	2.7	5.0	
	Male	569	4.5	2.6	5.0	0.53
Dyspnea	Total	1073	2.1	2.8	1.0	
	Female	488	2.3	2.9	1.0	
	Male	585	2.0	2.7	1.0	0.19

[1] symptom severity range = 0-10; 0 = minimum symptom distress, 10 = worst symptom distress
[2] p-value was obtained by univariate logistic regression of gender (Female vs. Male) on ESAS item (significance level <0.05)

In the secondary analysis, breast and prostate primary cancer sites were excluded and 641 patients were analysed. Since other gender biased primary cancer sites (gynaecological and testicular cancer) were rarely observed in the evaluated population (<1%), they were not excluded in the secondary analysis. Additionally, other primary cancer sites were not significantly related to gender (lung, p=0.18; gastrointestinal (GI), p=0.17; other gastrourinary (GU), p=0.12). In the population excluding breast and prostate primary cancer sites, females were observed to report significantly more distress for anxiety (3.5 ± 3.2 versus 2.9 ± 3.1; p=0.039) and drowsiness (3.8 ± 3.3 versus 3.2 ± 30; p=0.038) (Table 3).

Table 3. Mean and median severity of 9 ESAS items excluding breast/prostate primary cancer site[1] (n= 641).

ESAS Symptom	Population	n	Mean	Standard deviation	Median	p-value2
Pain	Female	269	4.8	3.6	5.0	0.96
	Male	371	4.6	3.3	5.0	
Tired	Female	264	5.3	3.1	5.0	0.055
	Male	367	4.7	3.0	5.0	
Nausea	Female	264	1.4	2.5	0.0	0.20
	Male	368	1.1	2.3	0.0	
Depression	Female	261	2.7	3.0	2.0	0.19
	Male	358	2.3	2.8	1.0	
Anxious	Female	261	3.5	3.2	3.0	0.039
	Male	360	2.9	3.1	2.0	
Drowsy	Female	262	3.8	3.3	4.0	0.038
	Male	361	3.2	3.0	3.0	
Appetite	Female	264	4.3	3.5	5.0	0.69
	Male	368	4.3	3.4	4.0	
Wellbeing	Female	255	4.6	2.8	5.0	0.19
	Male	355	4.7	2.6	5.0	
Dyspnea	Female	262	2.5	3.1	1.0	0.67
	Male	363	2.3	2.9	1.0	

[1] symptom severity range = 0-10; 0 = minimum symptom distress, 10 = worst symptom distress

[2] p-value was obtained by univariate logistic regression of gender (Female vs. Male) on ESAS item (significance level <0.05)

Discussion

In this study, we observed females to suffer greater distress due to tiredness, nausea and anxiety when evaluated using ESAS. When gender biased primary cancer sites were excluded from the statistical analysis, females were observed to report higher distress scores for anxiety and drowsiness. Similar to our results, other studies have also reported that in outpatients with advanced stage cancer, females are more likely to experience anxiety (8-10). Furthermore, women tend to suffer depression (8,11), nausea (8), early satiety and vomiting (8, 10) more than men. Additionally, Chiu et al (12) observed that females with bone metastases reported more severe worst pain as compared to men (Table 4).

Some researchers have explained these gender differences in symptom distress by differences in physiology between the sexes (13). For instance, Donnelly and Walsh (9) observed that GI symptoms (nausea, vomiting, early satiety and dyspepsia) affect women more severely and are more prominent in women with gynaecological cancers. The authors hypothesized that in pregnancy and during the luteal phase of normal menstruation, increases in progesterone and estradiol may slow GI transit and dispose women to experience nausea, early satiety and vomiting (9). Secondly, it has been observed that women report more effective and prolonged analgesia than males with kappa-opioids (such as, pentazocine, butorphanol, nalbuphine) (13, 14). The gender difference in analgesia has been attributed to differences in the interaction of gonadal hormones with opioid transmitters (14). However, there is no concrete evidence to support these hypotheses and the exact etiology behind gender differences in symptom experience of oncology patients remains unclear.

Table 4. Review of literature on gender differences in symptom experience in advanced cancer

Reference	Cancer diagnosis	Population size	Assessment questionnaire	Results
Chow et al. (20)	Brain Metastases	170	Edmonton Symptom Assessment Scale (ESAS)	No gender difference in prevalence of ESAS symptoms prior to radiotherapy
Harris et al. (19)	Brain Metastases	170	Edmonton Symptom Assessment Scale (ESAS)	No gender difference in prevalence of ESAS symptoms prior to radiotherapy. Significantly more deterioration in women as compared men post whole brain radiotherapy
Fan et al. (8)	Metastatic cancer (bone, brain, tumour mass, other)	1296	Edmonton Symptom Assessment Scale (ESAS)	Females with advanced stage cancer more likely to be anxious, depressed and nauseated than men
Chow et al. (11)	Bone metastases	518	Edmonton Symptom Assessment Scale (ESAS)	Females more likely to be depressed than males
Edrington et al. (21)	Bone Metastases	187	Brief Pain Inventory (BPI)	No gender difference in pain experience, analgesic prescription or consumption
Chiu et al. (12)	Bone Metastases	199	Brief Pain Inventory (BPI)	Females suffer more severe worst pain than males. No gender difference in functional interference, analgesic consumption, response to radiation treatment
Donnelly & Walsh (9)	Advanced cancer	1000	38-item assessment tool	Females more likely to suffer nausea, anxiety, vomiting, early satiety. Males tended to develop dyspnea, hoarseness, dysphagia, hiccough
Walsh et al. (10)	Advanced cancer	1000	38-item assessment tool	Females tended to experience more early satiety, nausea, vomiting, anxiety. Males experienced more hoarseness, dysphagia, >10% weight loss, sleep problems

From a psychosocial point of view, women may be better able or more willing to fully report and describe their symptoms leading to a response bias (2,13,15-17). Also, women tend to utilize health care more often and report more return visits than men (13,16). Therefore, these differences in expressiveness and health care utilization may bias the symptom assessments towards women. Secondly, according to the gendered response theory, males and females may differ in their emotional responses to distress. For instance, women may respond to stress with anxiety and depression while males express stress through anger and agitation (2). If the gendered response view is correct then questionnaires that contain questions typical of women's responses may falsely report women to be more distressed (2). Nevertheless, in a survey of the general population controlling for response bias and gendered response, Mirowsky and Ross (2) concluded that women genuinely suffer more distress than men.

Alternatively, the structural strain view hypothesizes that gender differences in symptom distress may be due to different social positions and role expectations of men and women (2). Women's role as the homemaker and caregiver could impose responsibility and stress that is manifested in higher levels of distress (2). Hagedoorn et al (18) examined the relative importance of both an individual's gender and his or her status as the patient versus partner in explaining differences in distress within couples coping with cancer. In their meta-analysis, it was observed that women reported more distress than men, regardless of whether women were the individuals with cancer or the partners. The structural strain view may also explain higher rates of distress (2) and depression (3) in women in the general population.

Additionally, Miaskowski (13) discussed the results of several epidemiological studies on common clinical pain problems, suggesting that women report greater pain (with the same pathology or similar degree of tissue injury), greater number of painful sites, use analgesics more frequently and are more likely to develop a chronic pain syndrome after equivalent trauma. These observations warrant further research on psychosocial and biological differences between the sexes.

Contrary to our findings, two studies performed in brain metastases patients at baseline found no significant gender differences in the prevalence of ESAS symptoms (19,20) (see table 5). Similarly, Edrington et al (21) reported the absence of gender difference in pain experience, analgesic prescription and analgesic consumption in patients with bone metastases (see table 4).

Table 5. Review of literature on gender differences in symptom experience in patients with lung cancer

Reference	Cancer diagnosis	Population size	Assessment questionnaire	Results
Gift et al. (22)	Lung Cancer (elderly patients, newly diagnosed)	220	Physical Symptom Experience tool, Medical Outcomes Study tool, SF-36	No gender difference in physical functioning and pain
Kurtz et al. (23)	Lung Cancer (geriatric patients)	129	36-item Short Form Health survey (SF-36)	No effect of gender, cancer stage, treatment modality on physical performance. Prior physical ability, symptom severity, patient age predict loss of physical functioning
Degner & Sloan (24)	Lung cancer (newly diagnosed)	434	13-item symptom distress scale	Females report more symptom distress than males.

Importantly, studies that have controlled for gender biased in the cancer site by examining gender neutral primary cancers have reported contradictory results for differences in symptom prevalence or intensity between the sexes (see table 5). For instance, two studies in lung cancer populations failed to find any significant gender difference in physical functioning (22, 23), symptom severity (23) or pain (22). However, Degner and Sloan (24) reported that in newly diagnosed lung cancer patients, women reported more symptom distress than men on the 13-item symptom distress scale. Furthermore, they found that this gender difference was unrelated to men's unwillingness to use the entire range of the symptom assessment scale (24). On the whole, very few studies have investigated gender neutral cancers, such as lung and GI. Further research on gender differences will benefit from analysing these populations by avoiding the possibility of a primary cancer site gender bias confounding the symptom experience.

This study was limited to only English speaking patients. Additionally, since other advanced cancer symptoms such as constipation, dry mouth, dysphagia are not included in the ESAS, gender differences in these symptoms could not be investigated. Several other factors such as occupation, education, marital status, and ethnicity could also influence the symptom distress reports of advanced cancer patients. The influence of these factors on symptom experience and disease burden should be explored in further studies.

Finally, the overall clinical significance of our findings must be investigated in larger studies. Nevertheless, our study observed a gender difference in ESAS symptoms in advanced cancer patients. These findings should be considered in future studies and clinical trials with oncology populations.

Acknowledgments

This study was supported by the Michael and Karyn Goldstein Cancer Research Fund. We would like to thank Tammy Lilien, Special Projects Administrator, Sunnybrook Health Sciences Centre for her assistance with data extraction and Rene E. Harrison, PhD, Department of Biological Sciences, University of Toronto for her comments. We would also like to thank Stacy Lue for her secretarial assistance.

References

[1] Dibble SL, Padilla GV, Dodd MJ, Miaskowski C. Gender differences in the dimensions of quality of life. Oncol Nurs Forum 1998;25(3):577-83.

[2] Mirowsky J, Ross CE. Sex differences in distress: real or artefact. Am Sociol Rev 1995;60(3):449-68.

[3] Weissman M, Bland R, Canino G, Faravelli C, Greenwald S, Hwu, HG et al. Cross-national epidemiology of major depression and bipolar disorder. JAMA 1996;276(4):293-9.

[4] Paice JA. Assessment of symptom clusters in people with cancer. J Natl Cancer Inst Monogr 2004;32:98-102.

[5] Bruera E, Kuehn N, miller MJ, Selmser P, Macmillan K. The Edmonton Symptom Assessment System (ESAS): a simple method for the assessment of palliative care patients. J Palliat Care 1991;7(2):6-9.

[6] Barsevick AM, Whitmer K, Nail LM, Beck SL, Dudley WN. Symptom cluster research: Conceptual, design, measurement, and analysis issues. J Pain Symptom Manage 2006;31(1):85-95.
[7] Cancer Care Ontario. Leading Practices Display Presentation: The interactive symptom assessment and collection (ISAAC) tool. Accessed 2008 December 28. URL: http://cancercareontario.org/english/home/pcs/palliative/provpallcare/
[8] Fan G, Hadi S, Chow E. Symptom clusters in patients with advanced-stage cancer referred for palliative radiation therapy in an outpatient setting. Support Cancer Ther 2007;4(3):157-62.
[9] Donnelly S, Walsh D. The symptoms of advanced cancer. Semin Oncol 1995;22(2, supp 3):67-72.
[10] Walsh D, Donnelly S, Rybicki L. The symptoms of advanced cancer: relationship to age, gender, and performance status in 1,000 patients. Support Care Cancer 2000;8:175-179.
[11] Chow E, Fan G, Hadi S, Filipczak L. Symptom clusters in cancer patients with bone metastases. Support Care Cancer 2007;15(9):1035-43.
[12] Chiu HH, Chow E, Li K, Bradley N, Doyle M, Harris K, Sinclair E, Barnes T, Tsao M, Danjoux C. Is there a gender difference in painful bone metastases? A review of experience at an outpatient palliative radiotherapy clinic. J Cancer Pain Sympt Palliat 2005;1(4):15-24.
[13] Miaskowski C. Women and Pain. Crit Care Nurs Clin North Am 1997; 9(4):453-8.
[14] Kest B, Sarton E, Dahan A. Gender differences in opioids-mediated analgesia. Anesthesiology 2000;93:539-47.
[15] Lawlis GF, Achterberg J, Kenner L, Kopetz K. Ethnic and sex differences in response to clinical and induced pain in chronic spinal pain patients. Spine 1984;9(7):751-4.
[16] Unruh AM. Gender variations in clinical pain experience. Pain 1996;65:123-167.
[17] Puntillo K, Weiss SJ. Pain: Its mediators and associated morbidity in critically ill cardiovascular surgical patients. Nurs Res 1994;43(1):31-6.
[18] Hagedoorn M, Sanderman R, Bolks HN, Tuinstra J, Coyne JC. 2008. Distress in couples coping with cancer: A meta-analysis and critical review of role and gender effects. Psychol Bull 134(1):1-30.
[19] Harris K, Chow E, Davis L, Chiu HH, Bradley NME, Doyle M et al. Gender differences in patient-rated symptoms following whole brain radiotherapy for brain metastases. J Cancer Pain Sympt Palliat 2006;2(1):11-5.
[20] Chow E, Fan G, Hadi S, Wong J, Kirou-Mauro A, Filipczak L. Symptom clusters in cancer patients with brain metastases. Clin Oncol 2008;20:76-82.
[21] Edrington JM, Paul S, Dodd M, West C, Facione N, Tripathy D et al. No evidence for sex differences in the severity and treatment of cancer pain. J Pain Symptom Manage 2004;28(3):225-32.
[22] Gift AG, Jablonski A, Stommel M, given CW. Symptom clusters in elderly patients with lung cancer. Oncol Nurs Forum 2004;31(2):203-9.
[23] Kurtz ME, Kurtz JC, Stommel M, Given CW, Given BA. Symptomatology and loss of physical functioning among geriatric patients with lung cancer. J Pain Symptom Manage 2000;19(4):249-56.

[24] Degner LF, Sloan JA. Symptom distress in newly diagnosed ambulatory cancer patients and as a predictor of survival in lung cancer patients. J Pain Symptom Manage 1995;10(6):423-31.

[25] Karnofsky DA, Abelmann WH, Craver LF, Burchenal JH. The use of the nitrogen mustards in the palliative treatment of carcinoma. With particular reference to bronchogenic carcinoma. Cancer 1948; 1(4):634-56.

In: Advanced Cancer. Pain and Quality of Life
Editors: E. Chow, J. Merrick, pp. 177-189
ISBN: 978-1-61668-207-1
© 2010 Nova Science Publishers, Inc.

Chapter XVI

Is It Possible to Predict the Survival of Patients with Advanced Metastatic Cancer?

Edward Chow, MBBS*, George Hruby, MBChB, Kristin Harris, BSc, Katherine Enright, MD, Emily Sinclair, MRT (T) and Grace Chan, RN

Rapid Response Radiotherapy Program, Odette Cancer Centre, Sunnybrook Health Sciences Centre, Toronto, Canada

To compare the clinician predicted survival (CPS) with the actual survival (AS) of patients with advanced cancer we asked participants to estimate the median survival as well as the upper and lower range of expected survival in whole months from the time of referral to the outpatient radiotherapy clinic for five real cases presented in the survey. Secondly, the participants were asked to rank the five most important prognostic factors they considered in answering the previous questions. Finally they were asked to provide some basic information concerning time spent in their field of expertise so one could compare and contrast the survival estimates according to different disciplines, and according to their years of experience. Results: The response rates to the survey from physicians, nurses and radiation therapists were 50%, 53% and 59% respectively. In general, the survival prediction from all disciplines was not accurate. The predictions tended to be optimistic in patients with short-lived survival (= 6 months) and pessimistic in patients with longer survival (= 9 months). There did not appear to be significant differences in the direction of survival prediction among the three disciplines. The accuracy of survival prediction did not depend on the experience of the health care professionals. Conclusions: Survival predictions are important, but, given the poor predictions of the clinicians, it is necessary to develop better predictive models for

* Correspondence: Edward Chow, MBBS, PhD, FRCPC, Department of Radiation Oncology, Odette Cancer Centre, Sunnybrook Health Sciences Centre, 2075 Bayview Avenue, Toronto, ON M4N 3M5 Canada. Tel: 416-480-4998; Fax: 416-48-6002; E-mail: Edward.Chow@sunnybrook.ca

survival using clinical parameters rather than relying on intuition and clinical judgment alone.

Introduction

Patients with advanced cancer and their families often request an estimate of the life expectancy to plan end-of-life issues and remaining time together. Medical professionals also rely on such estimates to guide appropriate clinical decisions, plan supportive care, and allocate resource use (1).

Clinicians tend to be overly optimistic in the survival prediction of terminally ill cancer patients (2-4). This may result in delaying referral to hospice and other end-of-life care (5,6). The choice of dose fractionation in palliative radiotherapy or the use of chemotherapy may also depend on the survival prediction.

The primary purpose of this study was to compare the clinician predicted survival (CPS) with the actual survival (AS) of patients with advanced cancer. The secondary objectives were to examine whether the CPS improved with clinician experience and the impending death of the patient.

A survey was conducted to determine the ability to predict survival in patients with advanced metastatic cancer among health care professionals including nursing staff, oncologists, palliative care physicians and radiation therapists. The objectives were to enhance our understanding of health care professionals' (HCP) predictions of survival in patients with metastatic cancer; to compare and contrast the survival estimates among the various disciplines; and to examine the impact of prognostic factors which are readily available in the out-patient/ hospice setting on the HCPs' quantitative assessment of survival for each patient.

Our study

The Rapid Response Radiotherapy Program at Odette Cancer Centre provides quick access to radiotherapy to relieve suffering and improve the quality of life of patients with advanced cancer. Patients referred have a pathologic diagnosis of cancer and documentation of metastatic disease by pathologic confirmation, clinical examination, or imaging studies. Five real cases were presented in the survey (see appendix 1). The time to death from any cause was the outcome. The survival time was measured from the date of the first consultation at the Rapid Response Radiotherapy Program. Participants were asked to estimate the median survival as well as the upper and lower range of expected survival in whole months from the time of referral to the outpatient radiotherapy clinic. A summary of the Karnofsky Performance Status (KPS) was supplied in appendix 2.

Whole month of remaining life span was chosen in order to quantify any differences between the estimated and observed survival in each of the 5 cases. Secondly, the participants were asked to rank the five most important prognostic factors they considered in answering each of the cases. Finally they were asked to provide some basic information concerning time spent in their particular field of expertise so one can compare and contrast the survival estimates according to different disciplines, and to their years of experience. This project was approved by the research ethics board at Odette Cancer Centre.

Findings

The response rates to the survey from physicians, nurses and radiation therapists were 50%, 53% and 59% respectively (see table 1). Their years of licensure are listed in table 2.

Table 1. Return rates of the survey

Discipline	Surveys Sent	Surveys Completed	Return Rate
Physicians	48	24	50%
Oncology Nurses	62	33	53%
Radiation Therapists	98	58	59%

Table 2. The year of licensure

Disciplines	Before 1970	1970-1979	1980-1989	1990-1999	After 1999
Physicians(n=24)	0	2 (8%)	4 (17%)	9 (38%)	9 (38%)
Oncology Nurses(n=33)	7 (21%)	11 (33%)	7 (21%)	6 (18%)	2 (6%)
Radiation Therapists [a] (n=58)	0	6 (10%)	16 (28%)	22 (38%)	13 (22%)

[a] 1 missing

Table 3. Survival prediction

Case No.	Actual Survival (in months)	Survival Prediction	Disciplines (median and range in months)					
			Physicians		Nurses		Radiation Therapists	
1	< 1	ES	4	(2 – 8)	6	(2 – 36)	6	(2 – 24)
		LR	2	(0 – 4)	3	(1 – 12)	3	(0 – 18)
		UR	8	(3 – 12)	9	(2 – 24)	9	(3 – 36)
2	6	ES	12	(1 – 48)	12	(2 – 60)	10	(1 – 48)
		LR	6	(0 – 12)	6	(0 – 24)	6	(1 – 36)
		UR	24	(4 – 120)	15	(3 – 84)	14	(5 – 60)
3	9	ES	6	(1 – 24)	8	(1 – 24)	5	(1 – 36)
		LR	3	(0 – 12)	4	(0 – 14)	2	(0 – 24)
		UR	12	(3 – 60)	12	(2 – 36)	8	(2 – 48)
4	16	ES	12	(6 – 72)	12	(2 – 60)	16	(3 – 118)
		LR	6	(0 – 36)	10	(1 – 48)	10	(1 – 36)
		UR	24	(8 – 108)	24	(3 – 54)	24	(6 – 60)
5	12	ES	6	(1 – 12)	9	(2 – 120)	6	(1 – 48)
		LR	2	(0 – 6)	5	(1 – 60)	4	(0 – 24)
		UR	12	(5 – 24)	12	(3 – 100)	11	(2 – 72)

Note: ES = Estimated survival

LR = Lower range of expected survival

UR = Upper range of expected survival

The estimated survival with the lower and upper ranges of expected survival of the five cases from the health care professionals is detailed in table 3. In general, the survival prediction from the disciplines was not accurate. The prediction tended to be optimistic in patients with short-lived survival (= six months) and pessimistic in patients with longer survival (= nine months). There did not appear to be a significant difference in the direction of survival prediction among the three disciplines. The accuracy of survival prediction did not depend on the experience of the health care professionals either.

When asked to rank the most important factors (in descending order of importance) in estimating the patient's survival, physicians listed Karnofsky Performance Status (KPS), primary cancer site, site of metastases, weight loss and age of the patients. The responses from nurses were primary cancer site, histologic grade of the tumor, site of metastases, time of onset of metastases and KPS whereas those from the radiation therapists were site of metastases, histological grade of tumor, time of onset of metastases, primary cancer site and KPS.

Discussion

Accurate prediction of survival is very important in advanced cancer and the management and especially in the pain management of these cases in final stages. Patients and families can set appropriate goals and plan end-of-life issues. It enables clinicians to make appropriate treatment decisions and recommendations, researchers to select relevant patient groups for clinical trials, and health care administrators to allocate resources in end-of-life care.

It has been observed that clinicians consistently overestimate survival (2,7). A systematic review of physicians' survival predictors in terminally ill cancer patients suggested that survival of patients was typically 30% shorter than predicted (8). The authors emphasized that doctors need to be aware of their tendency to overestimate prognosis in cancer patients who are approaching death. This optimism may have serious implications for the patients in terms of inappropriate application of disease controlling treatment and delay referral to a hospice, and or supportive or palliative care. The steering Committee of the European Association for Palliative Care has recently published evidence based clinical recommendations on prognostic factors in advanced cancer patients. They caution that clinical prediction of survival should not be based on experience alone, but in conjunction with other prognostic factors (9). Our survey revealed the prediction tended to be optimistic in patients with short-lived survival and pessimistic in patients with longer survival. We cannot be confident of this observation whether this may be due to the small sample size or the use of the survey. However the range provided by the clinicians included the actual survival time. This supports what often occurs in clinical practice that clinicians feel more comfortable and are more accurate when providing ranges. The various disciplines reported using primary cancer site, site of metastases and KPS when formulating survival. These factors are known to be predictive of survival. Future studies may try to develop a predictive model based on these factors and we are trying to do so in our centre.

Some studies have concluded that, toward the end of the patient's life, physicians became better at anticipating the timing of death (10,11). This is analogous to what meteorologists call the "horizon effect" in that short-term forecasts are usually more accurate than long-term forecasts (12). However, this effect was not apparent in our study nor in others reported in the literature (13-15). Other studies have observed that doctors in the upper quartile of practice experience were the most accurate in their prediction of patient survival (16,17). We also did not observe such a trend in our study. However, our study was limited to a single institution and compliance was < 60% for all disciplines. Furthermore, the number of cases may have been too small to demonstrate small differences within the disciplines and between the disciplines. Our study employed a survey to assess clinician predicted survival which may not be a valid method of measuring the accuracy of health care professionals in predicting the survival of patients with advanced metastatic cancer. They were not provided of the opportunity of face to face contact with the patients.

Life expectancy is an important factor in decision-making. It may play a role when radiation oncologists decide on radiation dose fractionation schemes, transition from prolonging life to controlling symptoms and improving quality of life, and hospice referral. Excessive optimism may have a negative impact on all of these decisions. Parkes, in his recent commentary, aired his disappointment that doctors are still no better at predicting the length of survival of our terminally ill patients than they were 27 years ago. He also stated that if all predictions had been divided by 2, they would have been marginally more accurate (18).

Survival predictions are important, but, given the poor predictions of the clinicians, it is necessary to develop good predictive models for survival using clinical parameters rather than relying on intuition and clinical judgment alone. Research instruments such as Morita's palliative prognostic index (19-21) and Maltoni's palliative prognostic score (22,23) have had recent success, both of which were shown to predict short-term survival reasonably well. We employed ESAS as the instrument tool in our survey. There are also limitations in the prognostic models that they tend to do better when predicting survival in populations rather than individuals and they may not be much better and accurate than clinical judgment alone. Some of the models such as palliative prognostic score also include clinical predicted survival as one of the indices. Furthermore, our study was intended to be exploratory. Hopefully, with further research, we can fine-tune these models, including the one developed at our clinic (24) and make more reliable clinical predictions. Until that time, we would do better to stop guessing and, when predictions are needed, to make use of the available predictive instruments. Prognoses should be based on proven indexes and not intuition (18).

In practice, if asked to provide survival estimates, we need to inform patients and their families that, in general, clinicians' estimates are far from accurate. It may also be more useful to provide a range rather than discuss median survival figures. If discussing median survival, patients and their families need to understand the limitations of this statistical construct.

- In a study from Sydney, 11 medical oncologists were asked to estimate survival in 86 cases. The survival predictions were well calibrated but imprecise. Almost two-thirds (61%) of patients had actual survivals that fell between half and double that of their predicted survivals. Therefore ranges based on simple multiples of the predicted survival time convey both prognosis and its uncertainty (25).

- Finally, it may be important to switch patient and family focus on the quality, rather than the quantity, of their remaining time.

Acknowledgments

We thank Ms Stacy Lue for the secretarial support, Michael and Karyn Goldstein Cancer Research Fund and all participants in completing the survey. We declare no conflicts of interest.

References

[1] Maher EJ. How long have I got doctor? Eur J Cancer 1994;3:283-4.

[2] Chow E, Harth T, Hruby G, et al. How accurate are physicians' clinical predictions of survival and the available prognostic tools in estimating survival times in terminally ill cancer patients? A systematic review. Clin Oncol 2001;13:209-18.

[3] Heyse-Moore LH, Johnson-Bell VE. Can doctors accurately predict the life expectancy of patients with terminal cancer? Palliat Med 1987;1:165-6.

[4] Parkes CM. Accuracy of predictions of survival in later stages of cancer. BMJ 1972;2:29-31.

[5] Demer C, Johnston-Anderson AV, Tobin R, et al. Cost of hospice care: Late versus early entry [Abstract]. Proc ASCO 1992;11:392.

[6] National Hospice Organization (NHO) Newsline, 1992. Stats show continued growth in programs and patients. NHO Newsline 1993; 3:1–2.

[7] Vigano A, Dorgan M, Buckingham J, et al. Survival prediction in terminal cancer patients: A systemic review of the medical literature. Palliat Med 2000;14:363-374.

[8] Glare P, Virik K, Jones M, et al. A systemic review of physicians' survival predictions in terminally ill cancer patients. BMJ 2003;327 (7422):1048-9.

[9] Maltoni M, Caraceni A, Brunelli C, et al. Prognostic factors in advanced cancer patients: evidence-based clinical recommendations – a study by the steering committee of the European Association for Palliative Care. J Clin Oncol 2005;23(25):6240-8.

[10] Mackillop WJ, Quirt CF. Measuring the accuracy of prognostic judgments in oncology. J Clin Epidemiol 1997;50:21-9.

[11] Oxenham D, Cornbleet MA. Accuracy of prediction of survival by different professional groups in a hospice, Palliat Med 1998;12:117-8.

[12] Stanski HR, Wilson LJ, Burrows WR. Survey of common verification methods in meteorology. Downsview, ON: Environment Canada Atmospheric Environment Service Research Report (MSRB) 1989:89-95.

[13] Bruera E, Miller MJ, Kuehn N, et al. Estimate of survival of patients admitted to a palliative care unit: A prospective study. J Pain Symptom Manage 1992;7:82–86.

[14] Evans C, McCarthy M. Prognostic uncertainty in terminal care: Can the Karnofsky index help? Lancet 1985;1:1204-6.

[15] Vigano A, Dorgan M, et al. The relative accuracy of the clinical estimation of the duration of life for patients with end of life cancer. Cancer 1999;86:170-6.

[16] Christakis NA, Lamont EB. Extent and determinants of error in doctors' prognoses in terminally ill patients: Prospective cohort study. BMJ 2000;320:469-73.

[17] Maltoni M, Nanni O, Derni S et al. Clinical prediction of survival is more accurate than the Karnofsky performance status in estimating life span of terminally ill cancer patients. Eur J Cancer 1994;6: 761-6.

[18] Parkes CM. Commentary: Prognoses should be based on proved indices not intuition. BMJ 2000;19:473.

[19] Morita T, Tsunoda J and Inoue S et al. Prediction of survival of terminally ill cancer patients. A prospective study. Jap J Cancer Chemother 1998; 25:1203-11.

[20] Morita T, Tsunoda J, Inoue S, et al. Survival prediction of terminally ill cancer patients by clinical symptoms: Development of a simple indicator. Jap J Clin Oncol 1999;29:156-9.

[21] Morita T, Tsunoda J, Inoue S, et al. The palliative prognostic index: A scoring system for survival prediction of terminally ill cancer patients. Support Care Cancer 1999;7:128-33.

[22] Maltoni M, Nanni O, Pirovano M, et al. Successful validation of the palliative prognostic score in terminally ill cancer patients. Italian Multicenter Study Group on Palliative Care. J Pain Symptom Manage 1999;7:240-7.

[23] Pirovano M, Maltoni M, Nanni O, et al. A new palliative prognostic score: A first step for the staging of terminally ill cancer patients. J Pain Symptom Manage 1999;17:231-9.

[24] Chow E, Fung KW, Panzarella T, et al. A predictive model for survival in metastatic cancer patients attending an out-patient palliative radiotherapy clinic. Int J Radiat Oncol Biol Phys 2000;53: 1291-1302.

[25] Stockler MR, Tattersall MH, Boyer MJ et al. Disarming the guarded prognosis: predicting survival in newly referred patients with incurable cancer. Br J Cancer 2006:94:208-12.

Appendix 1

Case 1

Small cell lung cancer, extensive disease at diagnosis with bilateral intra-pulmonary nodules and multiple bone metastases. Reason for referral to the Outpatient Radiotherapy Clinic: post surgical decompression of spinal cord C7-T2.

Clinical Status at time of referral to the Outpatient Radiotherapy Clinic

- 67 year old male
- No liver, brain, adrenal or lymph node involvement.
- Small intra-pulmonary nodules on chest radiograph, no pleural effusion

Significant symptoms: (0 = absence of symptom, 10 = worst possible symptom)

- Pain 5/10
- Fatigue 5/10
- Dyspnoea 3/10
- Loss of appetite 9/10
- Sensation of well being 7/10

KPS:	40
Weight Loss (>10% in last 6/12):	Yes
Analgesia:	Tylenol as required
Date of initial cancer diagnosis:	8 months previously
Chemotherapy:	cis-platinum + etoposide 4 cycles completed 4 months ago

Please provide your survival estimates in whole months (0,1,2,3…) from the time of referral to the Outpatient Radiotherapy Clinic.

My estimated survival for this patient is [ ] months

His lower range of expected survival is [ ] months

His upper range of expected survival is [ ] months.

Case 2

Metastatic ductal breast cancer

Reason for referral to the Outpatient Radiotherapy Clinic: post-surgical fixation of pathological fracture of the left hip.

Clinical status at time of referral to the Outpatient Radiotherapy Clinic

- 67 year old female
- Sites of metastases: lung nodules, mediastinal lymphadenopathy, multiple bony sites including pelvis, femurs, ribs, cervical and thoracic spine. No liver or brain metastases.

Significant symptoms: (0 = absence of symptom, 10 = worst possible symptom)

- Pain 0/10
- Fatigue 8/10
- Loss of appetite 9/10
- Dyspnoea 0/10

- Sensation of well being 8/10

KPS:	50
Weight Loss (>10% in last 6/12):	No
Analgesia:	Morphine 90 mg daily Amitryptiline 75 mg daily
Date of initial cancer diagnosis:	35 months previously Estrogen receptor positive (ER+) at diagnosis.
Treatment	modified radical mastectomy then adjuvant cyclophosphamide, methotrexate and fluorouracil (CMF x 6) 34-27 months ago adjuvant tamoxifen, commenced 27 months ago
Date metastases first diagnosed	2 weeks ago (fractured hip).

Please provide your survival estimates in whole months (0,1,2,3…) from the time of referral to the Outpatient Radiotherapy Clinic.

My estimated survival for this patient is [ ] months

Her lower range of expected survival is [ ] months

Her upper range of expected survival is [ ] months

Case 3

Metastatic Lobular Breast Cancer

Reason for referral to the Outpatient Radiotherapy Clinic: tender lytic sacral metastasis

Clinical status at time of referral to the Outpatient Radiotherapy Clinic

- 78 year old female
- Sites of metastases: multiple bony sites, diffuse metastases to stomach, right colon, para-aortic lymph nodes and ileum (the bulky metastases were excised)

Significant symptoms: (0 = absence of symptom, 10 = worst possible symptom)

- Pain 5/10
- Fatigue 8/10
- Dyspnoea 5/10
- Loss of appetite 10/10
- Sensation of well being 8/10

KPS:	60
Weight Loss (>10% in last 6/12):	Yes
Analgesia:	Tylenol 3, 6 tablets daily
Date of initial cancer diagnosis:	4 months previously Presented with metastatic disease ER (+) at diagnosis.

Treatment	Surgical excision of abdominal metastases 4 months ago. Tamoxifen, commenced after surgery Clodronate, commenced 1 month ago.

Please provide your survival estimates in whole months (0,1,2,3…) from the time of referral to the Outpatient Radiotherapy Clinic.

My estimated survival for this patient is [ ] months

Her lower range of expected survival is [ ] months

Her upper range of expected survival is [ ] months

Case 4

Prostate cancer with bone metastases

Reason for referral to the Outpatient Radiotherapy Clinic: painful cervical spine and left hip

Clinical Status at time of referral to the Outpatient Radiotherapy Clinic

- 69 year old male
- Sites of metastases: Cervical spine, skull, pelvis and femurs

Significant symptoms: (0 = absence of symptom, 10 = worst possible symptom)

- Pain 3/10
- Fatigue 0/10
- Dyspnoea 0/10
- Loss of appetite 1/10
- Sensation of well being 1/10

KPS:	80
Weight Loss (>10% in last 6/12):	Yes
Analgesia:	100 mg of morphine equivalent per day
Date of initial cancer diagnosis:	16 months previously (PSA 54 ng/dL). Prostatic biopsy confirmed Gleason Score 8 prostatic carcinoma.
Treatment	Orchiectomy and casodex 11 months ago PSA dropped to 34 ng/dL(7 months ago) but has risen steadily to 107ng/dL at time of referral for XRT
Date metastatic disease diagnosed	12 months ago Bone scan revealed increased uptake in the lumbar spine and pelvis, not present at diagnosis.

Please provide your survival estimates in whole months (0,1,2,3...) from the time of referral to the Outpatient Radiotherapy Clinic.

My estimated survival for this patient is [ ] months

Her lower range of expected survival is [ ] months

Her upper range of expected survival is [ ] months

Case 5

Breast cancer with brain metastases

Reason for referral to the Outpatient Radiotherapy Clinic: 2 brain metastases.

Clinical status at time of referral to the Outpatient Radiotherapy Clinic

- 62 year old female
- Sites of metastases: brain and lung.

Significant symptoms: (0 = absence of symptom, 10 = worst possible symptom)

- Pain 2/10
- Fatigue 3/10
- Dyspnoea 4/10
- Loss of appetite 4/10
- Sensation of well being 4/10

KPS:	90
Weight Loss (>10% in last 6/12):	No
Analgesia:	450 mg daily morphine equivalent
Date of initial cancer diagnosis:	33 months previously T2N1, ER+, high grade
Treatment	Left modified radical mastectomy, 33 months ago CMF x 6 completed 27 months ago Tamoxifen started 27 months ago
Date metastatic disease diagnosed	18 months previously (lung metastases) Treated with: Arimidex (from 18 to 9 months ago), Megace, commenced 9 months ago due to further progression of the 3 lung nodules

Please provide your survival estimates in whole months (0,1,2,3…) from the time of referral to the Outpatient Radiotherapy Clinic.

My estimated survival for this patient is [   ] months

Her lower range of expected survival is [   ] months

Her upper range of expected survival is [   ] months

Questionnaire

A. In which year did you gain your fellowship/ certification ________ *date*

Specialty (please put X on one of the followings)

Medical Oncology ______

Radiation Oncology ______

Surgical Oncology ______

Palliative Care Physician ______

Other, please specify ________________________________

B. In which year did you gain your Nursing diploma / degree ________ *date*

In which year did you begin working in oncology ________ *date*

C. In which year did you gain your Radiation Therapy diploma / degree ________ *date*

Of the following 9 items, please rank the 5 you consider the most important (in descending order of importance) in helping you estimate the patient's survival

1. Age of patient
2. Primary Cancer Site
3. Histologic grade of disease
4. Time from initial cancer diagnosis to onset of metastatic disease (the disease free interval)
5. Site of metastases
6. Karnofsky Performance Status (KPS)

7. Weight loss >/= 10% over the last 6 months
8. Symptom Distress e.g. pain, appetite, dyspnoea, sense of "well being"
9. Analgesic intake

Please place the corresponding number (1-9) in the space provided below:

The most important factor is ______________________________
The second most important factor is ______________________________
The third most important factor is ______________________________
The fourth most important factor is ______________________________
The fifth most important factor is ______________________________

Appendix 2

Karnofsky Performance Status Index	
100	Normal, no complaints, no evidence of disease
90	Able to carry on normal activity, minor signs of symptoms of disease
80	Normal activity with effort, some signs or symptoms of disease
70	Cares for self, unable to carry on normal activity or to do work
60	Requires occasional assistance from others but able to care for most needs
50	Requires considerable assistance from others and Frequent medical care
40	Disabled, requires special care and assistance
30	Severely disabled, hospitalization indicated, death not imminent
20	Very sick, hospitalization necessary, active supportive treatment necessary
10	Moribund
0	Dead

In: Advanced Cancer. Pain and Quality of Life
Editors: E. Chow, J. Merrick, pp. 191-200

ISBN: 978-1-61668-207-1
© 2010 Nova Science Publishers, Inc.

Chapter XVII

Projected Referral for an Out-Patient Palliative Radiotherapy Clinic

Roseanna Presutti, BSc(C), Liying Zhang, PhD, May Tsao, MD, Elizabeth A Barnes, MD, Cyril Danjoux, MD, Arjun Sahgal, MD, Gunita Mitera, MRT(T), Emily Sinclair, MRT(T) and Edward Chow, MBBS*

Rapid Response Radiotherapy Program, Department of Radiation Oncology,
Odette Cancer Centre, Sunnybrook Health Sciences Centre,
University of Toronto, Canada

The purpose of this chapter was to investigate the potential practice of referral to non-radiation oncology health care professions in patients with advanced cancer. Methods: Patients referred to the Rapid Response Radiotherapy Program (RRRP) for palliative radiotherapy between July 2007 and October 2008 were evaluated. Basic demographic information was collected for all patients including age, primary cancer site and Karnofsky Performance Status (KPS). The Edmonton Symptom Assessment System (ESAS) was completed by all patients prior to consultation with the health care team. The ESAS evaluates the intensity of nine symptoms on a scale of zero (minimum distress) to ten (maximum distress). As part of the analysis, the numeric scale was converted into a categorical scale of none (score 0), mild (score 1-4), moderate (score 5-6) and severe (score 7-10). Patients with moderate to severe pain, lack of appetite, anxiety or depression were identified as potential referrals to other health care professionals for the purpose of symptom management. Results: Approximately 50% of patients reported moderate to severe pain and lack of appetite, and would need referral for symptom management. About 30% experienced moderate to severe anxiety or depression, and would need to be referred for psychosocial intervention. Conclusion: Cancer symptoms are complex and a multidisciplinary approach should be taken to provide timely symptom

* Correspondence: Edward Chow, MBBS, PhD, FRCPC, Department of Radiation Oncology, Odette Cancer Centre, Sunnybrook Health Sciences Centre, 2075 Bayview Avenue, Toronto, Ontario, Canada M4N 3M5. Tel: 416-480-4998; Fax: 416-480-6002; E-mail: Edward.Chow@sunnybrook.ca

management for palliative patients. This may pose a burden to our existing health care system.

Introduction

Patients with advanced cancer often present with multiple symptoms, impacting both physical and psychosocial well-being (1, 2). The symptom experience differs among patients and is multifactorial in nature arising from disease progression, cancer treatment or a combination of these factors (3,4). In the palliative setting, maintaining the patient quality of life (5) and functional status are vital end points to consider, and is emphasized by the World Health Organization stating "The goal of palliative care is achievement of the best possible quality of life for patients and their families"(6). One way to reach this goal is to ensure sufficient symptom management in palliative settings.

Before symptom management can occur, valid assessment scales must be used to adequately evaluate symptom severity. Several reliable and valid instruments have been developed to investigate the prevalence and intensity of symptoms in cancer patients. Commonly used tools include the MD Anderson Symptom Inventory (MDASI), the Memorial Symptom Assessment Scale (MSAS), the Rotterdam Symptom Checklist (RSC), the Symptom Distress Scale (SDS), Functional Assessment Cancer Therapy (FACT-G), and the Edmonton Symptom Assessment System (ESAS) (7, 8).

In Ontario, there are several ongoing projects aimed at improving the delivery of care for cancer patients. In particular, Cancer Care Ontario (CCO) launched the Palliative Care Program in 2004 to ensure optimal symptom management for all individuals diagnosed with cancer. As part of this initiative, the Provincial Palliative Care Integration Project (PPCIP) was implemented two years later with the aim of improving quality of care through evidence-based symptom screening and collaborative care plans for patient care (9). The PPCIP uses the ESAS as a screening tool to identify patient symptoms, thereby allowing patients to communicate their symptoms with their health care team in a standardized fashion (10, 11). Furthermore, CCO recently implemented the Psychosocial Oncology Program in 2008, in which a holistic patient care approach may be considered for cancer care management, encompassing services from a variety of health care professions, including psychology, psychiatry, social work and nutrition (12).

The purpose of this study was to determine the potential for referrals to other health care professionals based on ESAS scores of patients referred for palliative radiotherapy (RT).

Our Study

The Odette Cancer Centre (OCC) is one of the regional cancer centres participating in the PPCIP. The OCC, formerly the Toronto Regional Sunnybrook Cancer Centre, established the Rapid Response Radiotherapy Program (RRRP) in 1996 to provide expedited consultation, planning and delivery of RT to patients with metastatic cancer for the purpose of symptom relief. The present study evaluated the ESAS scores of patients referred to the RRRP for palliative RT between July 2007 and October 2008.

Prior to consultation (baseline), basic demographical information was collected for all patients including age, gender and primary cancer site. The Karnofsky Performance Scale (KPS) was used to assess performance status (Appendix 1). At baseline, patients were also asked to complete the ESAS, either electronically via a touch-screen kiosk or in paper-format. Patients were encouraged to complete the assessment independently, but if they were unable to do so a research assistant would assist.

The ESAS is a validated, self-administered tool for use in palliative care settings (1). Patients rate the severity of nine symptoms—pain, tiredness, nausea, depression, anxiety, drowsiness, appetite, sense of well being and dyspnea—on an 11-point (0-10) scale, with zero indicating the absence of symptom and 10 representing maximum symptom severity (13). A total distress score is obtained by adding the scores for each of the nine symptoms.

In the present study, demographics were expressed as mean, standard deviation (SD) and median (range) for continuous variables, and as proportion (%) for categorical variables. The mean, SD and median values were calculated for each ESAS item as well. The numeric scale of the ESAS was converted into a categorical scale of none (score 0), mild (scores 1-4), moderate (scores 5-6) and severe (scores 7-10) for each item (14). The total number and percentage of patients belonging to each symptom category was determined. For this study, patients categorized as having moderate or severe symptom distress (scores $\geq$5 on the ESAS) are identified as potential referrals. All results were analyzed by Statistical Analysis Software (SAS Institute, version 9.1 for Windows).

Our findings

Prior to consultation, a total of 588 patients completed the ESAS. The median age was 70 years (range: 21-95). Both genders were similarly represented in the study population, with slightly more males (55%) than females (45%). The majority (54%) of patients were referred for painful bone metastases, followed by brain metastases (24%) and a combination of others (22%). Patients with lung, breast and prostate primary cancers were referred most frequently representing 38%, 19% and 19% of the study population, respectively. The remaining 24% of the population had gastrointestinal, genitourinary and other sites of primary cancer. Baseline performance status scores were available for 578 patients in which the median KPS score was 60 (range: 10-100) and the mean (± SD) KPS was 62.1(± 16.9) (see table 1).

The mean, SD and median values for each ESAS item is outlined in table 2. Fatigue, impaired well-being and pain were the most distressing symptoms with a mean ± SD score of 4.79 ± 3.18, 4.69 ± 2.83 and 4.09 ± 3.43, respectively. Nausea (1.13 ± 2.42) was the least distressing symptom reported.

Table 3 lists each ESAS item when analyzed using the categorical scale of none, mild, moderate or severe. Similar to the numeric scale, fatigue, impaired well-being and pain had the highest reports of symptom intensity with 57%, 57% and 49% of patients, respectively, being categorized as having moderate or severe symptom distress. Furthermore, moderate to severe distress was reported in 45% of patients for appetite, 33% for anxiety and 24% for depression.

Table 1.Baseline Demographics (n=588)

Age (years)		
N	588	
Mean ± SD	68.2 ± 12.9	
Median (Range)	70 (21 – 95)	
KPS		
N	578	
Mean ± SD	62.1 ± 16.9	
Median (Range)	60 (10 – 100)	
Gender		
Male	321	(54.6%)
Female	267	(45.4%)
Primary cancer site		
Lung	223	(37.9%)
Breast	111	(18.9%)
Prostate	111	(18.9%)
Gastrointestinal	56	(9.5%)
Other Genitourinary	47	(8.0%)
Others	40	(6.8%)
Reason of referral		
Bone Metastases	319	(54.3%)
Brain Metastases	138	(23.5%)
Others	78	(13.2%)
Mass	41	(7.0%)
Cord Compression	12	(2.0%)

Table 2.ESAS items in all Patients

	n	Mean	SD	Median*
Pain	587	4.09	3.43	4
Tired	587	4.79	3.18	5
Nausea	588	1.13	2.42	0
Depression	588	2.20	3.03	0
Anxious	588	2.86	3.27	2
Drowsy	588	3.11	3.28	2.5
Appetite	588	3.95	3.32	4
Well-being	585	4.69	2.83	5
Dyspnea	588	2.05	2.97	0

* Range of 9 ESAS items are from 0 to 10.

Table 3.ESAS items by Category

ESAS	None (0) n (%)	Mild (1-4) n (%)	Moderate (5-6) n (%)	Severe (7-10) n (%)	Total
Pain	178 (30.3%)	121 (20.6%)	120 (20.5%)	168 (28.6%)	587

ESAS	None (0) n (%)	Mild (1-4) n (%)	Moderate (5-6) n (%)	Severe (7-10) n (%)	Total
Tired	102 (17.4%)	149 (25.4%)	138 (23.5%)	198 (33.7%)	587
Nausea	448 (76.2%)	74 (12.6%)	26 (4.4%)	40 (6.8%)	588
Depression	337 (57.3%)	108 (18.4%)	70 (11.9%)	73 (12.4%)	588
Anxious	265 (45.1%)	132 (22.4%)	86 (14.6%)	105 (17.9%)	588
Drowsy	247 (42.0%)	132 (22.4%)	92 (15.7%)	117 (19.9%)	588
Appetite	161 (27.4%)	160 (27.2%)	125 (21.3%)	142 (24.1%)	588
Well-being	67 (11.5%)	186 (31.8%)	179 (30.6%)	153 (26.1%)	585
Dyspnea	343 (58.3%)	118 (20.1%)	56 (9.5%)	71 (12.1%)	588

Discussion

In the present study, patients that were referred for palliative RT were evaluated using the ESAS. Patients reporting moderate to severe symptom distress for pain, anxiety or depression, and lack of appetite are identified as potential referrals to other health care disciplines for symptom management.

Cancer related pain is one of the most feared and common consequences for patients, with approximately 80% of patients suffering from pain before death (15). However, due to inconsistencies in assessment tools, the reported prevalence of pain in oncology patients greatly varies and ranges from 14-100% (4). In the present study, 70% of patients reported some degree of pain when evaluated using the ESAS. These findings are consistent with Bradley et al. in which the prevalence of pain was reported as 77% in patients referred to the RRRP (16). Similar studies in the RRRP have indicated that pain is prevalent in 84% and 61% of patients with bone and brain metastases, respectively (17, 18).

In terms of categorical symptom severity, approximately 50% of our study population reported moderate to severe pain. Whelan et al. used the SDS in cancer patients attending a regional cancer centre, evaluating symptom distress for 13 items on a five point scale of one (no distress) to five (extreme distress). Each symptom was further categorized as “no”, “moderate” or “intense” distress. Similar to the present study, 42% of patients reported moderate to intense pain frequency, with 27% reporting moderate pain intensity (19). Furthermore, Cleeland et al. used the MDASI to measure the severity of 26 symptoms on a scale of zero to ten; with ten representing maximum distress. Using the same definitions for moderate and severe symptom intensity as in the present study, 34% of their oncology outpatients had moderate to severe pain (1).

Cancer related pain is multidimensional and management often involves oral analgesics, adjuvant therapies as well as non-pharmacological treatments (15, 20, 21). The type of oral analgesic used depends on the severity of pain reported. Mild opioid agonists including codeine are often used for moderate pain, whereas severe pain requires more potent opioids, such as morphine (15, 20, 22). However, when a rapid onset is required, the oral route may not be as effective and analgesics are often administered intravenously or subcutaneously (15, 22). Cancer pain is complex and often involves adjuvant therapies such anti-depressants or anti-convulsants for the treatment of neuropathic pain, which responds poorly to opioids (15, 22).

From a non-pharmacological perspective, Otis-Green et al. propose a psychosocial-spiritual model, encompassing the emotional, cognitive, social, behavioural and spiritual domains in order to tackle cancer related pain. They suggest that a multidisciplinary team including social workers, psychologists, psychiatrists, spiritual leaders, nurses and physicians is used for comprehensive pain management (21). Furthermore, cognitive-behavioural interventions may be beneficial for some patients to relieve pain (22). In a study by Anderson et al. audiotapes containing positive mood, relaxation or distraction techniques were given to cancer patients suffering from pain. It was found that the use of relaxation and distraction audio tapes provide immediate improvement in pain intensity (23). Although the benefit of cognitive-behavioural intervention may not be long-lived, in the palliative setting short-term improvements are of greater importance.

The prognosis for patients with metastatic cancer is poor. Even with advanced cancer treatments resulting in improved survival, death is imminent for most individuals. In light of this, these patients are at high risk of developing psychosocial distress including anxiety and depression (24). The prevalence of anxiety and depression varies greatly; however, some studies suggest the prevalence to be approximately 20% (4, 25, 26). In the present case, 43% and 55% of patients presented with some degree of symptom distress for depression and anxiety, respectively, with moderate to severe anxiety being reported by 33% and 24% for depression. Similar levels of severity were reported by Cleeland et al. when patients were evaluated using the MDASI. They reported that 34% of patients suffered from moderate to severe nervousness, and 32% from moderate to severe sadness (1). Although the ESAS and MDASI are validated instruments for assessing symptom distress, they are not suitable for evaluating clinically relevant levels of psychological distress. In a study by Frick et al. the Hospital Anxiety and Depression Scale (HADS) was used to assess mental health status of outpatients receiving RT. Only 8% of patients suffered from clinically relevant depression, and 13% from anxiety (27). While the reported level of clinical anxiety and depression for cancer patients are relatively low; the number of patients experiencing subjective symptoms of distressing depression and anxiety may be more relevant and certainly a greater prevalence is reported in this series.

Psychosocial intervention can be useful for relieving feelings of depression and anxiety in cancer patients and to improve quality of life. Commonly used interventions include counselling, cognitive-behavioural therapy, guided imagery, support groups and music therapy (28). In a meta-analysis conducted by Rehse et al (29) psychosocial interventions including education programs, professionally guided social support groups, coping skills training and psychotherapy were found to be effective for enhancing quality of life in adult cancer patients. Andersen et al (30) randomized breast cancer patients to weekly support group sessions or a control group, and found that the interventional group had higher functional status and lower levels of overall symptom distress. Graves et al (31) conducted a meta-analysis of Social Cognitive Theory (SCT)-based psychosocial interventions which emphasize self-efficacy, outcome expectation and self-regulation as key factors for improving quality of life in cancer patients. When SCT-based interventions are used, global quality of life, as well as depressive symptoms improved, however, anxiety was unchanged (31).

The metabolism of cancer patients is significantly altered. Accelerated proteolysis and lipolysis along with depressed protein synthesis inevitably lead to a loss of lean body mass and fat tissue (32). Despite the increase in metabolic activity, food intake often does not follow the same pattern. In combination with tumor effects at both the systemic and local level, as well as cancer treatments, these factors can lead to significant weight loss, malnutrition and the development of cachexia (32, 33). The incidence of malnutrition in cancer patients ranges from 40-80% and is more common in individuals with gastrointestinal cancers, the elderly and those with metastatic spread. Poor nutritional status is associated with decreased response to treatment, functional status and most importantly, a reduced quality of life (33,34).

Various forms of nutritional support are often offered to cancer patients in order to improve nutritional status and quality of life. Bauer et al (35) investigated the effect of nutritional supplementation and dietary counselling on quality of life, nutritional status, and performance status in cachetic cancer patients receiving chemotherapy. Over an eight week period, it was found that improvement in nutritional status was significantly correlated with improvement in quality of life (35). In a study by Isenring et al (34) nutritional status and quality of life were evaluated in outpatients receiving RT using the Patient-Generated-Subjective Global Assessment tool (PG-SGA) and European Organization for Research and Treatment of Cancer's QLQ-C30 global index, respectively. Patients were randomized to receive individualized nutrition counselling by a dietician only, or were given nutritional advice by a nurse, an information booklet and oral nutrition supplements. Over a 12-week period, the mean quality of life improved from 67.7 to 72.7/100 in patients receiving dietary counselling compared to a decrease from 75.3 to 62.6/100 in those who did not, suggesting that individualized dietary counselling can improve quality of life in cancer patients (34). Furthermore, in a randomized control trial by Ravasco et al. colorectal cancer patients receiving RT were randomized to either receive dietary counselling, consume a liquid nutritional supplement twice daily or maintain their regular diet. After RT, all patients receiving nutritional counselling had improvement in all six functional scales on the EORTC-QLQ-C30. On the other hand, patients receiving nutritional supplementation had improvement in only three functional scores, with the control group having deterioration in all six categories (36). As demonstrated, nutritional counselling by a dietician may be a beneficial intervention to improve quality of life and functional status in cancer patients.

The present study was limited to English speaking patients. In our analysis, only patients reporting moderate to severe (i.e. symptom distress $\geq$5 on the ESAS) pain, anxiety or depression and lack of appetite were considered to be potential referrals. This cut off point is based on PPCIP recommendations that referrals should be made for patients reporting depression of 5 or above on the ESAS, and therefore, may not be applicable for referrals for pain, anxiety or lack of appetite (37). Furthermore, the ESAS was used as a general tool to screen for symptom distress and despite its validity in palliative patients, further assessment tools such as the PG-SGA for nutritional status may be necessary before referral to other health care professionals. Lastly, the categories of mild, moderate and severe symptom distress were obtained from a previous analysis by Li et al. in which the Brief Pain Inventory was used (14). Therefore, the categories of mild [1-4], moderate [5-6] and severe [7-10] may only be valid for assessing pain intensity.

In conclusion, alleviating symptom distress in palliative settings is vital for maintaining quality of life. Individuals reporting moderate to severe distress on the ESAS require adequate symptom management, and should be considered for referral to other health care professionals. Based on our findings, approximately 50% of patients would be referred for pain management or nutritional counselling and roughly 30% for psychosocial intervention. In the RRRP alone, the demand for services from other health care disciplines is quite substantial. Due to the nature of this patient population, it is essential that symptom distress is managed in a timely fashion to maximize quality of life at the end of life.

Acknowledgments

This project was funded by Michael and Karyn Goldstein Cancer Research Fund. We thank Stacy Lue for secretarial assistance. Conflicts of Interest Notification: None

References

[1] Cleeland CS, Mendoza TR, Wang XS, et al. Assessing symptom distress in cancer patients: The M.D. anderson symptom inventory. Cancer 2000;89(7):1634-46.

[2] Rosenbaum E, Gautier H, Fobair P, et al. Cancer supportive care, improving the quality of life for cancer patients. A program evaluation report. Support Care Cancer 2004;12(5):293-301.

[3] Palmer JL, Fisch MJ. Association between symptom distress and survival in outpatients seen in a palliative care cancer center. J Pain Symptom Manage 2005;29(6):565-71.

[4] Patrick DL, Ferketich SL, Frame PS, et al. National institutes of health state-of-the-science conference statement: Symptom management in cancer: Pain, depression, and fatigue, july 15-17, 2002.[see comment]. J Natl Cancer Inst 2003;95(15):1110-7.

[5] Kutner JS, Bryant LL, Beaty BL, Fairclough DL. Time course and characteristics of symptom distress and quality of life at the end of life. J Pain Symptom Manage 2007;34(3):227-36.

[6] Morasso G, Capelli M, Viterbori P, et al. Psychological and symptom distress in terminal cancer patients with met and unmet needs. J Pain Symptom Manage 1999;17(6):402-9.

[7] Paice JA. Assessment of symptom clusters in people with cancer. J Natl Cancer Inst Monogr 2004;32:98-102.

[8] Chang VT, Hwang SS, Feuerman M, Kasimis BS. Symptom and quality of life survey of medical oncology patients at a veterans affairs medical center: A role for symptom assessment. Cancer 2000;88(5):1175-83.

[9] Cancer Care Ontario. The Provincial Palliative Care Integration Project (PPCIP) Accessed 2009 Febr 25. URL: http://www.cancercare.on.ca/english/home /pcs/palliative/provpallcare/
[10] Cancer Care Ontario. Palliative Care Program. Accessed 2009 Febr 25.URL: http://www.cancercare.on.ca/english/home/pcs/palliative/pallcare/
[11] Dudgeon D. Provincial Palliative Care Integration Project (PPCIP): Enhancing the quality of palliative care services. 2007;9:2.
[12] Cancer Care Ontario. Psychosocial Oncology Program. Accessed 2009 Febr 25. URL: http://www.cancercareontario.ca/english/home/ocs/clinicalprogs/psychosocialonc/
[13] Chang VT, Hwang SS, Feuerman M. Validation of the Edmonton Symptom Assessment Scale. Cancer 2000: 88;2164-71.
[14] Li KK, Harris K, Hadi S, Chow E. What should be the optimal cut points for mild, moderate, and severe pain? J Palliat Med 2007;10(6):1338-46.
[15] Bruera E, Kim HN. Cancer pain. JAMA 2003;290(18):2476-9.
[16] Bradley N, Davis L, Chow E. Symptom distress in patients attending an outpatient palliative radiotherapy clinic. J Pain Symptom Manage 2005;30(2):123-31.
[17] Chow E, Fan G, Hadi S, Filipczak L. Symptom clusters in cancer patients with bone metastases. Support Care Cancer 2007;15(9):1035-43.
[18] Chow E, Fan G, Hadi S, Wong J, Kirou-Mauro A, Filipczak L. Symptom clusters in cancer patients with brain metastases. Clin Oncol (R Coll Radiol) 2008;20(1):76-82.
[19] Whelan TJ, Mohide EA, Willan AR, et al. The supportive care needs of newly diagnosed cancer patients attending a regional cancer center. Cancer 1997;80(8):1518-24.
[20] Quigley C. The role of opioids in cancer pain. BMJ 2005;331:825-9.
[21] Otis-Green S, Sherman R, Perez M, Baird P. An Integrated Psychosocial-Spiritual Model for Cancer Pain Management. Cancer Pract 2002;10(1):58-65.
[22] Cherny NI. The management of cancer pain. CA Cancer J Clin 2000;50(2):70-116.
[23] Anderson KO, Cohen MZ, Mendoza TR, Guo H, Harle MT, Cleeland CS. Brief cognitive-behavioral audiotape interventions for cancer-related pain: Immediate but not long-term effectiveness. Cancer 2006;107(1):207-14.
[24] Bramsen I, van der Linden MH, Eskens FJ, et al. Evaluation of a face-to-face psychosocial screening intervention for cancer patients: Acceptance and effects on quality of life. Patient Educ Couns 2008;70(1):61-8.
[25] Stark D, Kiely M, Smith A, Velikova G, House A, Selby P. Anxiety disorders in cancer patients: Their nature, associations, and relation to quality of life. J Clin Oncol 2002;20(14):3137-48.
[26] Skarstein J, Aass N, Fossa SD, Skovlund E, Dahl AA. Anxiety and depression in cancer patients: Relation between the hospital anxiety and depression scale and the european organization for research and treatment of cancer core quality of life questionnaire. J Psychosom Res 2000;49(1):27-34.
[27] Frick E, Tyroller M, Panzer M. Anxiety, depression and quality of life of cancer patients undergoing radiation therapy: A cross-sectional study in a community hospital outpatient centre. Eur J Cancer Care (Engl) 2007;16(2):130-6.

[28] Jacobsen PB, Jim HS. Psychosocial interventions for anxiety and depression in adult cancer patients: Achievements and challenges. CA Cancer J Clin 2008;58(4):214-30.

[29] Rehse B, Pukrop R. Effects of psychosocial interventions on quality of life in adult cancer patients: Meta analysis of 37 published controlled outcome studies. Patient Educ Couns. 2003;50(2):179-86.

[30] Andersen BL, Farrar WB, Golden-Kreutz D, et al. Distress reduction from a psychological intervention contributes to improved health for cancer patients. Brain Behav Immun 2007;21(7):953-61.

[31] Graves KD. Social cognitive theory and cancer patients' quality of life: A meta-analysis of psychosocial intervention components. Health Psychol 2003;22(2):210-9.

[32] Marin Caro MM, Laviano A, Pichard C. Nutritional intervention and quality of life in adult oncology patients. Clin Nutr 2007;26(3):289-301.

[33] Capra S, Ferguson M, Ried K. Cancer: Impact of nutrition intervention outcome--nutrition issues for patients. Nutrition 2001;17(9):769-72.

[34] Isenring EA, Capra S, Bauer JD. Nutrition intervention is beneficial in oncology outpatients receiving radiotherapy to the gastrointestinal or head and neck area. Br J Cancer 2004;91(3):447-52.

[35] Bauer JD, Capra S. Nutrition intervention improves outcomes in patients with cancer cachexia receiving chemotherapy--a pilot study. Support Care Cancer 2005;13(4):270-4.

[36] Ravasco P, Monteiro-Grillo I, Vidal PM, Camilo ME. Nutritional deterioration in cancer: The role of disease and diet. Clin Oncol 2003;15:443-50.

[37] Cancer Care Ontario. Ontario's Palliative Care Integration Project. Accessed 2009 Mar 16. URL: http://www.cancercare.on.ca/documents/OHA_ErinHughes AndSusanKing_Palliative Care_May7_Final.pdf

Appendix 1: karnofsky performance scale

Index	Specific Criteria
100	Normal, no complaints, no evidence of disease
90	Able to carry on normal activity, minor signs of symptoms of disease
80	Normal activity with effort, some signs or symptoms of disease
70	Cares for self, unable to carry on normal activity or to do work
60	Requires occasional assistance from others but able to care for most needs
50	Requires considerable assistance from others and frequent medical care
40	Disabled, requires special care and assistance
30	Severely disabled, hospitalization indicated, death not imminent
20	Very sick, hospitalization necessary, active supportive treatment necessary
10	Moribund
0	Dead

In: Advanced Cancer. Pain and Quality of Life
Editors: E. Chow, J. Merrick, pp. 201-212

ISBN: 978-1-61668-207-1
© 2010 Nova Science Publishers, Inc.

Chapter XVIII

Utilization of Performance Scales in an Outpatient Palliative Radiation Oncology Clinic

Sarah Campos, BSc(C), Liying Zhang, PhD, Emily Sinclair, MRT(T), May Tsao, MD, Elizabeth A Barnes, MD, Cyril Danjoux, MD, Arjun Sahgal, MD, Philiz Goh, BSc, Shaelyn Culleton, BSc(C), Gunita Mitera, MRT(T) and Edward Chow, MBBS.*

Rapid Response Radiotherapy Program, Department of Radiation Oncology,
Odette Cancer Centre, Sunnybrook Health Sciences Centre,
University of Toronto, Toronto, Ontario, Canada

The Palliative Performance Scale (PPS) was developed in 1996 to modernize the Karnofsky Performance Scale (KPS), an established tool for measurement of patient performance status. Although the reliability of the KPS is well established, there has been little research done on the reliability of the PPS, despite its wide use in Canada. Furthermore, only limited research has been done correlating the PPS with other performance status tools such as the KPS. Purpose: To examine the correlation between the KPS and the PPS in patients with advanced cancer. Methods: KPS and PPS were recorded for 421 patients seen in the Rapid Response Radiotherapy Program (RRRP) at the Odette Cancer Centre in Toronto, Ontario, between July 2007 and March 2008. KPS and PPS scores of patients were then examined using the Pearson correlation. This study was approved by the research ethics board at Sunnybrook Health Sciences Centre. Results: Good overall correlation was observed between KPS and PPS of the patients enrolled in this study ($r = 0.87$). The correlation between KPS and PPS was higher when the performance status of the patient fell within the middle portion of the scales at 50-80

* Correspondence: Edward Chow, MBBS, PhD, FRCPC, Department of Radiation Oncology, Odette Cancer Centre, Sunnybrook Health Sciences Centre, 2075 Bayview Avenue, Toronto, ON M4N 3M5, Canada. Tel: 416-480-4998; Fax: 416-480-6002; E-mail: Edward.Chow@sunnybrook.ca

($r>0.5$; $p< 0.05$). Conclusion: PPS showed good correlation with the well-established KPS and thus is a reliable measure of patient performance status.

Introduction

Performance status is defined by the National Cancer Institute as "A measure of how well a patient is able to perform ordinary tasks and carry out daily activities" (1). Reliable measurement of performance status is useful for clinicians to quantitatively measure and track patients' disease and symptom progression to ensure appropriate treatment. Performance status can often determine a patient's eligibility for surgery or chemotherapy, as opposed to less aggressive palliative options. It is also used to determine the level of supportive care patients may require (especially for palliative patients) and is often a criterion for enrolment into clinical trials. Lastly, performance status can be a useful tool in predicting patient prognosis.

Karnofsky and Burchenal in 1949 recognized the need for a standard quantifier of performance status and developed the Karnofsky Performance Scale (KPS) (see figure 1) (2). The KPS has since been established as an accurate measure of performance status with good inter-rater reliability (3). Today, it is still considered a good predictor of survival in patients with advanced cancer (4-8) and thus is used very commonly in clinical practice.

Index	Specific Criteria
100	Normal, no complaints, no evidence of disease
90	Able to carry on normal activity, minor signs of symptoms of disease
80	Normal activity with effort, some signs or symptoms of disease
70	Cares for self, unable to carry on normal activity or to do work
60	Requires occasional assistance from others but able to care for most needs
50	Requires considerable assistance from others and frequent medical care
40	Disabled, requires special care and assistance
30	Severely disabled, hospitalization indicated, death not imminent
20	Very sick, hospitalization necessary, active supportive treatment necessary
10	Moribund
0	Dead

The KPS was developed in 1948 for the purpose of assessing performance status in patients with inoperable lung cancer undergoing palliative treatment.

Figure 1. The Karnofsky Performance Scale (2)

In 1996, the Victoria Hospice Society developed the Palliative Performance Scale (PPS, see figure 2) as a new tool designed to expand on and modernize the existing KPS. The PPS was developed for the purpose of accurately assessing and communicating a patient's functional level, describing the workload needed for their care, and assisting in prognosis (9). It includes several different categories, which cumulatively predict a patient's ability to carry out their activities of daily living (ADLs). The PPS assesses ambulation, activity, evidence of level of disease, self-care, intake, and consciousness (9). Like the KPS, the score is a quantitative measure with a scale ranging from 0 (death) to 100 (normal activity), but evaluates some clinically important criteria not included in the KPS, such as ambulation and nutritional intake. This additional information was designed specifically to provide a more accurate reflection of patient physical status and therefore overall performance status (10).

PPS Level	Ambulation	Activity & Evidence of Disease	Self-Care	Intake	Conscious Level
100%	Full	Normal activity & work No evidence of disease	Full	Normal	Full
90%	Full	Normal activity & work Some evidence of disease	Full	Normal	Full
80%	Full	Normal activity *with* Effort Some evidence of disease	Full	Normal or reduced	Full
70%	Reduced	Unable Normal Job/Work Significant disease	Full	Normal or reduced	Full
60%	Reduced	Unable hobby/house work Significant disease	Occasional assistance necessary	Normal or reduced	Full or Confusion
50%	Mainly Sit/Lie	Unable to do any work Extensive disease	Considerable assistance required	Normal or reduced	Full or Confusion
40%	Mainly in Bed	Unable to do most activity Extensive disease	Mainly assistance	Normal or reduced	Full or Drowsy +/- Confusion
30%	Totally Bed Bound	Unable to do any activity Extensive disease	Total Care	Normal or reduced	Full or Drowsy +/- Confusion
20%	Totally Bed Bound	Unable to do any activity Extensive disease	Total Care	Minimal to sips	Full or Drowsy +/- Confusion
10%	Totally Bed Bound	Unable to do any activity Extensive disease	Total Care	Mouth care only	Drowsy or Coma +/- Confusion
0%	Death	-	-	-	-

The PPS was developed by the Victoria Hospice Society for the purpose of assessing performance status in palliative care patients in Victoria, B.C. This version replaces the original PPS, developed in 1996. This is reproduced with the permission of the Victoria Hospice Society.

Figure 2. The Palliative Performance Scale (PPSv2) (9)

Cancer Care Ontario (CCO), a Canadian provincial cancer authority, has recently implemented a plan to standardize patient assessment tools in order to improve integration and co-ordination of care across the province (11). As part of an initiative launched in 2006 to improve palliative care services in Ontario, CCO began collecting PPS data for patients seen in cancer clinics province-wide, using a common database (11). In a recent review of prognostication tools, Lau et al. remark on the value of the PPS as a communication, as well as prognostic tool for palliative patients. Lau et al. go as far as to suggest that the PPS may eventually replace the KPS as a component of other predictive tools (12).

In a palliative medicine review of prognostication, Glare et al. also suggest that the PPS may be better fit to measure performance status in today's contemporary health care system (13). Despite the remarkable enthusiasm in embracing the PPS as the standard performance status measurement tool instead of the well-established KPS, only one study to date has compared the two tools (14). The primary objective of this study was to determine the degree of correlation between these two measurement tools in an outpatient palliative radiation oncology clinic.

Our Study

Patients referred for palliative radiotherapy with a pathological diagnosis of cancer and documented evidence of symptomatic metastases were eligible. The patients' PPS scores were determined by the attending radiation oncologist upon initial patient evaluation, while the KPS score was determined concurrently by the research assistant. Demographic data was also collected, including reason for referral to the RRRP (Rapid Response Radiotherapy Program), primary cancer site, the location from which the patient came to the consultation from (i.e.: home, hospital) and whether or not they came by ambulance. Ethics approval for this study was obtained from the hospital research ethics board.

Correlation between PPS and KPS was calculated using Pearson correlation and a linear regression model. Correlation was also calculated between corresponding levels of KPS and PPS. Patients were also grouped by KPS level, and the Pearson correlation conducted for each group's KPS and PPS scores. For example, correlation between KPS and PPS scores of patients having KPS =20, =30, =40, =50, =60, =70, =80, =90 and =100 were calculated. Similarly, correlation between KPS and PPS of patients having KPS of <20, <30, <40, <50, <60, <70, <80, <90 and <100 were calculated to determine at which specific levels better correlation existed. Correlation coefficients with p values =0.05 were considered statistically significant results.

What We Found

Between July 2007 and March 2008, 421 patients were seen in the Rapid Response Radiotherapy Program (RRRP) at the Odette Cancer Center of the Sunnybrook Health Sciences Centre in Toronto, Ontario, Canada. Approximately 45% of assessments were done on female patients and approximately 55% on males. The median age was 69 years (range, 26-100 years). The majority of patients had either: lung (36%), prostate (19%), or breast cancer (17%) (see table 1). Patients varied in the reason for referral to RRRP, but were mostly referred for palliation of their painful bone metastases (55%), or brain metastases (21%) (see table 2). Most patients (72%) received radiotherapy after consultation; 8% of patients required further investigation before treatment, 6% were referred for treatment other than radiotherapy, 5% were asymptomatic, and 3% declined treatment. The majority of patients were outpatients living at home, and the minority of patients traveled to their appointments by ambulance (see table 1). Of the 421 patients, the mean KPS and PPS scores were both 60 with a standard deviation of 20. Similarly, median KPS and PPS scores were 60. Both sets of scores ranged from 10-100.

Pearson correlation of the relationship between KPS and PPS scores reported a highly significant, positive correlation ($r=0.84$; $p<0.0001$). Table 3 shows the cross-analysis of KPS and PPS scores. There is good correlation between KPS and PPS, as most patients fall on or near the diagonal of the table (bolded numbers) indicating identical KPS and PPS scores.

Table 1. Patient demographics (n = 421)

Age		
	Median	69 years
	Range	26 – 100 years
Sex		
	Female	191 (45 %)
	Male	230 (55 %)
Primary Cancer Site		
	Lung	152 (36 %)
	Prostate	80 (19 %)
	Breast	74 (18 %)
	Genitourinary	44 (11 %)
	Gastrointestinal	40 (10 %)
	Others	18 (4 %)
	Unknown	13 (3 %)
Patient from		
	Outpatient	314 (75 %)
	Inpatient in Hospital	103 (24 %)
	Others	4 (<1 %)
Ambulance		
	Yes	90 (21 %)
	No	329 (79 %)
	Unknown	2 (<1 %)

Table 2. Reason for referral to the Rapid Response Radiotherapy Clinic (n = 421)

Reason for Referral	N (%)
Painful Bony Metastases	232 (55%)
Brain Metastases	92 (22 %)
Others (i.e. Reduction of mass, spinal cord compression, fracture, bleeding)	97 (23%)

The correlation between KPS and PPS was further analyzed by comparing correlation of different levels of the tools. Patients were broken down into groups based on KPS score, and their KPS and PPS scores were subsequently correlated. The aim of this test was to determine whether correlation between the two tools varied according to patients' level of performance status. Table 4 shows correlation coefficients for patients grouped into separate KPS levels. KPS and PPS were best correlated at levels 50, 60, 70 and 80 ($r>0.5$; $p< 0.05$). When analyzing the correlation between the KPS and PPS of patients who fell within the KPS range of 10 to 40, inclusively ($n = 48$), no significant relationship was found. Similarly, no significant correlation was found in patients whose KPS fell within the range of 90 to 100, inclusively ($n = 53$). It should be noted, however, that KPS scores for this patient population were relatively centralized in the middle of both scales, so the lack of significant correlation could likely be due to the small sample of patients with either very high or very low performance status.

Table 3. Cross table of KPS and PPS

	PPS										Total
KPS	10	20	30	40	50	60	70	80	90	100	KPS
10	0	1	0	0	0	0	0	0	0	0	1
20	2	4	3	0	0	0	0	0	0	0	9
30	1	0	19	6	2	0	0	1	0	0	29
40	0	0	5	23	5	2	0	0	0	0	35
50	0	0	1	17	43	11	2	1	1	1	77
60	0	1	0	1	11	61	17	3	1	0	95
70	0	0	0	0	0	12	43	11	3	0	69
80	0	0	0	1	0	4	15	35	5	0	60
90	0	0	0	0	0	2	3	5	30	2	42
100	0	0	0	0	0	0	0	0	1	2	3
Total PPS	3	6	28	48	61	92	80	56	41	5	420

The above table shows the number of patients at each KPS level (rows), crossed with the number of patients at the corresponding PPS level (columns). The bolded numbers show the number of patients at each level who had identical KPS and PPS values.

Table 4. Pearson Correlation between KPS and PPS by level of KPS

	Correlation based on KPS above a certain level	Correlation based on KPS below a certain level
	KPS ≥ 20	**KPS < 20**
n	515	1
r (p-value)	0.87 (< 0.0001)	-
	KPS ≥ 30	**KPS < 30**
n	502	14
r (p-value)	0.86 (< 0.0001)	0.048 (0.90)
	KPS ≥ 40	**KPS < 40**
n	468	48
r (p-value)	0.84 (< 0.0001)	0.47 (0.0023)
	KPS ≥ 50	**KPS < 50**
n	424	92
r (p-value)	0.80 (< 0.0001)	0.58 (< 0.0001)
	KPS ≥ 60	**KPS < 60**
n	327	189
r (p-value)	0.75 (< 0.0001)	0.66 (< 0.0001)
	KPS ≥ 70	**KPS < 70**
n	216	300
r (p-value)	0.63 (< 0.0001)	0.76 (< 0.0001)
	KPS ≥ 80	**KPS < 80**
n	126	390
r (p-value)	0.55 (< 0.0001)	0.82 (< 0.0001)
	KPS ≥ 90	**KPS < 90**
n	53	463
r (p-value)	0.29 (0.055)	0.84 (< 0.0001)
	KPS ≥ 100	**KPS < 100**
n	4	512
r (p-value)	-	0.87 (< 0.0001)

The above table analyzes the correlation between KPS and PPS based on the level of KPS into which the patient falls. KPS and PPS were best correlated at levels 50, 60, 70 and 80 ($r>0.5$; $p< 0.05$).

Despite observed variation in correlation between levels of KPS and PPS, the overall relationship between these variables is a strongly positive one, as shown in the General Linear Model plotted in figure 3. Although a few outliers are present, the plot is generally well distributed on the regression line (PPS = 6.85 + 0.89(KPS)).

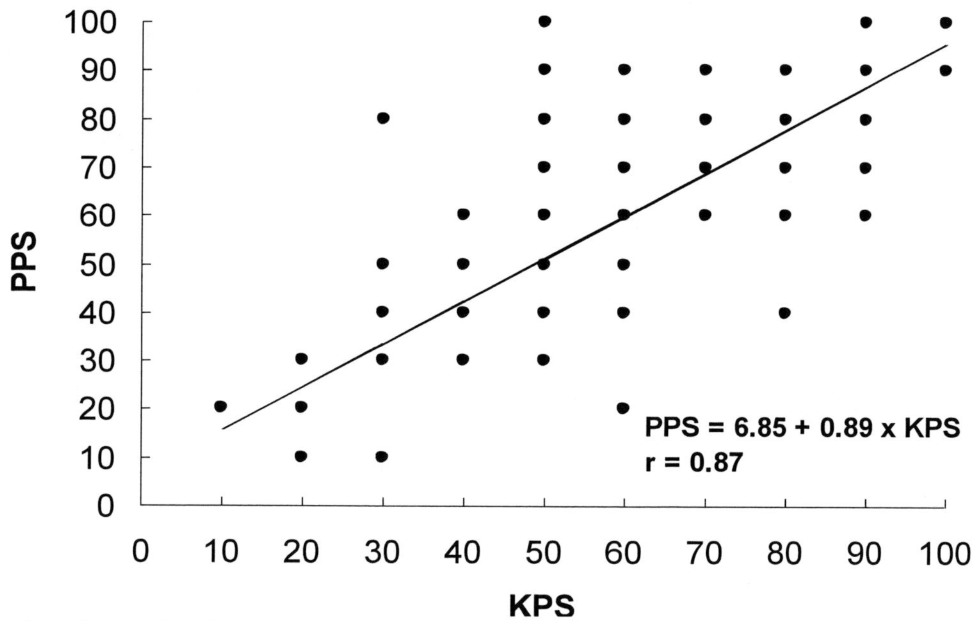

The above figure plots the regression model for the correlation between the KPS and PPS scales.

Figure 3. General Linear Model of Pearson Correlation between KPS and PPS

Discussion

Our study found an excellent correlation between KPS and PPS (r= 0.87), suggesting that both tools are similarly accurate in assessing performance status in our palliative cancer population. In a 2004 description of the PPS, Wilner and Arnold commented on the need for further studies analyzing the correlation of the PPS with other commonly used prognostic tools and symptom assessment scales (15). Although much research has been done on the KPS, only one study compared it with the PPS scale. Morita et al. undertook a study using PPS to predict survival in terminally ill cancer patients in Japan in 1999. The authors analyzed the relationship between KPS and PPS scores for 588 patient samples as a secondary objective of the study. They too found an excellent correlation between KPS and PPS (r = 0.93) (14), which supports the more detailed results obtained in this study.

An important difference to consider when interpreting the results obtained by Morita et al. when compared to our study lies in the patient demographics. The majority of our population consisted of outpatients, living in their own homes, not requiring ambulance services, and being treated with a palliative intent at the time of consultation. Patients included in the study by Morita et al. consisted of hospitalized terminally ill patients with a low performance status score (14). Eighty-one percent of patients in Morita et al.'s study had a PPS of =50 (14), compared to 35% in our study. Morita et al.'s study was able to correlate low PPS and KPS scores, whereas the patients in our population provided a wider scope of the two scales.

One apparent limitation of our study design lies in the method of assessment. KPS scores were rated by the research assistant, while PPS scores were formulated by the attending physician. This is a direct result of CCO's requirement that all PPS scores entered into their database be rated by a physician. The research assistant routinely rates KPS scores for all patients seen in the clinic, which are then entered into the clinical database. Furthermore, de Borja et al. studied the relationship between both KPS and ECOG scores assigned by various health care providers including physicians, nurses, radiation therapists and radiation therapy students (16). This study found moderate correlation of radiation therapist and physician scores ($r = 0.57$, $p = 0.002$), very good correlation of nurse and physician scores ($r = 0.77$, $p<0.0001$), and very good correlation of radiation therapy student and physician scores ($r = 0.81$, $p<0.0001$). Additionally, a study done by Liem et al. compared KPS assessments assigned by resident and attending physicians and found an excellent correlation ($r = 0.85$, $p<0.01$) between them (17). This demonstrates the similarity of performance status scores determined by all health care providers working with a particular patient. The research assistant, as a member of a multidisciplinary clinical team, was thereby named an accurate rater of performance status, and her KPS scores were deemed valid for the purpose of this study.

Despite the lack of research validating the PPS as a reliable performance status tool, much literature exists on the role of the PPS in predicting patient survival. PPS has been shown to be an independent prognostic factor in many studies (7,18-23), and is at least as good at predicting survival as the Eastern Co-operative Oncology Group (see figure 4) (24) and the KPS scales (19). Although the PPS is useful overall as a predictive tool, one study showed it to produce some discrepancies between patients of different performance status (21). Like the results produced by our study, suggesting different correlation of KPS and PPS at different levels of performance status, Lau and Downing reported the PPS to be better at calibrating expected survival of patients at 10, 20, 30 and 40%, as compared to higher levels of PPS (21). Correlation between KPS and PPS tended to be higher in patients with a better performance status, signifying that the PPS can isolate distinct changes in lower performance status patients that are not measured by the KPS scale. This suggests that the PPS is unique in grouping patients with low performance status, and can fairly reliably predict their survival accordingly. A systematic review of the literature by Lau and colleagues also suggests that the PPS is useful for predicting 1-6 month survival (12), which is the range typically expected for low performance status patients.

The PPS was developed by the Victoria Hospice Society with the intention of modernizing the KPS. The KPS, although well established, does not reflect the shift of resources to community and outpatient settings that have recently come into play in Canadian healthcare (10,25). Hospitalization is a vital part of KPS criteria, but is no longer an integral part of a patient's performance status given that many palliative patients are able to access adequate home care. Furthermore, many patients now choose available end-of-life care to allow them to die in their own homes. The PPS is advantageous in that it does not use information regarding patient hospitalization, but instead takes into account patients' levels of ambulation, oral intake and consciousness: criteria that clinical experience has shown to be very important in performance status evaluation (9).

ECOG PERFORMANCE STATUS	
Grade	ECOG
0	Fully active, able to carry on all pre-disease performance without restriction
1	Restricted in physically strenuous activity but ambulatory and able to carry out work of a light or sedentary nature, e.g., light house work, office work
2	Ambulatory and capable of all self-care but unable to carry out any work activities. Up and about more than 50% of waking hours
3	Capable of only limited self-care, confined to bed or chair more than 50% of waking hours
4	Completely disabled. Cannot carry on any self-care. Totally confined to bed or chair
5	Dead

The ECOG scale was developed in 1982 as part of criteria developed to assess toxicity and response to treatment. It is now widely used to assess performance status in cancer patients in clinical settings as well as in clinical trials and studies.

Figure 4. The Eastern Cooperative Oncology Group (ECOG) Scale (22)

In a study of survival predictors, Vigano and Bruera chose to measure performance status using the Eastern Co-Operative Oncology Group (ECOG) scale (see figure 4) (24) due to the incorporation of patient ambulation status (26). Had this study been performed after the PPS was released, the PPS might have been a more reliable choice due to the additional attention it gives to nutritional intake and consciousness. PPS is also the performance status tool used in the Palliative Prognostic Index: a tool developed by Morita that used performance status and the presence or absence of four symptoms to predict survival in terminally ill cancer patients (27).

Most research evaluating the PPS, as a survival tool or otherwise, involves patients in inpatient palliative care, hospice or hospital studies. Only one study evaluated PPS in patients from a tertiary care setting (22). Furthermore, the majority of studies in the literature look at patient populations with low median PPS. This suggests that PPS is only being analyzed in palliative care patients who have been admitted to hospice settings and are very near to death (20).

Conclusions

The PPS showed good correlation to the KPS overall in this primary outpatient palliative patient population. In particular, the PPS was highly correlated to the KPS for patients within the intermediate range of the scales (50-80), which applies to the majority of patients enrolled in the study. The PPS has the further advantage of accounting for clinically relevant variables applicable to modern outpatient palliative healthcare, and adequately assesses patients' ability to perform the activities of daily living.

PPS was reliable in assessing patients at intermediate levels of the scale, but shows some variance in measuring the performance status of nearly moribund patients. Studies evaluating the reliability of the PPS in populations with more evenly distributed performance status scores are necessary in determining the consistency of the scale as a whole.

Although we were able to measure the reliability of the PPS scale in terms of its correlation to the KPS, the value of this tool also greatly depends on its use in clinical practice. In light of the recent "closer to home" (25) shift in Canadian healthcare as well as the use of the PPS by Canadian authorities in cancer care, the usability of this tool by health care professionals and patients is crucial to its value. Further research is needed to ensure it is easy to understand and produces consistent, reliable results in a variety of settings.

Our study concludes that the PPS is reliable in predicting the performance status of outpatients with advanced cancer; however more research is needed to validate the PPS as a performance status tool in more heterogeneous populations.

Acknowledgments

This project was funded by Michael and Karyn Goldstein Cancer Research Fund. Conflicts of Interest Notification: None

References

[1] Definition of Performance Status - NCI Dictionary of Cancer Terms. 2008; Available at:http://www.cancer.gov/dictionary/?searchTxt=performance+status&sgroup=Starts+with&lang=&btnGo.x=9&btnGo.y=3. Accessed 2009 Jan 3.

[2] Karnofsky DA, Abelmann WH, Craver LF, Burchenal JH. The use of the nitrogen mustards in the palliative treatment of carcinoma. With particular reference to bronchogenic carcinoma. Cancer 1948; 1(4):634-56.

[3] Yates JW, Chalmer B, McKegney FP. Evaluation of patients with advanced cancer using the Karnofsky performance status. Cancer 1980;45(8):2220-4.

[4] Chow E, Harth T, Hruby G, Finkelstein J, Wu J, Danjoux C. How accurate are physicians' clinical predictions of survival and the available prognostic tools in estimating survival times in terminally ill cancer patients? A systematic review. Clin Oncol (R Coll Radiol) 2001;13(3):209-18.

[5] Chow E, Fung K, Panzarella T, Bezjak A, Danjoux C, Tannock I. A predictive model for survival in metastatic cancer patients attending an outpatient palliative radiotherapy clinic. Int J Radiat Oncol Biol Phys 2002;53(5):1291-1302.

[6] Maltoni M, Nanni O, Pirovano M, Scarpi E, Indelli M, Martini C, et al. Successful validation of the palliative prognostic score in terminally ill cancer patients. Italian Multicenter Study Group on Palliative Care. J Pain Symptom Manage 1999;17(4):240-7.

[7] Sloan JA, Loprinzi CL, Laurine JA, Novotny PJ, Vargas-Chanes D, Krook JE, et al. A simple stratification factor prognostic for survival in advanced cancer: the good/bad/uncertain index. J Clin Oncol 2001;19(15):3539-46.

[8] Wigren T. Confirmation of a prognostic index for patients with inoperable non-small cell lung cancer. Radiother Oncol 1997; 44(1):9-15.
[9] Downing GM, Wainwright W. Palliative Performance Scale (PPSv2) Version 2. Medical care of the dying, 4th ed. Victoria, BC: Victoria Hospice Society Learning Centre Palliat Care, 2006.
[10] Anderson F, Downing GM, Hill J, Casorso L, Lerch N. Palliative performance scale (PPS): a new tool. J Palliat Care 1996;12(1):5-11.
[11] Palliative care strategy: Improving the quality of palliative care services for cancer patients in Ontario. Toronto, ON: Cancer Care Ontario, 2006.
[12] Lau F, Cloutier-Fisher D, Kuziemsky C, Black F, Downing M, Borycki E, et al. A systematic review of prognostic tools for estimating survival time in palliative care. J Palliat Care 2007; 23(2):93-112.
[13] Glare PA, Sinclair CT. Palliative Medicine Review: Prognostication. J Palliat Med 2008;11(1):84-103.
[14] Morita T, Tsunoda J, Inoue S, Chihara S. Validity of the palliative performance scale from a survival perspective. J Pain Symptom Manage 1999;18(1):2-3.
[15] Wilner LS, Arnold RM. The Palliative Performance Scale #125. J Palliat Med 2006;9(4):994.
[16] de Borja MT, Chow E, Bovett G, Davis L, Gillies C. The correlation among patient and health care professionals in assessing functional status using the karnofsky and eastern cooperative oncolog group performance status scales. Support Cancer Ther 2004;2(1):59-63.
[17] Liem BJ, Holland JM, Kang MY, Hoffelt SC, Marquez CM. Karnofsky Performance Status Assessment: resident versus attending. J Cancer Educ 2002;17(3):138-41.
[18] de Miguel Sanchez C, Elustondo SG, Estirado A, Sanchez FV, de la Rasilla Cooper,C.G., Romero AL, et al. Palliative performance status, heart rate and respiratory rate as predictive factors of survival time in terminally ill cancer patients. J Pain Symptom Manage 2006; 31(6):485-92.
[19] Harrold J, Rickerson E, Carroll JT, McGrath J, Morales K, Kapo J, et al. Is the palliative performance scale a useful predictor of mortality in a heterogeneous hospice population? J Palliat Med 2005; 8(3):503-9.
[20] Head B, Ritchie CS, Smoot TM. Prognostication in hospice care: can the palliative performance scale help? J Palliat Med 2005; 8(3):492-502.
[21] Lau F, Downing GM, Lesperance M, Shaw J, Kuziemsky C. Use of Palliative Performance Scale in end-of-life prognostication. J Palliat Med 2006;9(5):1066-75.
[22] Olajide O, Hanson L, Usher BM, Qaqish BF, Schwartz R, Bernard S. Validation of the palliative performance scale in the acute tertiary care hospital setting. J Palliat Med 2007;10(1):111-7.
[23] Virik K, Glare P. Validation of the palliative performance scale for inpatients admitted to a palliative care unit in Sydney, Australia. J Pain Symptom Manage 2002;23(6):455-7.
[24] Oken MM, Creech RH, Tormey DC, Horton J, Davis TE, McFadden ET, et al. Toxicity and response criteria of the Eastern Cooperative Oncology Group. Am J Clin Oncol 1982;5(6):649-55.

[25] Seaton PD, et al. Closer to home. Report of the British Columbia Royal Commission on health care and costs. Victoria, BC: British Columbia Min Health, 1991.

[26] Vigano A, Bruera E, Jhangri GS, Newman SC, Fields AL, Suarez-Almazor ME. Clinical survival predictors in patients with advanced cancer. Arch Intern Med 2000;160(6):861-8.

[27] Morita T, Tsunoda J, Inoue S, Chihara S. The Palliative Prognostic Index: a scoring system for survival prediction of terminally ill cancer patients. Support Care Cancer 1999;7(3):128-33.

Section Four: Quality of Life

In: Advanced Cancer. Pain and Quality of Life
Editors: E. Chow, J. Merrick, pp. 215-223
ISBN: 978-1-61668-207-1
© 2010 Nova Science Publishers, Inc.

Chapter XIX

Can We Measure Quality of Life for Patients with Metastatic Spinal Cord Compression (MSCC)?

Gunita Mitera, MRT(T)*[*1], Nadil Zeiadin, BA[1], Arjun Sahgal, MD[1], Joel Finkelstein, MD[2], Edward Chow, MBBS[1] and Andrew Loblaw, MD[1]

[1]Rapid Response Radiotherapy Program, Department of Radiation Oncology, Odette Cancer Centre, Sunnybrook Health Sciences Centre, University of Toronto, Toronto, Ontario and
[2]Department of Orthopaedic Surgery, Sunnybrook Health Sciences Centre, University of Toronto, Toronto, Ontario, Canada

Patient morbidity from metastatic spinal cord compression (MSCC) includes back pain, paralysis/paresis, limb weakness, sensory loss, and bowel/bladder sphincter compromise. The goal of treatment with either surgery radiation or combined treatment is to improve the patient's quality of life (QOL) through palliation of pain and neurological recovery. QOL measures are important endpoints which are not well developed and infrequently measured. Objective: To identify clinical studies for patients with MSCC where QOL has been reported as either a primary or secondary endpoint. Furthermore, our aim was to report the specific measurement tools employed to capture QOL. Methods: A systematic literature review was conducted using the Ovid MEDLINE(R) 1950 to October 2008 database, Ovid Health and Psychosocial Instruments 1985 to October 2007 database, and EMBASE(R) 1980 to October 2008. Results: Five studies were identified. Two of the five (40%) studies employed the Schedule for Evaluation of Individualized Quality of

* Correspondence: Gunita Mitera MRT(T), Department of Radiation Therapy, Odette Cancer Centre, Sunnybrook Health Sciences Centre, 2075 Bayview Avenue, Toronto, ON M4N 3M5, Canada. Tel: 416-480-6100 ext 7543; Fax: 416-480-4672; E-mail: Gunita.Mitera@sunnybrook.ca

Life (SEIQoL-DW) tool to measure QOL. The Short Form 36 (SF36) Health Survey Questionnaire, the Pediatric Quality of Life Inventory (PedsQL) 4.0 Generic Core scale, and the Functional Assessment of Cancer Therapy (FACT-G) scales were generic QOL investigation tools that were used in the remaining three studies. Conclusions: Amongst the five studies that defined QOL as an endpoint, there was no consistency in the measure used. There appears to be no specific QOL survey tool for the MSCC population. Therefore, we identify the need to develop a tool specific for this population in order to generate meaningful data for future trials.

Introduction

Malignant spinal cord compression (MSCC) is defined as compression of the thecal sac that surrounds the spinal cord or cauda equina by an extradural tumour mass (1,2). This is a dreaded complication of advanced malignancy where neurological function may be compromised without immediate medical attention, hence, prioritizing it as an "oncological emergency" (3-5). The clinical incidence of MSCC is between 2.5% and 10% for all cancer patients (2-7), but this can be higher depending on factors such as primary cancer, disease stage and age (2). Population-based data reports that 2.5% of patients dying from cancer have at least one admission for MSCC (7). One study reports among the half a million patients who die from cancer each year, 12,700 will suffer from spinal cord compression (1) and therefore be at risk for back pain (1,3,4,8), sensory deficits, loss of mobility through paraplegia or paralysis (1,4,8-10) or incontinence (1,3,7,9).

Prognostic factors for MSCC have been reported in the literature to include the primary cancer, time interval from primary tumour diagnosis to the time of MSCC development, pre-treatment ambulatory function, time to developing motor deficits before radiation treatment, absence of visceral or other bony metastasis, and re-irradiation for in-field recurrences of MSCC (11,12-17). Life expectancy after MSCC is generally short with an expected median survival between three and six months (3,5); however, a small proportion of patients can live for years underscoring the importance of more aggressive treatment in patients with better prognosis. Radiation therapy and surgery are accepted as the primary modalities of treatment. Recently, a randomized trial has shown potential benefits in terms of neurologic recovery and survival for patients treated with a combined surgical and post-operative approach (17). However, poor performance status or surgical technical limitations render many patients ineligible for surgery and thus radiation therapy alone becomes the main treatment option. The goal of treatment is often considered to be palliation of pain, neurological recovery, and quality of life (2,3,5,9,15,18). Consequently, given the short life expectancy for these patients, it is important for them to maintain the best possible quality of life (QOL) for their remaining lifespan.

Most studies investigating treatment outcomes for spinal cord compression emphasize physical parameters, such as mobility and sphincter disturbances (8). However, according to patient reports, poor physical function is not directly associated or predictive of poor quality of life (8,20). Consequently, an increasing emphasis has been placed on QOL as an endpoint in clinical investigations. The World Health Organization defines health as "a state of complete physical, mental and social well-being and not merely the absence of disease or infirmity" (21). This multi-dimensional definition of health has encouraged health care professionals and research investigators to incorporate all aspects of health in treatment including QOL. Over the last three decades there have been numerous studies on QOL in medical literature. A Medline search using "quality of life" as a keyword reveals a significant increase in the number of articles related to the topic over a period of 30 years, from 32 in 1973 to 31,522 in 2008 (22). Interestingly, more recent publications are emphasizing the importance of the patient's perspective on QOL. According to patients, this may encompass physical, social, and cognitive levels of functioning and may have varying degrees of importance unique to the individual (9,20,23,24).

Consequently, effectiveness of treatments for MSCC patients should be evaluated from the patient's perspective. While few studies focus on QOL as a primary or secondary endpoint, we believe that research should incorporate this important outcome. Additionally, QOL measures should incorporate the unique components important to a MSCC patient population. QOL instruments help health care professionals quantify the impact of new or existing treatments on various aspects of a patient's life. For example, site-specific QOL measures have been developed to target the specific needs of each population (23,24). However, to our knowledge there are no published QOL measures specific for a MSCC population. The objective of this study was to review and document the extent to which previous studies have considered quality of life (QOL) as either a primary or secondary endpoint in MSCC study populations and document the specific measurement tool employed to capture QOL.

Our Study

A literature review was conducted in October 2008 using the Ovid MEDLINE(R) 1950 to October 2008 database, Ovid Health and Psychosocial Instruments 1985 to October 2007 database, and EMBASE(R) 1980 to October 2008 database using the terms "spinal cord compression" or "spinal compression" and "quality of life" and "cancer or neoplasm or metastasis or tumor." In the MEDLINE and EMBASE databases, we combined the terms "spinal cord compression" or "cauda equina (compression or compressed)" or "metastatic spinal cord compression" or "malignant spinal cord compression" with "quality of life" and "cancer or neoplasm or metastasis or tumor." Relevant articles and abstracts were reviewed and references from these sources were also manually searched for additional relevant publications.

The following information was extracted from the studies: the primary and secondary outcome, type and number of QOL measures used, any additional tools used, number of patients, median age and median survival, and symptom palliation. Articles were included in the literature review based on the subsequent criteria. The study population was patients diagnosed with malignant spinal cord compression or cauda equina compression; all study intervention was acceptable; randomized control trials, prospective or retrospective cohort studies were included; quality of life (QOL) measure or symptom palliation as measure of QOL were all acceptable endpoints. Articles were excluded from the literature review if they were non-English publications; testing efficacy of a treatment at prolonging development of malignant spinal cord compression or cauda equina compression or equating QOL with absence of MSCC or cauda equina compression; used performance assessment tools only; Heterogeneous study populations i.e. not exclusively MSCC or cauda equina compression patients; Individual case reports, or qualitative studies were also excluded.

Our Findings

Of 322 published results that manifested using the literature search criteria, only 5 studies assessed QOL as a primary or secondary endpoint and also used a QOL measure for their MSCC study populations. These studies are listed in table 1.

Schedule for evaluation of individualized quality of life (SEIQoL-DW)

Two of the five (40%) studies (8,20) employed the Schedule for Evaluation of Individualized Quality of Life (SEIQoL-DW) to measure quality of life. The SEIQoL-DW is a three-stage semi-structured, individualized interview measure from 0 (worst) to 100 (best), and has been validated for use in patients with advanced cancer (8,20,25). The questionnaire asks patients to nominate five areas of their life, termed cues, which contribute most to their QOL (20,25). Next, patients are asked to judge at which level each nominated cue is functioning by rating against a vertical visual analog scale labeled at the upper and lower extremities by the terms ''as good as could possibly be'' and ''as bad as could possibly be'' (25). In the third stage, patients provide the relative importance of each cue by "weighing" each cue relative to each other (20,25) The third stage of the SEIQoL-DW varies from that of the SEQoL in the method participants use to weight the relative importance of each QoL aspect, with the DW (direct weighing) method being more simple and direct. The SEIQoL-DW provides a global quality of life score ranging from 0 (no quality whatsoever) to 100 (perfect quality of life) as well as a personal and prioritized list of important areas of life for each patient (20,25). The SEIQoL-DW achieves high internal validity (R2= 0.88) and high internal reliability (r=0.90) (25).

The median SEIQoL score in the Conway et al (8) sample (n=128) for patients at one month after diagnosis of spinal cord compression was 72/100 and a median Karnofsky performance status of 50. In a sample of 180 patients shortly after MSCC diagnosis, Levack et al. (20) found a median SEIQoL score of 66/100 and a median KPS of 40. Both studies found a significant correlation between SEIQoL and performance status, with higher KPS associated with better SEIQoL scores (8,20). Nonetheless, physical disability was not significantly associated with SEIQoL and the effect of the physical condition on quality of life was surprisingly small (8,20). In fact, ninety-one percent of patients nominated family life as an important contributor to their quality of life. The average level of functioning of family life was 95% while the average weighting for this aspect was 30%. This means that patients determined that one third of their quality of life was determined by the level of functioning of their family life. On the other hand, health was nominated by only 44% and had an overall poor level of functioning and weighting of 20% (20).

Author, Year, Trial Type	Study Purpose	N	Median Survival	QoL Assessment Tools	Performance Assessment Tool	Other Assessment Tools/ Measures	Number of instruments used to measure QoL
Conway R, Graham J, Kidd J, Levack P. 2007 P	To present further findings from the Scottish Cord Compression Study, diagnosis, management and outcome of MSCC were examined.	128	59 days (i.e. approx 2 months)	Schedule for Evaluation of Individual Quality of Life (SEIQoL – Dw)	Karnofsky Performance Status	Hospital Anxiety and Depression Scale, Visual Analogue Scale for Pain, Mobility	1
Levack P, Graham J, Kidd J. 2004 P	Examine QoL in recently diagnosed MSCC patients	180	59 days.	Schedule for the Evaluation of Individual Quality of Life (SEIQoL-Dw)	Karnosky Performance Status	Barthel Disability Index, Hospital Anxiety and Depression Scale	1
Mannion RJ, Wilby M, Godward S, Lyratzopoulos G, Lain RJC2007 P	Prospective cohort study of metastatic cord or cauda equina compression patients treated with surgical decompression and fixation	62	13 Months	SF-36	N/A	Visual analogue pain scores, Roland Morris back pain scores.	1
Poretti A, Zehnder D, Boltshauser E, Grotzer MA 2008 P	Document effect of neurological deficits on social and psychological adjustment and quality of life of pediatric MSCC patients	28	The 10-year overall survival rate was 96%	PedsQL (Pediatric Quality of Life Inventory) 4.0 Generic Core to measure health related (HR) QoL	Functional Independence Measure (FIM) and WeeFIM	Youth Self Report (YSR) and Child Behavior Check List (CBCL)	1
Sundaresan N, Sachdev VP, Holland JF, Moore F, Sung M, et al. 1995 R	Determine results and outcome (incl. QoL) of patients with spincal metastasis treated with surgery	110	16 Months	Functional Assessment of Cancer Therapy Scale (FACT-G)	N/A	N/A	1

Notes: P – Prospective R - Retrospective

SF36

The remaining three studies employed different quality of life measures. In one study by Mannion et al. (27), the Short Form 36 (SF36) Health Survey Questionnaire was employed as a quality of life measure in a spinal cord compression patient population. The SF36 is a widely employed general outcome measure (26,27). It attempts to capture important health dimensions common to all patients. The SF36 assesses 8 health scales to measure 3 aspects of health, functional status, well being and overall evaluation of health, and assigns individual and an overall quality of life score from 0 to 100. The SF-36 has high internal consistency, with Crohnbach alphas exceeding 0.80 and correlation coefficients of 0.55 - 0.78. Clinical validity was also established through clear and predictable differences between general and patient populations (26). Furthermore, the questionnaire has been shown to be sensitive enough to detect changes in population health. For example, a significant improvement in SF-36 scores was shown in patients three months post-surgical decompression treatment. Improvements were seen in physical function, role limitation and bodily pain (27).

Pediatric Quality of Life Inventory (pedsQL) 4.0 Generic Core

Poretti et al (28) employed the Pediatric Quality of Life Inventory (PedsQL) 4.0 Generic Core scales to measure quality of life in a pediatric population of patients with intraspinal tumors with spinal cord compression. The PedsQL is a generic health related QOL measure that can be utilized with children and adolescents between the ages of 2 and 18 across different patient populations. It is a child self-report or parent proxy-report measure. The 23-items of the PedsQL 4.0 Generic Core assess the central physical, mental and social health dimensions as defined by the World Health Organization. Additionally, it assesses school functioning. The questionnaire has been shown to be valid and reliable, with alpha scores of 0.88 for child self-report and 0.90 for parent proxy-report (28). A sample of 20 pediatric MSCC patients scored lower on the PedsQL compared to healthy controls, 79.35 and 83.00, respectively. Nonetheless, the difference was not significant. In fact, emotional functioning was the only QOL aspect significantly impaired, while social and school functioning showed no significant impairments. The quality of life scores of the PedsQL were significantly correlated with functional independence scores, paresis and neurogenic bladder and bowel dysfunction (9).

Functional Assessment of Cancer Therapy (FACT-G)

The Functional Assessment of Cancer Therapy (FACT-G) scale was employed by Sundaresan et al (29). The 33-items of the FACT-G are divided into five subscales: physical well-being, social well-being, emotional well-being, functional well-being and relationship with doctor. The FACT-G is reliable and valid given the internal consistency of the FACT-G score had an alpha value of 0.89 and test-retest correlation coefficient of 0.92. Additionally, the questionnaire is able to differentiate patients according to stage of disease ECOG performance status rating and hospitalization status. Furthermore, the questionnaire allows patients to assign personal weights to each of the five subscales, which provides an evaluation of the objective functional impairment and the perceived effect of the impairment on quality of life (29). In the Sundaresan et al (29) study, in which they analyzed the post-surgical outcome of 110 MSCC patients, the mean post-surgery score on the FACT-G was 83, corresponding to a positive outcome in terms of quality of life.

Discussion

Malignant spinal cord compression (MSCC) is an oncologic emergency and represents a major cause of morbidity in advanced cancer patients (3-5). Consequently, MSCC requires prompt diagnosis and treatment in order to preserve quality of life (4). Prognosis for MSCC patients is proven to be poor (2) and the aim of treatment is generally palliative (3-5). As such, a central aim of palliative treatment is to incorporate a combined approach of direct management of the physical symptoms as well as improving quality of life (3). However, what healthcare providers consider to be a patient's QOL may not in fact correspond to what the patient them self define as QOL (20).

The concept of QOL is inherently complex since it purposely incorporates a multitude of factors. However, the emphasis on holistic patient care which incorporates QOL has increased. This is evident by the number of health-related QOL measures that have been published in recent times (20, 22,25,26,28,30). In particular, in cancer related study populations the EORTC QLQ-C30 is the most frequently used QOL tool. This measure is a general QOL measure that uses 30 core questions in attempt to assess overall QOL (20,31).

However, studies measuring the efficacy of treatment for MSCC often do not incorporate quality of life as an endpoint (8). Most studies of treatment outcome focus on physical parameters such as motor function, functional status, local tumor control, ambulatory status and survival (12,13, 15,29). Additionally, it has been reported that healthcare providers associate a patient's physical health to their quality of life, however, from the patient's perspective this may not be true (8). For example, in three of the five studies which examined multiple components of QOL, the physical condition had an unremarkable effect on quality of life (8,9,20). Indeed, patients which had major physical disability such as decreased mobility and neurological dysfunction rated their quality of life scores as good (8,20) or not significantly different from their healthy counterparts (9). Therefore, to ensure patients continue to have both quality and meaning during their remaining life, it is important to consider improvements in quality of life from the patient's perspective when measuring treatment outcome (27).

Physical functioning is only one component of quality of life. Other main components assessed by the quality of life measures used on the MSCC patient population include social well-being, mental well-being and emotional well-being (26,28,29). As such, it is important to incorporate a more holistic approach to the study of quality of life in general and specifically in the MSCC research field. Furthermore, in order to account for the individualistic property of quality of life, QOL measures should also incorporate a subjective component to allow patients to report their perceived level of QOL. Our analysis revealed only two measures that have been applied in the MSCC patient population which incorporate an individualistic approach to QOL (5,8,20).

The SEIQoL questionnaire allows patients to nominate their own components of QOL as well as report the level of functioning and importance of each component (8,20,25). Congruent with the idea that physical functioning is not the most important aspect of QOL; family life was most frequently nominated and was generally given the highest importance for determining QOL (20). The FACT-G questionnaire allows patients to assign personal importance to each QOL components assessed in the measure, which allows for a simultaneous evaluation of functional impairment and its perceived effect (29).

Due to the complexities of the concept of QOL (20), it is important to approach the assessment of QOL in a multi-dimensional manner which incorporates the subjective dimension. However, it is also important to employ a measure which is easy to administer in the MSCC population. For example, only a fraction of patients were able to complete the SEIQoL (64% of sample alive at one month follow-up) (8) or the SF-36 (29% of sample alive at one month follow-up) (27), because of the burden of their disease. Overall, we found that all of the QOL measures used in the MSCC patient population were general QOL measures and assessed multiple components of QOL that may or may not be relevant to this population (5,8,9,20,27). Furthermore, we also found that MSCC patients have a better level of QOL than would be assumed based on the physical condition (8,9,20). Finally, our analysis revealed that QOL is important to this population and can be measured from the patients' perspective using appropriate QOL tools (5,9, 27). Consequently, considerations should be given to develop a QOL module specific for MSCC patients to be used in future studies incorporate quality of life as a primary endpoint when assessing treatment efficacy.

Conclusions

Our findings show that despite the increased attention in recent years on quality of life of patients, only a small amount of research has investigated QOL in malignant spinal cord compression patients. Also, no consistent QOL measure was used across the studies for this group, which makes it difficult to compare findings or understand the relative meaning of a score on a measure. Furthermore, the concept of QOL must be expanded beyond just the physical condition to include cognitive and emotional aspects as well as unique subjective components of the patient. Only two measures incorporated all of these aspects (5,8,20). However, these measures tended to be quite demanding on patients to complete (8,20) and did not capture the unique, disease-specific components of this patient population. As such, future research should focus on designing an assessment tool for QOL in the MSCC patient population that is both easy to administer and incorporates physical, emotional, social, cognitive and subjective dimensions.

References

[1] Abrahm, JL. Assessment and treatment of patients with malignant spinal cord compression. J Support Oncol 2004;2(5): 377-401.

[2] Prasad D, Schiff D. Malignant spinal-cord compression. Lancet Oncol 2005;6(1):15-24.

[3] Aass N, Fossa SD. Pre- and post-treatment daily life function in patients with hormone resistant prostate carcinoma treated with radiotherapy for spinal cord compression. Radiat Oncol 2005; 74:259-65.

[4] Penas-Prado M, Loghin ME. Spinal cord compression in cancer patients: Review of diagnosis and treatment. Curr Oncol Rep 2008; 10(1):78-85.

[5] Sundaresan N, Sachdev VP, Holland JF, Moore F, Sung M, et al. Surgical treatment of spinal cord compression from epidural metastasis. J Clin Oncol 1995;13(9): 2330-5.

[6] Jawahar A, Ampil F, Reddy PK, Harman GH, Sathyanarayana S, Nanda A. Analysis of outcome and prognostic factors in metastatic cauda equina compression: A 20-year single institution experience. Neurosurg Quart 2002;12(2):108-13.

[7] Loblaw DA, Laperriere NJ, Mackillop WJ. A Population-based study of malignant spinal cord compression in Ontario. Clin Oncol 2003; 15:211-7.

[8] Conway R, Graham J, Kidd J, Levack P. What happens to people after malignant spinal cord compression? Survival, function, quality of life, emotional well-being and place of care 1 month after diagnosis. Clin Oncol 2007;19:56-62.

[9] Poretti A, Zehnder D, Boltshauser E, Grotzer MA. Long-term complications and quality of life in children with intraspinal tumors. Pediatr Blood Cancer 2008;50(4):844-8.

[10] Tang V. Harvey D. Park Dorsay J. Jiang S. Rathbone MP. Prognostic indicators in metastatic spinal cord compression: using functional independence measure and Tokuhashi scale to optimize rehabilitation planning. Spinal Cord 2007;45(10):671-7.

[11] Helweg-Larsen S, Sorensen P, Kreiner S. Prognostic factors in metastatic spinal cord compression: A prospective study using multivariate analysis of variables influencing survival and gait function in 153 patients. Int J Radiat Oncol Biol Phys 2000;46(5):1163-9.

[12] Rades D, Fehlauer F, Veninga T, Stalpers LJ, Basic H, et al. Escalation of radiation dose beyond 30Gy in 10 fractions for metastatic spinal cord compression. Int J Radiat Oncol Biol Phys 2007;67(2):525-31.

[13] Rades D, Fehlauer F, Veninga T, Stalpers LJ, Basic H, et al. Functional outcome and survival after radiotherapy of metastatic spinal cord compression in patients with cancer of unknown primary. Int J Radiat Oncol Biol Phys 2007;67(2):532-7.

[14] Rades D, Heidenreich F, Bremer M, Karstens J. Time of developing motor deficits before radiotherapy as a new and relevant prognostic factor in metastatic spinal cord compression: Final results of a retrospective analysis. Eur Neurol 2001;45:266-9.

[15] Rades D, Rudat V, Veninga T, Stalpers LJ, Hoskin PJ, Schild SE. Prognostic factors for functional outcome and survival after reirradiation for in-field recurrences of metastatic spinal cord compression. Cancer 2008;113(5):1090-6.

[16] Rades D, Stalpers LJA, Veninga T, Rudat V, Schults R, Hoskin PJ. Evaluation of functional outcome and local control after radiotherapy for metastatic spinal cord compression in patients with prostate cancer. J Urol 2006;175:552-6,9.

[17] Venkitaraman R, Barbachano Y, Dearnaley DA, Parker CC, Khoo V, Huddart RA, Eeles R, Horwich A, Sohaid A. Outcome of early detection and radiotherapy for occult spinal cord compression. Radiother Oncol 2007;85:469-72.

[18] Patchell RA, Tibbs PA, Regine WF, Payne R, Saris S, Kryscio RJ, Mohiuddin M, Young B. Direct decompressive surgical resection in the treatment of spinal cord compression caused by metastatic cancer: a randomised trial. Lancet 2005;366(9486):643-8.

[19] Kovner F, Shulem S, Rider I, et al. Radiation therapy of metastatic spinal cord compression. J Neurooncol 1999;42:85-92.

[20] Levack P, Graham J, Kidd J. Listen to the patient: Quality of life of patients with recently diagnosed malignant cord compression in relation to their disability. Palliat Med 2004;18(7):594-601.

[21] World Health Organization. http://www.who.int/en/

[22] Schoeggl A, Reddy M, Matula C. Neurological outcome following laminectomy in spinal metastases. Spinal Cord 2002;40:363-6.

[23] Tharmalingam S, Chow E, Harris K, Hird A, Sinclair E. Quality of life measurement in bone metastases: A literature review. J Pain Res, in press.

[24] Wong J, Hird A, Kirou-Mauro A, Napolskikh J, Chow E. Quality of life in brain metastases radiation trials: a literature review. J Curr Oncol 2008;15(5):25-45.

[25] Waldron D, O'Boyle CA, Kearney M, Moriarty M, Carney D. Quality-of-life measurement in advanced cancer: Assessing the individual. J Clin Oncol 1999;17(11):3603-11.

[26] Garratt AM, Ruta DA, Abdalla MI, Buckingham JK, Russell IT. The SF36 health survey questionnaire: an outcome measure suitable for routine use within the NHS? BMJ 1993;306(6890):1440-4.

[27] Mannion RJ, Wilby M, Godward S, Lyratzopoulos G, Lain RJC. The surgical management of metastatic spinal disease: Prospective assessment and long-term follow-up. Br J Neurosurg 2007;21(6): 593-8.

[28] Varni JW, Seid M, Knight TS, Uzark K, Szer IS. The PedsQL 4.0 Generic Core Scales: Sensitivity, responsiveness, and impact on clinical decision-making. J Behav Med 2002;25(2):175-93.

[29] Cella DF, Tulsky DS, Gray G, Sarafian B, Linn E, et al. The functional assessment of cancer therapy scale: Development and validation of the general measure. J Clin Oncol 1993;11(3):570-9.

[30] Rades D, Walz J, Schild SE, Veninga T, Dunst J. Do bladder cancer patients with metastatic spinal cord compression benefit from radiotherapy alone?. Urology 2007; 69(6):1081-5.

[31] Aaronson NK, Ahmedzai S, Bergman B, et al. The European Organisation for Research and Treatment of Cancer. QLQ-C30: a quality of life instrument for use in international clinical trials in oncology. J Natl Cancer Inst 1993;85:365-76.

In: Advanced Cancer. Pain and Quality of Life
Editors: E. Chow, J. Merrick, pp. 225-232

ISBN: 978-1-61668-207-1
© 2010 Nova Science Publishers, Inc.

Chapter XX

The European Organization for Research and Treatment of Cancer Quality-of-Life Group Bone Metastases Module (EORTC QLQ-BM22) questionnaire

*Candi J. Flynn, MSc(C)[1], Mark Clemons, MD[2], Liying Zhang, PhD[1] and Edward Chow, MBBS[*1]*

[1]Rapid Response Radiotherapy Program, Radiation Oncology, Odette Cancer Centre, Toronto, Ontario and [2]Medical Oncology, Princess Margaret Hospital and Campbell Family Institute for Breast Cancer Research, Toronto, Ontario, Canada

Clinical trials in palliative care settings require reliable and brief quality-of-life (QOL) assessment tools in order to obtain valid results with minimal burden on participants. Traditionally, patients with bone metastases in clinical trials have completed general QOL instruments, which did not cover the key issues pertinent for this specific population. The EORTC QLQ-BM22 was developed to supplement the EORTC QLQ-C30 core questionnaire as a bone metastases specific qualify-of-life instrument with cross-culture relevance. Methods: One hundred and fourteen patients at the Odette Cancer Centre and Princess Margaret Hospital were enrolled. Patients completed the EORTC QLQ-BM22 questionnaire in person at baseline during their clinic appointment, and completed the follow-up BM22 questionnaire one week later by telephone. A follow-up report was completed at the time of the one week follow-up to record any changes in clinical conditions and/or treatments. Results: Employing a 95% confidence interval, an intraclass correlation coefficient (ICC) was used to assess agreement between the baseline and follow-up responses for each BM22 item. The ICC values (median = 0.80;

* Correspondence: Edward Chow, MBBS, PhD, FRCPC, Department of Radiation Oncology, Odette Cancer Centre, Sunnybrook Health Sciences Centre, 2075 Bayview Avenue, Toronto, ON M4N 3M5, Canada. Tel: 416-480-4998; Fax: 416-480-6002; E-mail: Edward.Chow@sunnybrook.ca

range of 0.55-0.89) for the 22 items revealed 'moderate' (2 items), 'good' (10 items), and 'very good' (10 items) reliability. Conclusion: Based on the overall consistent agreement between the baseline and follow-up interview results, the EORTC QLQ-BM22 appears to be a reliable instrument for cancer patients with bone metastases.

Introduction

Bone metastases are common in patients with advanced cancers (1). Breast and prostate carcinomas are the most common to spread to bone, with an incidence of 75% and 68%, respectively (1). In addition, lung, thyroid, and renal carcinomas metastasize to bone in approximately 40% of cases (1).

Advances in effective systemic treatment and supportive care have substantially improved survival of patients with bone metastases. In fact, the prevalence of bone metastases in cancer patients is estimated to be double the number of new cases (2). For certain subsets of patients with bone metastases (e.g. breast and prostate cancer with predominately bone or bone-only metastases) life expectancies have increased to a range of approximately 2-5 years (3). With this increased survival, effective management of bone metastases has become essential in order to reduce skeletal complications and maximize patient quality-of-life (QOL).

A number of indicators of the need for reassessment of management strategies in patients with bone metastases have been identified (4). Such indicators include: i) pain arising from bone metastases is the most common symptom requiring treatment in cancer patients; ii) the symptoms of bone metastases are often severe; 50 to 75% of patients with bone metastases suffer from severe pain (1); iii) complication of skeletal metastases are common and can seriously impair patient QOL and function. Pain and impaired mobility occur in 65-75% of patients with bone metastases. Fractures of weight-bearing long bones occur in 10-20%; hypercalcaemia occurs in 10-15%; and spinal cord or nerve root compression occurs in 5%; iv) increasing incidence of bone metastases and longer survival duration of patients with bone metastases and v) increasing emphasis to assess the efficacy and side effects of existing and new interventions, as well as QOL from the patient's perspective.

According to the World Health Organization, health is described as 'a state of complete physical, mental and social well-being, and not merely the absence of disease or infirmity' (5). In palliative trials, symptom control as well as QOL is a major endpoint. Quality-of-life measurement is subjective in nature and is a multidimensional construct which reflects functional status, psychosocial well-being, health perceptions, and disease- and treatment-related symptoms from the patient's perspective (6). Quality-of-life incorporates a patient's expectations, satisfaction, value system and the other important aspects of his or her life. Since palliative interventions are unlikely to lead to survival prolongation and significant tumour regression, QOL is a more meaningful endpoint when compared with the traditional endpoints, such as survival times and local control. Thus, any palliative interventions should primarily aim to improve the QOL of patients with advanced cancer.

Some trials have employed the European Organization for Research and Treatment of Cancer QOL Group core questionnaire (EORTC QLQ-C30), version 3. There are a number of advantages to using this instrument, including extensive validation, available reference data, standardized procedures for scoring and translation, and a large number of published studies that have utilized this tool (7). However, it was not specifically designed to address the QOL issues relevant for cancer patients with bone metastases. There was, therefore, a need to develop a disease-specific QOL questionnaire for bone metastases patients to supplement the validated EORTC QLQ-C30. Consequently, the Bone Metastases Module (EORTC QLQ-BM22; from now on referred to as BM22) was created to address this need. This module addresses QOL issues that are particularly important to patients with bone metastases and are not sufficiently covered by the EORTC QLQ-C30. The instrument contains a total of 22 questions with 19 items that form three scales: Painful Sites (questions 1-5), Pain Characteristics (questions 6-8), Functional Interference (questions 9-15), and Psychosocial Aspects (questions 16-22).

The BM22 is presently undergoing large scale international field testing (Phase IV) as part of its development and validation. This phase of development aims to determine the test-retest reliability, validity and cross-cultural applicability of the module by testing the questionnaire in a large, international group of patients. The primary objective of the present study was to examine the test-retest reliability of the EORTC QLQ-BM22, and in doing so determine the degree to which the instrument is free from random measurement error. The secondary objective was to verify the relevance of the 22 items to patients diagnosed with bone metastases.

Our Study

Patients attending palliative radiation and medical oncology clinics at the Odette Cancer Centre and Princess Margaret Hospital in Toronto, Ontario between January and March 2008 were considered for study eligibility. Patients exhibiting radiological evidence of osseous metastases who were able to comprehend the survey and provide informed consent were approached to participate. Those who were not fit to complete the questionnaire or were unavailable for follow-up were excluded. In total, 114 patients were able to complete the study.

Once a patient was deemed eligible for study participation by their treating oncologist, he or she was approached by the clinical research assistant to discuss the study during his or her regularly scheduled appointment. All agreeable patients provided written informed consent and completed the EORTC QLQ-BM22 questionnaire (Figure 1) by rating their general pain and the degree of provocation of their symptoms and emotions by various activities. The clinical research assistant was available to assist the patients if necessary and was responsible for collecting patient demographics, disease information and treatment history as baseline measurements. Patients were contacted for follow-up via telephone one week after their initial interview. At this point they were asked to complete the EORTC QLQ-BM22 questionnaire again, and a follow-up report was compiled to record any changes in clinical condition and/or treatments. A one week period was selected as the appropriate time interval due to the recommendation that within this time frame patients are unlikely to both recall their previous responses and to experience significant changes in their condition relating to their bone metastases (7).

The statistical methodology involved within this study included the Wilcoxon rank-sum test, the Fisher exact test, and Intraclass Correlation Coefficients. The Wilcoxon rank-sum test (for continuous variables) and the Fisher exact test (for categorical variables) were conducted to determine which variables predicted good concordance between both administrations of the questionnaire. Intraclass correlation coefficients (ICCs) were determined to assess the agreement between each BM22 item on the test and retest questionnaires. Intraclass correlation coefficient values range from 0.00 to 1.00 and measure inter-rater reliability. Intraclass correlation coefficients are classified as belonging to one of five categories: Poor (range 0-0.20), fair (range 0.21-0.40), moderate (range 0.41-0.60), good (range 0.61-0.80), or very good (range 0.81-1.00). Statistical Analysis Systems (SAS, version 9.1) Macro was employed to calculate the ICCs with 95% confidence intervals. Results were considered significant at the 5% critical level (two sided p-value < 0.05). The study proposal and consent forms were reviewed and approved by the institutional Research Ethics Boards at both of the participating centres.

Our Findings

Patient characteristics are summarized in table 1. In total, 71 patients were female (62%) and 43 (38%) were male. The median age was 61 years with a range of 32-87 years. Breast and prostate cancers were most prevalent at 61% and 30%, respectively. Lung (4%) and renal cell (2%) carcinomas, as well as multiple myeloma (2%) were less common primaries. In general, patients were most often interviewed within medical oncology clinics (75%). This was followed by radiation oncology (17%) and multidisciplinary clinics (7%). With regards to the extent of patient metastases, the majority of those surveyed had two separate organ systems with metastatic disease (48%), with three (44%) and four (8%) metastatic locations being less frequently witnessed.

Concordance between test and re-test responses

Good concordance is defined as having the absolute difference between the test and the re-test responses equal to zero. The number of patients who obtained good concordance between the initial and follow-up questionnaires is shown in table 2. Overall, concordance ranged from 56.6% to 75.5% with a median value of 65.1%. Items 16 (felt isolated from those close to you?), 5 (pain in your buttocks?) and 4 (pain in your chest/ribs?) demonstrated the best concordance with 75.5%, 74.5% and 71.7% of responding patients obtaining good concordance, respectively. The worst concordance was demonstrated by items 7 (intermittent pain?), 17 (thinking about your illness?), and 22 (felt positive about your health?) with only 56.6%, 58.1% and 59.2% of responding patients obtaining good concordance, respectively. Percentages were based on the number of respondents as not all participants answered each item on the questionnaire.

Few demographic variables were successful at consistently predicting good concordance. Only eight items on the questionnaire had significant predictive variables, including items 5 (pain in your buttocks?), 8 (pain not relieved by pain medications?), 9 (pain while sitting or lying down?), 11 (pain while walking?), 14 (pain interfered with your sleeping at night?), 16 (felt isolated from those close to you?), 19 (worried about becoming dependent on others?), and 20 (worried about your health in the future?). Predictors of good concordance for each of the items were as follows: item 5 - the clinic in which the patient was received ($p = 0.0001$) and their primary cancer site ($p = 0.0020$); item 8 – clinic ($p = 0.0269$) and previous radiotherapy treatment ($p = 0.0370$); item 9 – previous chemotherapy treatment ($p = 0.0120$); item 11 – previous radiotherapy treatment ($p = 0.0037$); item 14 – clinic ($p = 0.0120$); item 16 – age ($p = 0.0244$); item 19 – previous radiotherapy treatment ($p = 0.0494$); and item 20 – previous chemotherapy treatment ($p=0.0171$). The remaining items failed to demonstrate any significant predictors of good concordance.

Agreement between test and re-test items

The ICC values and their respective 95% confidence intervals for each item of the BM22 questionnaire are available in Table 3. Of the 22 items, 10 (45%) demonstrated 'very good' agreement, 10 (45%) demonstrated 'good' agreement, and 2 (9%) demonstrated 'moderate' agreement between the test and retest questionnaires. The ICC values ranged from 0.55 to 0.89 with a median value of 0.80. In general, items related to future perspectives, patient concerns or the impact of osseous metastases on activity demonstrated 'very good' agreement. Items that dealt with the characteristics or location of the pain often demonstrated 'good' agreement. The only location of pain that demonstrated moderate agreement was the buttocks. One's degree of social isolation also only demonstrated moderate agreement.

Discussion

The European Organization for Research and Treatment of Cancer (EORTC) QOL Group has endorsed a modular approach to the evaluation of QOL in cancer patients involved in clinical trials since 1986. The development and validation of the C30 core questionnaire initiated this improvement in QOL assessment, and subsequent cancer- and site-specific modules have continued this advancement (9,10). Detailed guidelines, published to ensure scientific rigour of module development, were strictly followed during the creation of the BM22 (11). The module development process consists of four phases, including: (I) Generation of the relevant QOL issues; (II) Operationalization; (III) Pretesting; and (IV) Large scale international field testing. Phase I includes a literature search and semi-structured interviews with patients and health care professionals to generate a list of potential QOL issues. Phase II involves operationalizing the list of QOL issues into questions while using the format and time frame of the C30 core questionnaire. Phase III aims to identify and solve potential problems in the questionnaire's administration (e.g. the phrasing of questions, the sequence of questions), as well as to determine the need for additional questions or the elimination of others. Phase IV, as previously mentioned, involves testing the module questionnaire in a larger, international group of patients in order to determine its test-retest reliability, validity and cross-cultural applicability. Once a module has been developed, it is administered along with the C30 core questionnaire (or the C15-PAL for palliative patients with low performance status) to obtain a comprehensive QOL assessment in cancer patients.

The present study served to determine the reliability of the BM22 questionnaire. Concordance or percent agreement was calculated for each item of the module and determined the proportion of all patients whom provided identical responses to test and retest questions (12). Overall, good concordance was consistently demonstrated by a majority of patients for each item of the questionnaire. The best concordance was obtained by items dealing with pain locations and social isolation. This finding is intuitive, as pain is expected to be found in the location of osseous lesions, which are unlikely to change within a week's time. In addition, a patient's interpreted level of social interaction is also anticipated to remain constant within the initial and follow-up interviews. The worst concordance occurred in the items dealing with intermittent pain and psychosocial aspects. These findings are also not unexpected, as intermittent pain, by definition, is presumed to vary, and future concerns may be altered in tune with these bodily changes. Not all participants answered each item on the questionnaire, and so percentages were merely based on the number of respondents. This may have affected the results obtained within the study. However, as the questions were generally answered by a great majority of the participants, it is unlikely that the results have been altered to any significant degree.

Good concordance was successfully predicted by few demographic variables. The clinic in which the patient was interviewed and having previous radiotherapy treatment both significantly predicted good concordance in three items each. Previous chemotherapy treatment was a successful predictor in two items, and age and primary care site both only predicted good concordance in one item of the questionnaire. Despite these significant findings, it is unlikely that these demographic variables are relevant for maximizing concordance in future module development, as no single variable was a consistent predictor throughout the entirety of the BM22 questionnaire. In addition, a large proportion of the interviewed sample was breast cancer patients. Therefore, it is possible that this heavily weighted group of individuals may have induced statistical significance of variables relevant to their own condition (e.g. clinic and previous treatment). For this reason, it is suggested that these findings be interpreted with due caution until future research can confirm their significance.

An important potential limitation when employing concordance is that this measure fails to account for agreement that chance alone could predict (12). Therefore, ICC's, which correct for chance agreement, may be a more suitable measure for determining the test-retest reliability of the BM22. As the majority of items demonstrated either 'very good' or 'good' reliability, it appears as if the module is a reliable instrument. No specific ICC cut-offs for identifying module reliability is available within the EORTC guidelines (11). Therefore, the results and conclusions of previously published EORTC studies were employed as a measure of which to compare our results and draw conclusions in regards to our own module's reliability (10,13,14).

The two items that only expressed moderate reliability may have been influenced by the varying circumstances under which the initial and follow-up questionnaires were administered. The baseline measures were acquired following regularly scheduled appointments in comparison to the telephone interviews that were conducted for the follow-up portion of the study. For example, pain may have been exacerbated in a patient's buttocks after traveling to the hospital and waiting in the clinic for his or her appointment. This pain may have been less severe when they were interviewed in the comfort of their home one week later by telephone. In addition, patients are often accompanied by their family or friends to their clinic appointments. This may have enhanced their feelings of social support and reduced their feelings of isolation. Consequently, one week after their appointment they have been alone in their home when contacted for follow-up. This may have altered their perception of their own personal isolation from their opinions the previous week.

To ensure the most accurate reliability of the measure, perhaps patients should have been interviewed in the same atmosphere for each administration of the questionnaire. However, in order to obtain informed consent, the patients had to be approached in person, and it would not be appropriate to insist that patients travel back to the clinic one week later to simply fill out the questionnaire again. This limitation may have served to reduce the true reliability of the BM22, but seems worthwhile to minimize the burden on those participating in the study. Failure to accept this slight limitation may have resulted in a significant reduction of the number of patients agreeable to participate, or may have increased the number of individuals lost to follow-up. Therefore, it would seem as if this was a worthwhile sacrifice to make. The BM22 has undergone slight modification since the completion of our accrual.

The development and validation of a QOL assessment tool specifically for patients with bone metastases is vital. Such an instrument will enable better patient management as an identifier of effective treatments for cancer patients in a clinical setting. Furthermore, the establishment of a standardized instrument will facilitate cross-study comparisons for the development of new treatments in patients with bone metastases. The successful determination of the module's test-retest reliability within the present study will assist in achieving EORTC validation. However, completion of Phase IV large scale international field testing of the module is required before the module can be finalized for use in future clinical trials.

Based on the overall consistent agreement that was witnessed between the baseline and follow-up interviews, the EORTC QLQ-BM22 appears to be a reliable instrument and will be a brief and suitable tool in future clinical trials involving palliative patients with bone metastases.

Acknowledgments

This study was supported by Michael and Karyn Goldstein Cancer Research Fund and Novartis Oncology. We thank the research assistants in the accrual and Stacy Lue for her secretarial assistance.

References

[1] InSightec.com: InSightec Image Guided Treatment Ltd. Pain palliation of bone metastases – overview. Accessed 2009 Feb 23. URL: http://www.insightec.com/135-en-r10/BoneMetastases.aspx

[2] Harrington KD. The management of acetabular insufficiency secondary to metastatic malignant disease. J Bone Joint Surg Am 1981;63:653-4.

[3] Harrington KD. Prophylactic management of impending fractures. In: Harrington KD. Orthopedic management of metastatic bone disease. St Louis, MO: CV Mosby, 1988:283-307.

[4] Patrick DL, Ferketich SL, Frame PS, Harris JJ, Hendricks CB, Levin B, et al. National Institutes of Health state-of-the-science conference statemen t: Symptom management in cancer: Pain, depression, and fatigue, July 15-17, 2002. J Natl Cancer Inst 2003;95(15):1110-7.

[5] World Health Organization. Constitution of the World Health Organization. Geneva, Switzerland: WHO Basic Documents, 1948.

[6] Soni MK and Cella D. Quality of life and symptom measures in oncology: An overview. Am J Manag Care 2002;8(18):S560-73.

[7] Streiner DL, Norman GR. Health measurement scales: a practical guide to their development and use. New York: Oxford Univ Press, 2003:126-52.

[8] Nunnally JC, Bernstein IH. Psychometric theory. New York: McGraw-Hill, 1994:264-5.

[9] Aaronson NK,Ahmedzai S, Bergman B, Bullinger M, Cull A, Duez NJ, Filiberti A, Flechtner H, Fleishman SB, de Haes JC, et al. The European Organization for Research and Treatment of Cancer QLQ-C30: A quality-of-life instrument for use in international clinical trials in oncology. J Natl Cancer Inst 1993;85(5):365-76.

[10] Chie W-C, Chang K-J, Huang C-S, K W-H. Quality of life of breast cancer patients in Taiwan: Validation of the Taiwan Chinese version of the EORTC QLQ-C30 and EORTC QLQ-BR23. Psychooncology 2003;12:729-35.

[11] Blazeby J, Sprangers M, Cull A, Groenvold M, Bottomley A. EORTC quality of life group: guidelines for developing questionnaire modules. Third edition revised. Accessed 2009 Feb 23. URL: http://groups.eortc.be/qol/downloads/200208module_development _guidelines.pdf

[12] Koepsell TD, Weiss NS. Epidemiologic methods: studying the occurrence of illness. New York, New York: Oxford Univ Press, 2003.

[13] Sprangers MAG, te Velde A, Aaronson NK. On behalf of the European Organization for Research and Treatment of Cancer Study Group on Quality of Life. The construction and testing of the EORTC colorectal cancer-specific quality of life questionnaire module (QLQ-CR38). Eur J Cancer 1999;35(2):238-47.

[14] Bloechle C, Izbicki JR, Knoefel WT, Kuechler T, Broelsch CE. Quality of life in chronic pancreatitis .Results after duodenum-preserving resection of the head of the pancreas. Pancreas 1995;11(1):77-85.

In: Advanced Cancer. Pain and Quality of Life
Editors: E. Chow, J. Merrick, pp. 233-246
ISBN: 978-1-61668-207-1
© 2010 Nova Science Publishers, Inc.

Chapter XXI

Quality of Life Issues in Patients with Bone Metastases

Sarah Campos, BSc(C), Liying Zhang, PhD and Edward Chow, MBBS*
Rapid Response Radiotherapy Program, Department of Radiation Oncology,
Odette Cancer Centre, Sunnybrook Health Sciences Centre,
University of Toronto, Toronto, Ontario, Canada

The purpose of this chapter was to test the reliability of patient perceptions in important bone metastases quality of life (QOL) items. A secondary objective was to determine whether changes in disease progression or changes in treatment affected the reliability of their responses. Methods: Twenty seven patients were asked to complete the EORTC – QLQ BM61 Bone Metastases Module upon visiting the Odette Cancer Centre on two occasions between 2005 and 2008. Patients were asked to complete 61 items assessing quality of life, ranking each item on a scale of 1 to 4 based on their own experience, then indicating whether they would recommend inclusion on the final questionnaire for each item. Basic demographic information was collected from each patient on first and re-approaches, as well as information regarding patients' condition and treatment regimens. New complications and changes in therapies were recorded. Results: Patient perception of the important bone metastases QOL issues was overall reliable over time, but was found to be related to changes in treatment and complications of disease. Conclusion: The finding should be kept in mind when developing QOL measurement tools based on patient perceptions of generated QOL issues, and when assessing the reliability of QOL measurement tools over time.

---

* ***Correspondence:*** Edward Chow, MBBS, PhD, FRCPC, Department of Radiation Oncology, Odette Cancer Centre, Sunnybrook Health Sciences Centre, 2075 Bayview Avenue, Toronto, ON M4N 3M5, Canada. Tel: 416-480-4998; Fax: 416-480-6002; E-mail: Edward.Chow@sunnybrook.ca

Introduction

Metastases of cancer to the bone are a complication that occurs frequently in a wide population of individuals diagnosed with advanced cancer. Bone metastases are also much more common than primary bone tumors (1). Approximately 75% of breast cancer patients will develop bone metastases (2-4), along with 68% of those affected by prostate cancer (2,3). The incidence in renal, thyroid and lung cancer is slightly lower, but still amounts to about 40% of cases (2,3). Some cancers have relatively low incidence rates, such as gastric cancer with only 5% (4), however bone metastases has been identified in 70-80% of cancer patients on autopsy (2,3).

Patients with predominantly bone only disease can survive from 2-5 years after diagnosis, which is a marked improvement in recent years due to the use of more effective systemic therapies (3). Survival has thus been discarded as a primary endpoint for clinical trials of bone metastases, in favor of improved quality of life (QOL) (3,5). The importance of QOL is in fact, underscored by the increased survival times of these patients, as end of life care is often not imminent.

One of the most common symptoms of bone metastases is pain (2,3, 6,7), affecting at least 50-75% of bone metastases patients (3), with 50% of all cancer pain due to bone metastases (4), and severe pain reported in 45% of patients assessed in one study (8). Pain is frequently under treated (8,9) and this poses a major public health concern (9), as pain can significantly hinder patients' QOL and ability to carry out daily activities. A recent study found that of those patients complaining of moderate or severe pain, 34% were either only prescribed weak opiates, non opiates or no analgesics at all (8). Other frequent complications include pathological fractures (4,10), occurring in 25% of patients on average (11). These fractures also affect many aspects of QOL causing unmanageable pain, motor impairment, neurological complications (12), and even negatively affecting survival (13). Other prevalent symptoms reflecting QOL include fatigue, drowsiness and a poor sense of well being (2).

Following the World Health Organization's definition of health as the complete state of physical, mental and social well being, notwithstanding the absence of disease or infirmity (14), QOL is a well accepted outcome for patients in clinical settings, including trials (5). The EORTC- QLQ- 30 is a widely available QOL measurement tool used in the cancer population that focuses on common symptoms and concerns faced by all cancer patients, including those of physical, emotional, social, and cognitive concern. It is supplemented by different modules applying to sub populations of cancer patients, including those affected by lung, and breast cancer. The EORTC- QLQ – C-30 has been validated in various populations internationally, and has been demonstrated to be a reliable tool (15).

More recently, a bone metastases module to supplement the EORTC- QLQ C-30 has been developed, after extensive interviews with bone metastases patients and health care professionals to determine the most commonly faced issues impacting patient QOL. Development of this module was done in several stages. Stage I involved the generation of a tentative 61 item questionnaire, later to be refined in Stage II, for a final product at Stage III of an internationally validated 22 item questionnaire. The 61 item questionnaire, or EORTC – QLQ BM61, was administered to patients in 2005 to obtain feedback on the most important items to be included in the final questionnaire. The purpose of this study was to use that data, and re-approach patients at a later date to test the reliability of patients' responses, as well as their perception of the most important items on the questionnaire. A secondary objective was to determine whether changes in disease progression of patients during the interval between both approaches, as well as changes in treatment, affected the reliability of their responses.

Our Study

In 2005, 130 patients were asked to complete the newly compiled EORTC – QLQ BM61 Bone Metastases Module (see appendix I): a 61 item precursor to the EORTC – QLQ BM22 (BM22) questionnaire. The BM22 was designed to meet the need for a QOL measurement tool specifically for cancer patients with metastases to the bone. The BM22 has demonstrated reproducibility and validity, and has been validated on an international basis (16). This questionnaire, having been refined for a lower patient burden, and validated in clinical settings, is a useful tool for helping clinicians uncover patient concerns and symptoms. The patients were approached upon visiting the Rapid Response Radiotherapy clinic, or other clinics at the Odette Cancer Centre in Toronto, Ontario. All patients were asked to complete the 61 items assessing QOL, rating each on a scale of 1 to 4, based on their own experience for that item. Patients were also asked to indicate, for each item, whether they considered that particular item relevant enough to be included on a final, condensed version of the questionnaire.

Between 2007 and 2008, 27 of these patients were re-approached upon a visit to a clinic at the Odette Cancer Centre. The follow ups were conducted on the basis of patient attendance to clinics, and thus varied in their intervals from baseline. Patients were again asked to complete the EORTC- QLQ BM61, ranking each item on a scale of 1 to 4 based on their own experience, then indicating whether they would recommend inclusion on the final questionnaire for each item. Written consent was obtained from patients both at first approach and re-approach, and the purpose, benefits and risks of the study was clearly explained to them at both times.

Outcomes and statistical analysis

Results were expressed as mean, standard deviation (SD), median and range for continuous variables, as proportion (%) for categorical variables. Basic demographic information was collected from each patient on first and re-approaches, as well as information regarding patients' condition and treatment regimens. Performance status, date of primary cancer diagnosis, date of bone metastasis diagnosis, time between original cancer diagnosis and diagnosis of bone metastasis, as well as primary cancer site and sites of metastasis were recorded both at baseline and at re-approach. Skeletal related events include spinal cord compression, cauda equina syndrome, pathological fractures, hypercalcaemia, surgical intervention to bone, or radiotherapy (RT) to bone. Dates of all skeletal related events were recorded for each patient at baseline and on re-approach. Patients' systemic therapy regimens included their use of hormonal therapy, bisphosphonates and chemotherapy. The type of treatment and specific drug was recorded at both time points, as were the start and stop dates. Any RT was recorded, including the sites of RT, the doses received and the dates of treatment. This information was then compared at analysis to determine which patients had developed new sites of metastasis and/or new skeletal related events since baseline. Changes in all therapies between baseline and re-approach were also noted. Fisher exact test was used to compare the QOL change (or Final Questionnaire FQ change) on the new complications and treatments. QOL or FQ change was considered as zero change or non-zero change between baseline and re-approach. Two-sided p-value of less than 0.05 was considered as statistical significance. Statistical Analysis Software (SAS Institute, version 9.1 for windows) was used in the study.

Findings

The demographics of the 27 patients re-approached, including their ages, gender, performance status (measured by KPS), duration of cancer diagnosis, duration of cancer diagnosis before diagnosis of bone metastases, and primary cancer sites are given in table 1. Information regarding the clinic in which the patients were re-approached can also be found in table 1. Patients' complications and treatment regimens are listed in Table 2.

Using the Fischer exact test, patients' responses to the 61 QOL items on the EORTC-QLQ BM61 at baseline in 2005 and at re-approach in 2007-2008 were compared. Any changes in these responses reflect patients' perception of change in their QOL in that time period. Of 61 items, item #1 assessing the patient's chronic pain, item #18, their ability to perform self-care, and item #43, their emotional stress related to receiving a diagnosis of advanced, incurable cancer, showed significant change. In terms of the items patients wished to include on the final questionnaire, no significant change was observed for all of the items.

Changes in patients' response to QOL items were significantly correlated to new complications or changes in treatments in 9 of 61 items (see table 3). Changes in response to item #15, difficulty planning activities outside the home, and in item #23, difficulty in standing up, and changes in response to item #55, worry about running out of medical treatments were related to new sites of RT. Item # 25, difficulty sitting, showed correlation to new sites of metastasis; item #27, difficulty lying flat was related to changes in hormonal therapy; and item #29, the presence of drowsiness was related to the incidence of new skeletal related events and new sites of RT. QOL responses to item #42, mood changes and item # 44, increased focus on spiritual issues were related to changes in bisphosphonates and chemotherapy, respectively.

Patients' selection of items for the final questionnaire was related to new complications and treatment in 10 of 61 items (see table 4). Changes in all ten items either showed correlation ($p<0.05$) to new skeletal related events, new RT, changes in chemotherapy or new sites of metastasis. Changes in selection of item #20, difficulty in completing daily tasks, #30, dizziness, # 34, strength of relationship to family and friends, #35, the presence of a clear, alert mind, were only shown to be related to new skeletal related events. Changes in selection of item #52, worry about the future were only related to new RT. Changes in selection of item #38, reluctance to use pain medicines were related to changes in chemotherapy. Changes in items #29, drowsiness, and item #30, confusion were related to both new skeletal events and new RT. Changes in selection of item #41, frustration, for the final questionnaire was shown to be related to new sites of metastasis.

Table 1. Patient baseline demographics

Sex	
Male	9 (33.3%)
Female	18 (66.7%)
Age (years)	
n	27
Mean ± SD	60.5 ± 10.5
Median (range)	61 (41 – 82)
KPS	
n	26
Mean ± SD	78.8 ± 14.2
Median (range)	80 (50 – 100)
Duration of primary cancer diagnosis (years)	
n	26
Mean ± SD	6.22 ± 6.31
Median (range)	4.31 (0.003 – 18.4)
Duration of bone metastasis diagnosis (year)	
n	19
Mean ± SD	1.44 ± 1.13
Median (range)	1.33 (0 – 3.44)
Duration from cancer diagnosis to BM (year)	
n	19
Mean ± SD	5.08 ± 5.99
Median (range)	3.77 (0 – 17.4)
Location of re-approach	
Inpatient ward	2 (7.4%)
Medical Oncology Clinic	18 (66.7%)
Palliative Pain Outpatient Clinic	3 (11.1%)
Palliative Radiation Outpatient Clinic	2 (7.4%)
Radiation Oncology Clinic	2 (7.4%)
Primary cancer site	
Breast	15 (55.6%)
Prostate	2 (7.4%)
Lung	1 (3.7%)
Renal cell	2 (7.4%)
Multiple myeloma	4 (14.8%)
Others	3 (11.1%)

Table 2. Changes in patient disease complications and treatment

New sites of metastases	
No	19 (70.4%)
Yes	8 (29.6%)
New skeletal related events	
No	14 (51.9%)
Yes	13 (48.2%)
New pathological fracture	
No	24 (88.9%)
Yes	3 (11.1%)
Surgery since baseline	
No	26 (96.3%)
Yes	1 (3.7%)
New Radiotherapy	
No	15 (55.6%)
Yes	12 (44.4%)
Changes in Bisphosphonate therapy	
No	22 (81.5%)
Yes	5 (18.5%)
Changes in Chemotherapy	
No	9 (33.3%)
Yes	18 (66.7%)
Changes in Hormone therapy	
No	20 (74.1%)
Yes	7 (25.9%)
New sites of Radiotherapy	
No	15 (55.6%)
Yes	12 (44.4%)

Table 3. Comparison of QOL changes with new complications and treatments*:

Item #	New site of metastases	New Skeletal events	New pathological fracture	Surgery since baseline	New Radiotherapy	Changes in Bisphosphonates	Changes in Chemo	Changes in Hormone therapy	New sites of radiation
11	0.3981	0.1283	0.5692	0.4444	**0.0071**	0.9999	0.2172	0.1850	0.2576
15	0.9999	0.2087	0.9999	0.9999	**0.0433**	0.9999	0.3748	0.9999	**0.0433**
23	0.4048	0.9999	0.9999	0.4074	0.9999	0.3705	0.0969	0.6618	**0.0473**
25	**0.0433**	0.7036	0.5692	0.9999	0.7068	0.3419	0.1266	0.6618	0.4408
27	0.6776	0.7064	0.9999	0.4815	0.1283	0.1647	0.6946	**0.0329**	0.7036
29	0.0687	**0.0138**	0.5385	0.3846	0.6891	0.3402	0.0873	0.6680	**0.0426**
42	0.9999	0.9999	0.9999	0.9999	0.9999	**0.0391**	0.4110	0.9999	0.4283
44	0.9999	0.2519	0.9999	0.4074	0.4517	0.6185	**0.0417**	0.0840	0.1302
55	0.9999	0.6483	0.5453	0.9999	**0.0200**	0.9999	0.9999	0.9999	0.6618

* Fisher exact test was used to compare QOL change (zero change vs. non-zero change) on new complications and treatments. The Item was not listed in the table if there is no any statistical significance on all complications and treatments.

Table 4. Comparison of patient selection for final questionnaire (FQ) and new complications and treatments*

Item #	New site of metastases	New Skeletal events	New pathological fracture	Surgery since baseline	New Radiotherapy	Changes in Bisphosphonates	Changes in Chemotherapy	Changes in Hormone therapy	New sites of radiation
20	0.5165	**0.0440**	0.5165	0.2000	0.5253	0.9999	0.5055	0.9999	0.2418
29	0.9999	**0.0319**	0.9999	0.3846	**0.0319**	0.9999	0.0754	0.9999	0.9999
30	0.9999	**0.0150**	0.5055	0.9999	**0.0150**	0.9999	0.2208	0.9999	0.0949
31	0.9999	**0.0030**	0.9999	0.3571	0.0909	0.9999	0.0859	0.9999	0.2657
32	0.1084	0.5105	0.4231	0.9999	**0.0350**	0.2308	0.9999	0.2028	0.2028
34	0.5604	**0.0256**	0.4762	0.2667	0.2352	0.9999	0.2308	0.5165	0.9999
35	0.5604	**0.0256**	0.4762	0.2667	0.2352	0.9999	0.2308	0.9999	0.2352
38	0.5055	0.0909	0.9999	0.3571	0.0909	0.9999	**0.0310**	0.5804	0.2657
41	**0.0410**	0.2448	0.5055	0.2857	0.9999	0.9999	0.2208	0.2507	0.5804
52	0.1538	0.9999	0.5165	0.9999	**0.0440**	0.3714	0.9999	0.5253	0.9999

* Fisher exact test was used to compare FQ change (zero change vs. non-zero change) on new complications and treatments. The Item was not listed in the table if there is no any statistical significance on all complications and treatments.

Discussion

QOL depends largely on many factors, including health status, financial status, job satisfaction, and living conditions. QOL that depends solely on an individual's health is known as Health Related Quality of Life (HR-QOL). In cancer patients, the morbidities associated with the disease often have such a huge impact on their lives that as symptoms worsen, QOL can be considered equivalent to HR-QOL (17). This is especially true for patients with bone metastases, where symptom control is often the primary goal of treatment. In the current study, bone metastases patients were asked about their QOL perceptions over three years, and it is almost certain that they would suffer from new complications due to disease progression during that time. These may take the form of new sites of metastasis, skeletal related events or increased pain. Systemic treatments, such as hormonal therapy or chemotherapy are initiated in certain patients, depending on other disease related factors, but these therapies can only slow disease progression (4). It is therefore important to consider QOL as an endpoint for these patients.

QOL fluctuates frequently in bone metastases patients over time, as complications and their treatments can easily diminish or improve it. Treatments such as RT and bisphosphonates are used for symptom palliation and prevention of skeletal related events, which are a main cause of diminished QOL in these patients. RT has been shown to significantly improve pain, and help local control at sites of metastasis (9,18,19). One study compared symptom distress of patients before and after RT. Patients who responded to RT, generally had decreased symptoms, including pain and fatigue as soon as two weeks after baseline, while symptoms in patients who did not respond stayed constant (2). Pathological fractures are another serious complication of bone metastases, and can cause pain, motor impairment, and neurological complications (6,7,20). The use of bisphosphonates can delay and prevent pathological fractures in many bone metastases patients (11,21, 22), thereby preventing further impaired QOL.

Significant change in QOL was observed in two of the 61 items on the EORTC–QLQ BM61, over nearly three years between baseline and re-approach, which is expected given the nature of our bone metastases population. One of those items was the ability to perform self care (item #18), which is very reflective of a patient's performance status and QOL. We also found that of the 61 items, change in QOL responses for 9, were correlated to new complications or altered treatment regimens, which is not surprising since those factors greatly influence QOL. This relationship is not an indication of the reliability of patients' perceptions, as it likely reflects real changes in their QOL as a result of treatment.

There was no significant change in the items that patients selected for the final questionnaire between baseline and re-approach. This indicates that their perceptions of relevant QOL items did not change over time. This shows good reliability of patient perceptions of important QOL issues, which is very important since most QOL measurement tools are developed from patient perceptions. Accurate QOL measurement based on patient perception is therefore the most meaningful evaluation of patient QOL.

When assessing the relationship of the change in items patients selected for the final questionnaire and complications and treatment, we found that 10 of the 61 items showed a significant value. This indicates that increased complications of disease and changes in treatment, can affect patients perceptions of important QOL items. Patient perceptions of any disease endpoint are not static, and change according to their own disease experiences. This means that the experience of new complications and treatments likely affect patient perceptions on QOL. For example, early in their disease, a patient may not assign importance to QOL items regarding mobility, but once immobilized by a fracture their importance becomes clear. This weakens the reliability of patient perceptions, but uncovers important information regarding patients' ever-evolving perceptions of QOL.

A limitation of the current study is the relatively small sample size. It is likely that if all the patients who were originally sampled had been re-approached, the results would have varied significantly. However, due to the longitudinal nature of our study, and the short lifespan of our patient population, it is likely that the patients re-approached are representative of those patients who survived since baseline. Furthermore, the performance status of this sample was considerably high (median 70), for a population of palliative cancer patients. This is again, likely a survival bias, as most patients who survived during the study period would be expected to have a low burden of disease. Nevertheless, high performance status is reflective of high QOL, and therefore perceptions related to that endpoint may be skewed.

QOL is considered a meaningful endpoint partially because it accounts for patient perspective, as well as responsiveness and change over time (3). This study was able to provide insight into how QOL is perceived by patient and how it evolves over time. Furthermore, it indicated the reliability of the BM61 in assessing patient QOL. Although the BM61 is not used on a large scale for this purpose, it represents a precursor to a validated QOL questionnaire developed through patient perceptions. Many QOL measurement tools are developed in this way, and assessing the reliability of the BM61 ultimately provides insight on how patients perceive QOL in their own lives, as well as those of patients with similar conditions.

Conclusions

Patient perception of the importance of particular QOL issues was overall reliable over time, but was found to be related to changes in treatment and complications of disease. This should be kept in mind when developing QOL measurement tools based on patient perceptions of generated QOL issues, and when assessing the reliability of QOL measurement tools over time.

Acknowledgments

This project was funded by Michael and Karyn Goldstein Cancer Research Fund and Novartis Oncology. We thank Stacy Lue of her secretarial assistance. Conflicts of interest notification: None

References

[1] American Cancer Society. Cancer facts and figures. Atlanta, GA: Am Cancer Society, 1997.

[2] Chow E, Fan G, Hadi S, Filipczak L. Symptom clusters in cancer patients with bone metastases. Support Care Cancer 2007; 15(9):1035-43.

[3] Chow E, Hoskin P, van der Linden Y, Bottomley A, Velikova G. Quality of life and symptom end points in palliative bone metastases trials. Clin Oncol 2006;18(1):67-9.

[4] Kanis JA. Bone and cancer: Pathophysiology and treatment of metastases. Bone 1995;17(2 Suppl):101S-5S.

[5] Soni MK, Cella D. Quality of life and symptom measures in oncology: An overview. Am J Manag Care 2002;8(18 Suppl):S560-73.

[6] Kanis JA, O'Rourke N, McCloskey EV. Consequences of neoplasia-induced bone resorption and the use of clodronate. Int J Oncol 1994;5:713-31.

[7] Paterson AH. Bone metastases in breast cancer, prostate cancer and myeloma. Bone 1987;8(Suppl 1):S17-22.

[8] Yau V, Chow E, Davis L, Holden L, Schueller T, Danjoux C. Pain management in cancer patients with bone metastases remains a challenge. J Pain Sympt Manage 2004;27(1):1-3.

[9] Patrick DL, Ferketich SL, Frame PS, Harris JJ, Hendricks CB, Levin B, et al. National institutes of health state-of-the-science conference statement: Symptom management in cancer: Pain, depression, and fatigue, july 15-17, 2002. J Natl Cancer Inst 2004;Monogr(32):9-16.

[10] Saad F. Impact of bone metastases on patient's quality of life and importance of treatment. Eur Urol Suppl 2006;5:547-50.

[11] Saad F, Gleason DM, Murray R, Tchekmedyian S, Venner P, Lacombe L, et al. Long-term efficacy of zoledronic acid for the prevention of skeletal complications in patients with metastatic hormone-refractory prostate cancer. J Natl Cancer Inst 2004;96(11):879-82.
[12] Harrington KD. Orthopedic surgical management of skeletal complications of malignancy. Cancer 1997;80(8 Suppl):1614-27.
[13] Oefelein MG, Ricchiuti V, Conrad W, Resnick MI. Skeletal fractures negatively correlate with overall survival in men with prostate cancer. J Urol 2002;168(3):1005-7.
[14] World Health Organization. Constitution of the world health organization. Geneva, Switzerland: WHO, 1948.
[15] Osoba D, Zee B, Pater J, Warr D, Kaizer L, Latreille J. Psychometric properties and responsiveness of the EORTC quality of life questionnaire (QLQ-C30) in patients with breast, ovarian and lung cancer. Qual Life Res 1994;3(5):353-64.
[16] Chow E, Hird A, Velikova G, Johnson C, Dewolf L, Bezjak A, et al. The european organisation for research and treatment of cancer quality of life questionnaire for patients with bone metastases: The EORTC QLQ-BM22. Eur J Cancer 2008 Dec 17 [Epub ahead of print].
[17] Guyatt GH, Feeny DH, Patrick DL. Measuring health-related quality of life. Ann Intern Med 1993;118(8):622-9.
[18] Hoskin PJ. Radiotherapy for bone pain. Pain 1995;63(2):137-9.
[19] Tong D, Gillick L, Hendrickson FR. The palliation of symptomatic osseous metastases: Final results of the study by the radiation therapy oncology group. Cancer 1982;50(5):893-9.
[20] Weinfurt KP, Li Y, Castel LD, Saad F, Timbie JW, Glendenning GA, et al. The significance of skeletal-related events for the health-related quality of life of patients with metastatic prostate cancer. Ann Oncol 2005;16(4):579-84.
[21] Coleman RE. Bisphosphonates: Clinical experience. Oncologist 2004;9(Suppl 4):14-27.
[22] van Holten-Verzantvoort AT, Kroon HM, Bijvoet OL, Cleton FJ, Beex LV, Blijham G, et al. Palliative pamidronate treatment in patients with bone metastases from breast cancer. J Clin Oncol 1993;11(3):491-8.

APPENDIX I: The EORTC-QLQ BM61 Tool

QUALITY OF LIFE ISSUES		i) Please indicate for each experience separately, the extent to which you have had it during your illness, on a scale of (1) "not at all" to (4) "very much."				ii) Include this issue on the final questionnaire? (circle Yes or No for each item)	
		Not At All (1)	A Little (2)	Quite a Bit (3)	Very Much (4)		
FUNCTION (continued)							
17	Difficulty in carrying out meaningful activity (including employment)	1	2	3	4	Yes	No
18	Able to perform self-care	1	2	3	4	Yes	No
19	Able to return to work promptly	1	2	3	4	Yes	No
20	Difficulty carrying out usual daily tasks (i.e. grocery shopping, work outside the home, housework)	1	2	3	4	Yes	No
21	Difficulty bending	1	2	3	4	Yes	No
22	Difficulty lifting	1	2	3	4	Yes	No
23	Difficulty standing up	1	2	3	4	Yes	No
24	Difficulty climbing stairs	1	2	3	4	Yes	No
25	Difficulty sitting	1	2	3	4	Yes	No
26	Difficulty lying in bed	1	2	3	4	Yes	No
27	Difficulty lying flat	1	2	3	4	Yes	No
28	Ability to have sex	1	2	3	4	Yes	No
SIDE EFFECTS FROM TREATMENT OF BONE METASTASES							
29	Drowsiness	1	2	3	4	Yes	No
30	Confusion	1	2	3	4	Yes	No
31	Dizziness	1	2	3	4	Yes	No
PSYCHOSOCIAL							
32	Able to perform role functioning (including domestic and family roles)	1	2	3	4	Yes	No
33	Feeling socially isolated	1	2	3	4	Yes	No

QUALITY OF LIFE ISSUES		i) Please indicate for each experience separately, the extent to which you have had it during your illness, on a scale of (1) "not at all" to (4) "very much."				ii) Include this issue on the final questionnaire? (circle Yes or No for each item)	
		Not At All (1)	A Little (2)	Quite a Bit (3)	Very Much (4)		
PSYCHOSOCIAL (continued)							
34	Strengthened relationships with family and friends	1	2	3	4	Yes	No
35	Have a clear, alert mind	1	2	3	4	Yes	No
36	Feel in control, positive, and confident	1	2	3	4	Yes	No
37	Hope to live as long as possible	1	2	3	4	Yes	No
38	Reluctance to use pain medication	1	2	3	4	Yes	No
39	Fear of addiction to pain medication	1	2	3	4	Yes	No
40	Anxiety	1	2	3	4	Yes	No
41	Frustration	1	2	3	4	Yes	No
42	Mood changes	1	2	3	4	Yes	No
43	Emotional stress of diagnosis of advanced, incurable cancer	1	2	3	4	Yes	No
44	Increased focus on spiritual issues	1	2	3	4	Yes	No
45	Loss of interest in activities you normally enjoy	1	2	3	4	Yes	No
46	Loss of interest in sex	1	2	3	4	Yes	No
47	Worry about pain	1	2	3	4	Yes	No
48	Worry about suffering	1	2	3	4	Yes	No
49	Worry about loss of mobility compromising independence	1	2	3	4	Yes	No
50	Worry about becoming dependent on others	1	2	3	4	Yes	No
51	Worry about current health status	1	2	3	4	Yes	No

QUALITY OF LIFE ISSUES		i) Please indicate for each experience separately, the extent to which you have had it during your illness, on a scale of (1) "not at all" to (4) "very much."				ii) Include this issue on the final questionnaire? (circle Yes or No for each item)	
		Not At All (1)	A Little (2)	Quite a Bit (3)	Very Much (4)		
SYMPTOMS							
1	Long-term (or chronic) pain	1	2	3	4	Yes	No
2	Short-term (or acute), severe pain	1	2	3	4	Yes	No
3	Pain at rest (i.e. when sitting)	1	2	3	4	Yes	No
4	Pain with activity (i.e. when walking)	1	2	3	4	Yes	No
5	Pain aggravation with movement or weight-bearing	1	2	3	4	Yes	No
6	Uncontrolled, unmanageable pain not relieved by pain killers	1	2	3	4	Yes	No
7	Pain at night preventing sleep	1	2	3	4	Yes	No
8	Aches and stiffness	1	2	3	4	Yes	No
9	Lack of energy	1	2	3	4	Yes	No
10	Numbness	1	2	3	4	Yes	No
11	Tingling	1	2	3	4	Yes	No
12	Burning Sensation	1	2	3	4	Yes	No
13	Postural problems	1	2	3	4	Yes	No
FUNCTION							
14	Limited movement due to pain	1	2	3	4	Yes	No
15	Difficulty planning activities outside the home	1	2	3	4	Yes	No
16	Difficulty traveling outside the home (i.e. using public transportation, driving, sitting in car)	1	2	3	4	Yes	No

QUALITY OF LIFE ISSUES		i) Please indicate for each experience separately, the extent to which you have had it during your illness, on a scale of (1) "not at all" to (4) "very much."				ii) Include this issue on the final questionnaire? (circle Yes or No for each item)	
		Not At All (1)	A Little (2)	Quite a Bit (3)	Very Much (4)		
PSYCHOSOCIAL (continued)							
52	Worry about the future	1	2	3	4	Yes	No
53	Worry about becoming bed-bound	1	2	3	4	Yes	No
54	Worry about disease progression, deterioration in condition, and future complications	1	2	3	4	Yes	No
55	Worry about running out of medical treatments	1	2	3	4	Yes	No
56	Worry about hospitalization	1	2	3	4	Yes	No
57	Worry about ending days in a hospital or nursing home	1	2	3	4	Yes	No
58	Worry about death	1	2	3	4	Yes	No
TREATMENT EXPECTATIONS							
59	Hope for sustained pain relief (reduce pain for as long as possible)	1	2	3	4	Yes	No
60	Hope treatment will reduce pain as much as possible	1	2	3	4	Yes	No
OTHER ISSUES							
61	Financial burden due to the illness	1	2	3	4	Yes	No

In: Advanced Cancer. Pain and Quality of Life
Editors: E. Chow, J. Merrick, pp. 247-259
ISBN: 978-1-61668-207-1
© 2010 Nova Science Publishers, Inc.

Chapter XXII

Bone Metastases Quality of Life Instrument Tool

Lying Zhang, PhD, Janet Nguyen, BSc (C), Amanda Hird, BSc (C) and Edward Chow, MBBS*

Rapid Response Radiotherapy Program, Department of Radiation Oncology, Odette Cancer Centre, Sunnybrook Health Sciences Centre, University of Toronto, Toronto, Ontario, Canada

Purpose was to shorten the 22-item bone metastases (BM22) quality of life (QOL) instrument tool for bone metastases patients with a low performance status. Methods: The BM22 was developed in patients with bone metastases from eight countries. It was divided into four scales: painful sites, pain characteristics, functional interferences, and psychosocial aspects. Differential item functioning (DIF), item response theory (IRT), and item information functions (IIFs) analyses were used to shorten the tool. A Bonferroni adjusted p-value of < 0.002 was considered statistically significant. Results: The data from four hundred and ninety four patients were analyzed in this study. There were 283 females (57%) and 211 males (43%). The median age was 62 years. The majority of patients had primary breast (46%), prostate (22%), or lung (12%) cancer. No significant DIF was found between translations of the questionnaire (62 patients) and the original English version (432 patients). Based on the IRT model and IIFs, eight items were removed from the original version. Both the shortened 14-item and the original 22-item versions predicted four scales with excellent agreement. Demographic group comparisons yielded the same conclusions on both the shortened and original versions with little or no loss of measurement efficiency. Conclusion: The BM22 can be condensed to 14 items, which may ease patient burden in completing baseline and follow-up quality of life assessments in future clinical trials.

* Correspondence: Edward Chow, MBBS, PhD, FRCPC, Department of Radiation Oncology, Odette Cancer Centre, Sunnybrook Health Sciences Centre, 2075 Bayview Avenue, Toronto, Ontario, Canada M4N 3M5. Tel: 416-480-4998; Fax: 416-480-6002; E-mail: Edward.Chow@sunnybrook.ca

Introduction

Proper and timely assessment of patients' subjective symptomatology in a palliative care setting is important to ensure good quality of care. Patient-based self-assessment is the gold standard to gather information about the symptoms, functional, and psychosocial problems patients are experiencing (1). However, because patients with advanced disease often present with low performance status and limited life expectancy, there is a strong need to reduce responder burden when completing quality of life (QOL) questionnaires (1,2).

In view of this, the European Organization for Research and Treatment of Cancer core questionnaire (EORTC QLQ-C30) has been shortened to a core palliative version (EORTC QLQ-C15-PAL) for cancer palliative patients using item response theory (IRT) (1, 3). IRT seeks to make scores from a shortened questionnaire compatible with the scores from the original questionnaire (2). Additionally, disease-specific modules have been developed to accompany either the EORTC QLQ-C30 or EORTC QLQ-C15-PAL. The 22-item Bone Metastases Module (BM22) has recently been developed to assess quality of life in patients with bone metastases (4). The BM22 was developed in accordance to the EORTC Module Development Guidelines, which consists of four stages of development (4, 5). The objective of this analysis was to determine if the BM22 can be shortened further to reduce patient burden and thus increase the duration by which patients are able to continue the quality of life follow-up assessment in a routine clinical or clinical trial setting, while retaining the ability to reliably capture the overall issues relevant to the patient.

In the present study, we used differential item functioning (DIF) analyses with regard to different translations. Several methods for analysis of DIF have been used (6-9), which include contingency tables, logistic regression and IRT. The major objective was to retain as few items as possible within each scale while still allowing for an accurate estimation (i.e. prediction) of the original score. For unidimensional scales consisting of two or more items with categorical response choices, IRT is a very efficient statistical technique for item selection and score estimation (10,11). This approach to shortening scales was first described in Bjorner et al (3) and was further developed, applied and evaluated from EORTC Quality of Life Group (1-2,12). In the current paper, IRT was used to shorten the BM22. The agreement between the original and the shortened scales was explored, and the potential loss of statistical power was illustrated in demographic group comparisons.

Study

Patients with bone metastases treated with chemotherapy, surgery, bisphosphonates, radiotherapy, and symptom management were eligible to participate. Patients were accrued in Argentina, Australia, China (Hong Kong), Canada, Germany, Greece, Spain and the United Kingdom. Five translations were presented in the study (English, Greek, Spanish, Chinese, and German). All patients provided written informed consent. Demographic variables including gender, age, and primary cancer site were collected, and all patients completed the BM22 questionnaire at baseline. Each item has four response categories: 1 = "Not at all", 2 =

"A little", 3 = "Quite a bit", and 4 = "Very much". Note that items 21 and 22 have inversed responses comparing to other psychosocial questions (i.e., items 17 – 20).

The BM22 was divided into four scales (0 – 100): painful sites (PS; items 1 – 5), pain characteristics (PC; items 6 – 8), functional interferences (FI; items 9 – 16), and psychosocial aspects (PA; items 17 – 22). The four scale scores were constructed by summation and linear transformation of the scores on the items. For instance, the average (XPS) of items 1 to 5 was calculated and the PS scale was then computed by a linear transformation to convert to a 0 – 100 scale, $\{(XPS - 1) / 3\} \times 100$. Scales were considered missing if fewer than 3 of the PS or PA items, fewer than 2 of the PC items, or fewer than 4 of the FI items were answered by patients. Patients were considered to have worse symptoms if the PS or PC scales were higher, and patients were classified to have better functioning if the FI or PA scales were higher.

Statistical analysis

Results were expressed as mean, standard deviation (SD), and median (range) for continuous variables, and proportion (%) for categorical variables. To compare other translations (German, Greek, Spanish or Chinese) versus English, three methods of differential item functioning (DIF) analyses were applied for each item of BM22 (6-9). Differential item functioning analyses include the Fisher exact test between the item responses and translations, ordinal logistic regression, and methods based on item response theory (IRT). All IRT-models predict the probability of choosing a particular response to an item as governed by characteristics of the item and characteristics of the person (the person's IRT score). We used the Generalized Partial Credit Model (GPCM) in the IRT analysis (13), which deals with two types of item characteristics (item parameters): threshold parameters and slope parameters. For example, Figure 1 shows the GPCM model predictions (response probability functions) for each response choice for item Q9 (pain while sitting?). The model has three threshold parameters due to four item responses (not at all, a little, quite a bit, very much). The slope parameter describes the item's ability to discriminate; the items with higher slope parameters are better at discriminating between people with good and poor QOL than items with lower slope parameters. The average of threshold parameters in other translations was compared to the average of thresholds in English for each BM22 item. In order to avoid many spurious positives, the Bonferroni adjusted p-value < 0.002 (0.05/22 items) was used as the significance criteria for the multiple comparisons. We considered the difference between translations if three DIF analyses have significant p-values for each BM22 item.

Based on the IRT model, we estimated the score distribution using the expected a posteriori (EAP) method and we calculated the item information functions (IIFs) for all items (14-16). The IIF can be seen as a function of the standard error of the latent score estimate and is a measure of how much information the item provides about the person score for various levels of the BM22 scales. By choosing the items with the largest information in the area where most patients were expected to be, we obtained the most accurate estimation of the IRT scores. The items with lower information in the area (lower slope parameters) were removed from the BM22 items, and the shortened scales were calculated. To evaluate the shortened scales, Cronbach's alpha and Spearman coefficient were calculated between the original and shortened scales, and the group comparisons of demographics (age = 60 vs. < 60, males vs. females, and primary cancer site of breast, prostate or lung) were performed on the original and shortened scales using Wilcoxon rank-sum test or Kruskal-Wallis test.

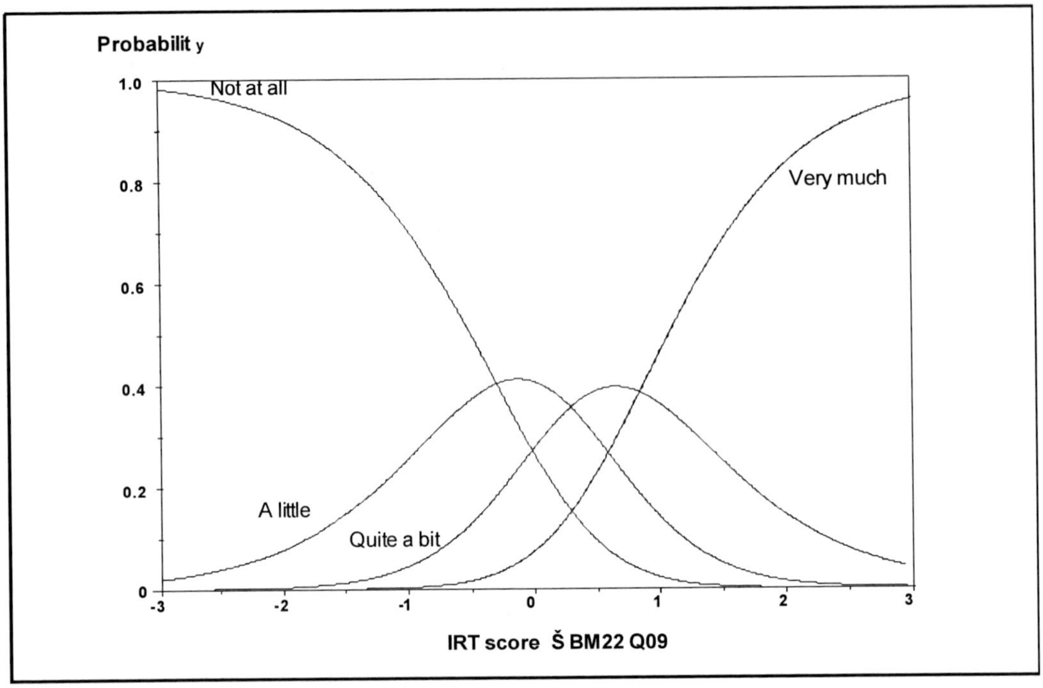

NOTE: The curved lines are the trace lines (response probability functions) for each response choice. The slope parameter describes the item's ability to discriminate; the items with higher slope parameters are better at discriminating between people with good and poor quality of life than items with lower slope parameters. The slope parameter for item 9 is 1.44.

Figure 1. Item trace lines – Generalized Partial Credit Model (GPCM) for item 9 (pain while sitting?).

IRT analyses were conducted using the PARSCALE (14, 17) computer program (version 4, Scientific Software International, Lincolnwood, IL). The item parameters were estimated using marginal maximum likelihood estimation. For all estimations, 75 quadrature points and a precision level for convergence of 0.01 were used. All observations with complete data on the four scales were used for estimation of the IRT model. Statistical Analysis Software (SAS, version 9.1 for Windows) was also used.

Findings

Patient characteristics

Patient characteristics are summarized in table 1. Among 494 patients with bone metastases, the median age was 62 years (range: 53 – 72 years). There were 283 females (57%) and 211 males (43%). The most common primary cancer sites were breast (46%), prostate (22%) and lung (12%) patients. Participants were accrued from eight countries: Canada, Greece, Australia, UK, Hong Kong (China), Germany, Argentina and Spain. The majority of patients were accrued in Canada (83%). Four hundred and thirty-two patients (87%) completed the original English version, and 62 patients (13%) completed the translated non-English versions (29 in Greek, 14 in Spanish, 10 in Chinese, and 9 in German).

Table 1. Demographics of the 494 patients

Age (years)		
n	486	
Mean ± SD	62.8 ±13.0	
Median (range)	62 (53 – 72)	
Gender		
Female	283	(57.3%)
Male	211	(42.7%)
Primary Cancer site		
Breast	225	(45.5%)
Prostate	107	(21.7%)
Lung	61	(12.3%)
Kidney	26	(5.3%)
Myeloma	22	(4.5%)
Bladder	12	(2.4%)
Colon	12	(2.4%)
Others	22	(4.5%)
Unknown	7	(1.4%)
Translations		
English	432	(87.5%)
Greek	29	(5.9%)
Spanish	14	(2.8%)
Chinese	10	(2.0%)
German	9	(1.8%)

The BM22 consists of 22 items and forms four scales which were transformed to a 0-100 scale. The average (± SD) and median for the PS scale were 31.3 (± 24.1) and 26.7; for the PC scale they were 37.2 (± 28.5) and 33.3. Functioning scales have higher scores than symptoms scales. The average (± SD) and median for the FI scale was 56.9 (± 29.2) and 61.1; for the PA scale they were 58.8 (± 22.8) and 55.6.

DIF analyses

Table 2 summarizes the results of the DIF analyses, comparing the p-values between non-English versions and the English version. BM22 items with non-significant DIF are not shown. Using the Fisher exact test, significant DIF was found in 3 items [items 5, 6 and 7] involving two non-English versions (Greek or Spanish). Using ordinal logistic regression of item response on translation subgroups, only one item (item 6) was found to be significant between Greek and English versions. There were more significant DIF found using IRT method [items 9, 10, 18 – 20]. However, none of the findings had significant DIF from three methods at the same time.

Table 2. Test for differential item functioning (DIF) between translations and the original English using Fisher exact test, ordinal logistic regression, and IRT analysis

QOL item	p-value* Fisher exact test	Ordinal logistic regression	IRT analysis
German vs. English			
9. pain while sitting or lying down?	0.804	0.424	**0.001**
Greek vs. English			
5. Pain in your buttock(s)?	**0.0008**	0.036	0.377
6. constant pain?	**0.0004**	**0.0004**	0.503
10. pain when trying to stand up?	0.070	0.195	**0.001**
Spanish vs. English			
7. intermittent pain?	**0.0001**	0.002	0.199
18. worried about loss of mobility?	0.055	0.564	**0.001**
19. worried about becoming dependent on others?	0.268	0.093	**0.001**
20. worried about your health in the future?	0.224	0.516	**0.001**
Chinese vs. English			
9. pain while sitting or lying down?	0.971	0.691	**0.001**
10. pain when trying to stand up?	0.945	0.795	**0.001**

* Bonferroni adjusted p-value < 0.002 was considered as significance for each test. We considered the difference between translations if three DIF analyses have significant p-values for each BM22 item. The non-significant BM22 items were not shown in the table.

IRT model and information functions

Table 3 shows the slope parameter (with standard error) in the IRT models for each BM22 item. This table illustrates the implications of the item parameters for the response probabilities for different levels of symptoms or functioning domain. Among 5 items from the painful site (PS) domain, item 3 (pain in the arm or shoulder) had a much smaller slope parameter than the four other items in the PS scale (0.331 for item 3; 0.406 for item 1; 0.523 for item 2; 0.460 for item 4 and 0.643 for item 5; respectively). This finding indicates that item 3 had a poorer ability to discriminate relative to the other items in the scale. Among 3 items from the PC domain, item 7 had a lower slope parameter than the other two items. Moreover, items 14 and 16 had lower slope parameters compared to the other items in the FI domain. Four items (17, 20, 21, and 22) had smaller slope parameters in the PA domain. The IIFs based on four different domains (PS, PC, FI, and PA) are shown in Figure 2a–d. Some BM22 items provided markedly less information than the other items, which had similar contributions to IRT model. For instance, Figure 2b shows that the item 7 provided less information on the Pain Characteristic (PC) score than other two items (Q6 and Q8).

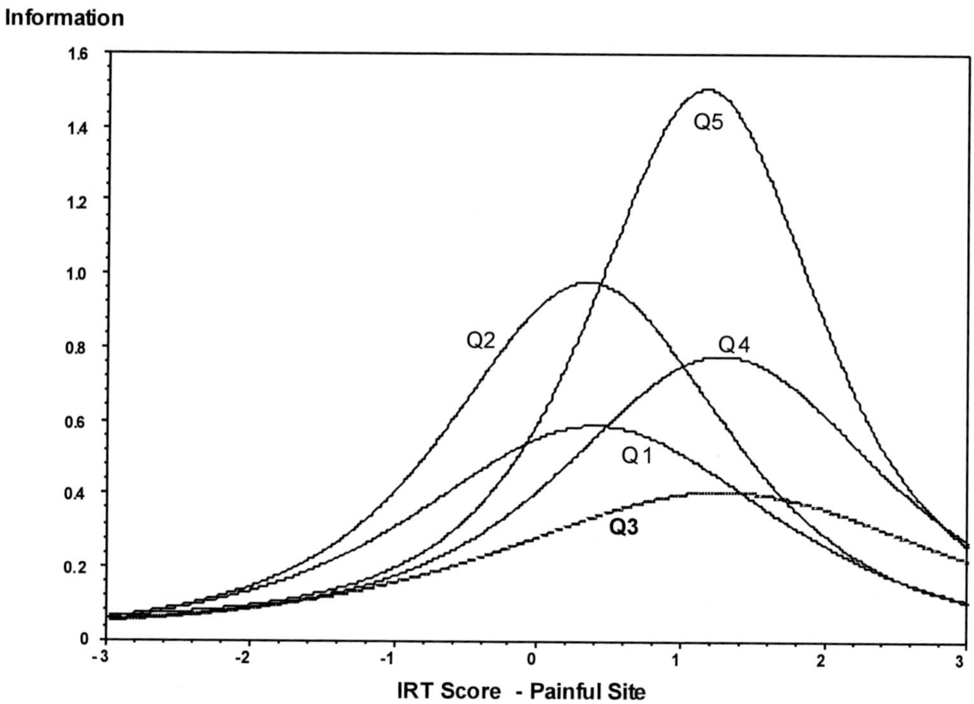

(a)

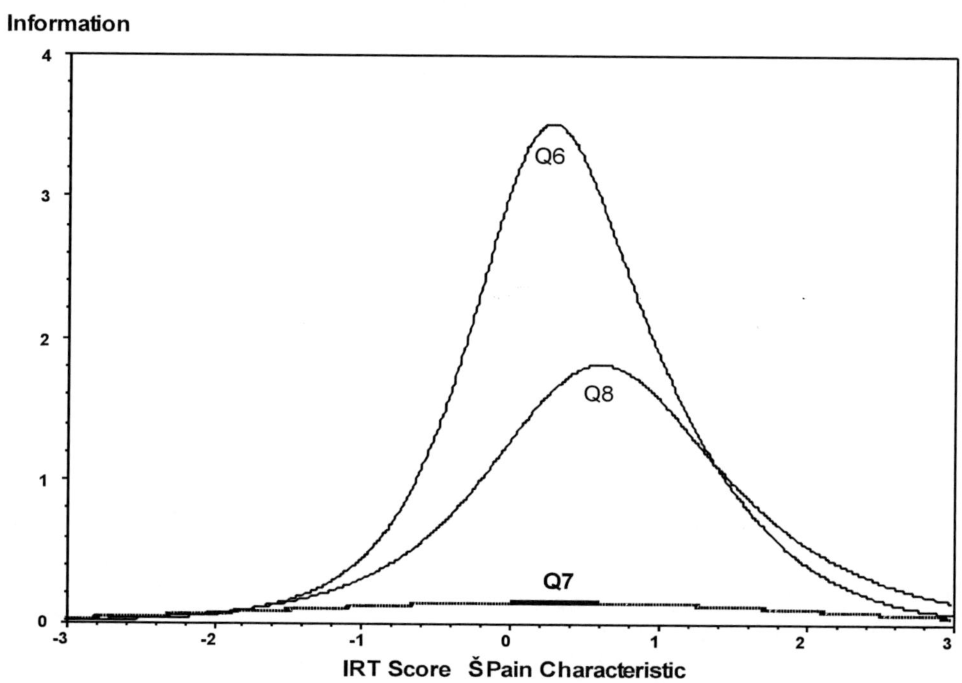

(b)

Figure 2. (continued)

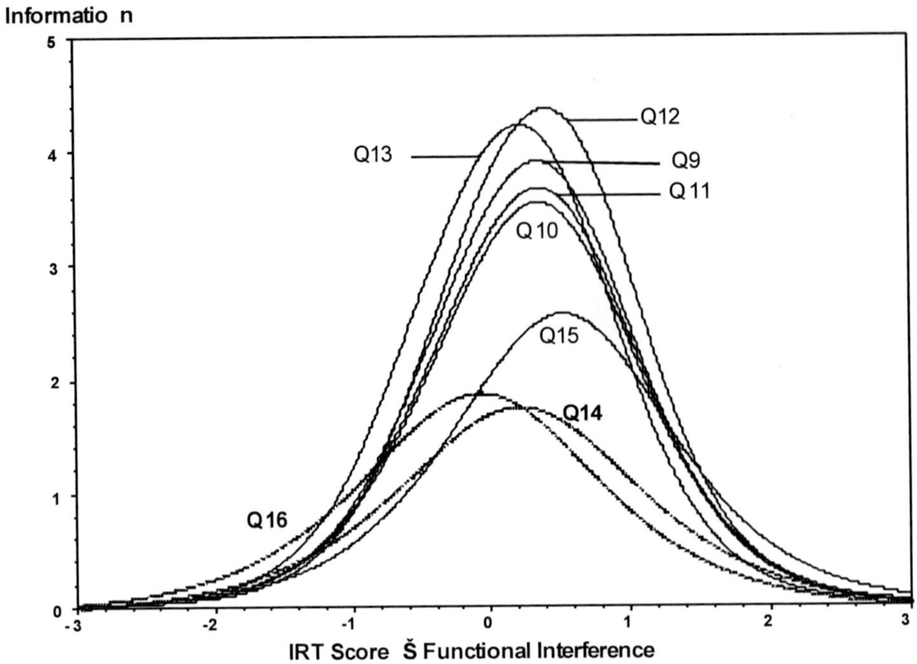

(c)

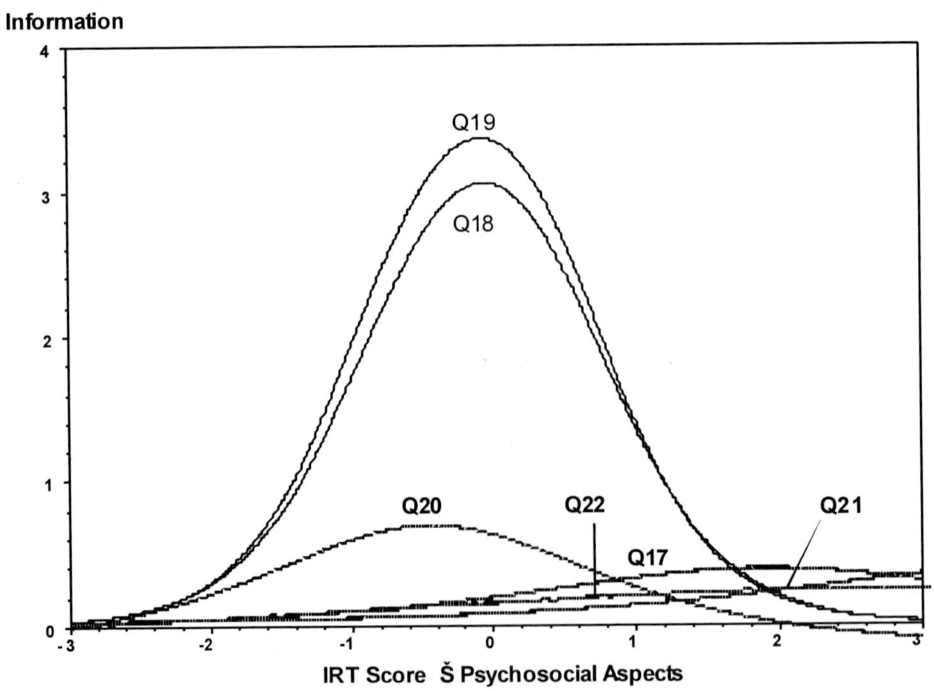

NOTE: An item with a high slope will generally provide more information than an item with a low slope. The items with low slope were removed from the original version for shortening the bone metastases quality of life tool.

Figures 2a to 2d. Estimated item information functions (IIF) for the a) Painful Site; b) Pain Characteristic; c) Functional Interference; and d) Psychosocial Aspects.

Table 3. Slope parameter and corresponding standard error (SE) from the Item response theory (IRT) model for each bone metastases QOL tool

BM22	Slope parameter	SE
Painful Site (PS)		
1. Pain in your back?	0.406	0.053
2. Pain in your leg(s) or hip(s)?	0.523	0.064
3. Pain in your arm(s) or shoulder(s)?	**0.331**	**0.047**
4. Pain in your chest or rib(s)?	0.460	0.062
5. Pain in your buttock(s)?	0.643	0.077
Pain Characteristics (PC)		
6. constant pain?	1.163	0.198
7. intermittent pain?	**0.239**	**0.041**
8. pain not relieved by pain medications?	0.795	0.123
Functional Interference (FI)		
9. pain while sitting or lying down?	1.444	0.200
10. pain when trying to stand up?	1.347	0.175
11. pain while walking?	1.377	0.148
12. pain with activities such as bending or climbing stairs?	1.571	0.158
13. pain with strenuous activity (e.g. exercise, lifting)?	1.532	0.188
14. pain interfered with your sleeping at night?	**0.852**	**0.079**
15. modify your daily activities?	1.073	0.105
16. isolated from those close to you (e.g. family, friends)?	**0.886**	**0.101**
Psychosocial Aspects (PA)		
17. thinking about your illness?	**0.361**	**0.042**
18. worried about loss of mobility?	1.309	0.172
19. worried about becoming dependent on others?	1.408	0.216
20. worried about your health in the future?	**0.559**	**0.042**
21. hopeful your pain will get better?	**0.350**	**0.030**
22. positive about your health?	**0.122**	**0.033**

Table 4. Summarization of shortened bone metastases QOL tool

QOL tool	Original version	Removed item	Shortened version: Remaining items	Shortened version: No. of items
Painful Site (PS)	Items 1 – 5	3	1, 2, 4, 5	4
Pain Characteristics (PC)	Items 6 – 8	7	6, 8	2
Functional Interference (FI)	Items 9 – 16	14, 16	9, 10, 11, 12, 13, 15	6
Psychosocial Aspects (PA)	Item 17 – 22	17, 20, 21, 22	18, 19	2

Based on the IRT model and IIFs, eight items would be removed from the original version of the BM22, namely items 3, 7, 14, 16, 17, 20, 21, and 22. Table 4 shows the remaining items in the "shortened version" of BM22 for each symptom or functioning domain. Therefore, the shortened version includes 14 items.

Evaluation of shortened BM22

The PS, PC, FI and PA scales were calculated based on the shortened version of the BM22. The average (± SD) and median value for the shortened PS scale were 32.1 (± 25.7) and 25.0; for the shortened PC scale they were 33.0 (± 33.6) and 33.3. Shortened functioning scales have higher scores than symptoms scales. The average (± SD) and median for the shortened FI scale was 59.8 (± 30.1) and 66.7; for the shortened PA scale they were 47.6 (± 36.5) and 50.0. The Cronbach's alpha and Spearman correlation coefficient between the original version and the shortened version of the BM22 were 0.98 and 0.95 for the PS scale, 0.96 and 0.92 for the PC scale, 0.99 and 0.98 for the FI scale, and 0.92 and 0.87 for the PA scale, respectively.

Table 5. Evaluation of shortened BM22 by group comparisons of demographics on painful site, painful characteristics, functional interference or psychosocial scales

		Original version		Shortened version	
Scale	Groups	Mean of scale	p-value*	Mean of scale	p-value*
Painful Site (PS)	Age ≥ 60	28.0	0.0144	34.3	0.0279
	Age < 60	33.5		28.9	
	Male	33.3	0.1511	33.7	0.1521
	Female	29.8		30.9	
	Breast cancer	25.5	**0.0001**	26.2	**0.0001**
	Prostate cancer	33.4		34.0	
	Lung cancer	38.6		40.2	
Painful Characteristics (PC)	Age ≥ 60	39.9	0.0064	35.2	0.0830
	Age < 60	32.8		29.3	
	Male	39.9	0.0643	35.4	0.1574
	Female	35.2		31.2	
	Breast cancer	30.2	**0.0001**	24.9	**0.0001**
	Prostate cancer	40.6		34.3	
	Lung cancer	48.3		48.6	
Functional Interference (FI)	Age ≥ 60	54.9	0.0504	57.8	0.0368
	Age < 60	59.9		63.1	
	Male	53.5	0.0235	56.6	0.0397
	Female	59.4		62.2	
	Breast cancer	64.7	**0.0001**	67.4	**0.0001**
	Prostate cancer	55.9		58.1	
	Lung cancer	45.2		49.3	
Psychosocial Aspects (PA)	Age ≥ 60	59.4	0.8176	48.1	0.8746
	Age < 60	58.5		47.3	
	Male	58.2	0.5395	45.5	0.2646
	Female	59.3		49.2	
	Breast cancer	62.0	0.0284	55.3	0.0138
	Prostate cancer	61.7		49.8	
	Lung cancer	53.2		40.2	

* Wilcoxon rank-sum statistic was used for comparing patients with age ≥ 60 vs. age < 60, or comparing males vs. females; Kruskal-Wallis statistic was used for comparing breast, prostate or lung primary cancer. Bonferroni adjusted p-value < 0.002 was considered as significance.

As the final step in the development of a shortened version, the group comparisons was performed on four original scales and on four shortened scales. The group comparisons included: age = 60 vs. age < 60; males vs. females; breast vs. prostate vs. lung primary cancer site (Table 5). The p-values were similar in original version and in shortened version. Primary cancer site had a significant difference on all scales. Age and gender had no difference on the scales for both versions. These findings indicate that the shortened version is able to detect a significant group difference with at least the same level of measurement efficiency as the original version of the BM22.

Discussion

The results of this study have shown that the BM22 can be shortened down to 14 items, while still maintaining the important QOL issues relevant to the patient and producing a QOL score comparable to that obtained using the original version. It is crucial that the items are correctly translated when comparing results from health status questionnaires across countries (18-20). Three methods were used to compare responses in translations: Fisher exact test of contingency tables, ordinal logistic regression of item responses, and IRT method. In each analysis, the translated item was compared against the English original. Due to the small sample size of item responses on translations (29 in Greek, 14 in Spanish, 10 in Chinese, and 9 in German, respectively), we considered a significant DIF when three tests have significant p-values for each item of the BM22. There was not any significant DIF between translations and the original English version; however, further validation of these findings in a larger sample of patients from different countries is necessary.

Several studies have used IRT methodology in recent years to shorten QOL questionnaires, such as the shortening of the EORTC QLQ-C30 core questionnaire to the EORTC QLQ-C15-PAL core questionnaire for palliative cancer patients (1-3,21-23). The results from the present study confirmed the analytical and theoretical advantages of IRT modeling for the development of a shortened BM22 questionnaire. This approach was successful in reducing the full 22–item questionnaire to 14 items. The shortened PS scale consists of items 1, 2, 4, and 5; the PC scale consists of items 6 and 8; the FI scale consists of items 9, 10, 11, 12, 13, and 15; and the PA scale consists of items 18 and 19. The differences between shortened scales and the original scales were small and their correlations (Cronbach's alpha and Spearman correlation) were also high. Separate group comparisons confirmed that our shortened symptom or functioning scales worked well as the original scales.

The BM22 was subsequently tested in an additional cohort of 170 patients from 9 different countries. This phase is critical to determine whether the module items compiled are comparable cross-culturally, as well as to make any amendments to the BM22 if necessary prior to undergoing large-scale field-testing. There was a consensus from participants to modify two items on the BM22. The first was item 9, "pain while sitting or lying down?", where 27 patients (16%) recommended this item be divided into two separate items. Many of the participants who suggested this modification only had pain during one of these activities. The second recommendation was to delete item 17, "thinking about your illness?", where five patients expressed that this was an obvious question, and two patients found this upsetting. The BM22 was amended in response to these issues prior to beginning ongoing large scale field-testing.

Readers are cautioned that the BM22 used in this study was the original version prior to the recommendation from the additional 170 participants. We recognize that this exercise of shortening needs to be repeated after the final version from the large scale field testing in light of the fact that there may be additional changes made to the questionnaire based on patient recommendations. However, the current study will provide methodology to shorten the final quality of life instrument tool, which may help ease patient burden in clinical trials, and allow for the comparison of QOL scores for patients with a better performance status to those of patients with a poor performance status.

Acknowledgments

This study was supported by the Michael and Karyn Goldstein Cancer Research Fund and Novartis Oncology. We would also like to thank Stacy Lue for her secretarial assistance.

References

[1] Groenvold M, Petersen MA, Aaronson NK, Arraras JI, Blazeby JM, et al. EORTC Quality of Life,Group. The development of the EORTC QLQ-C15-PAL: A shortened questionnaire for cancer patients in palliative care. Eur J Cancer 2006;42(1):55-64.

[2] Petersen MA, Groenvold M, Aaronson N, Blazeby J, Brandberg Y, et al. European Organisation for Research and Treatment of Cancer Quality of Life Group. Item response theory was used to shorten EORTC QLQ-C30 scales for use in palliative care. J Clin Epidemiol 2006;59(1):36-44.

[3] Bjorner JB, Petersen MA, Groenvold M, Aaronson N, Ahlner-Elmqvist M, et al. European Organisation for Research and Treatment of Cancer Quality of Life Group. Use of item response theory to develop a shortened version of the EORTC QLQ-C30 emotional functioning scale. Qual Life Res 2004;13(10):1683-97.

[4] Chow E, Hird A, Velikova G, Johnson C, Dewolf L, et al. European Organisation for Research and Treatment of Cancer Quality of Life Group. The European Organisation for Research and Treatment of Cancer Quality of Life Questionnaire for patients with Bone Metastases: The EORTC QLQ-BM22. Eur J Cancer 2008 Dec 17 [Epub ahead of print]

[5] Blazeby J, Sprangers M, Cull A, et al. EORTC Quality of Life Group: guidelines for developing questionnaire modules. 3rd ed. revised. August 2002. <http://groups.eortc.be/qol/downloads/2008module_development_guidelines.pdf>.

[6] Holland PW, Wainer H. Differential Item Functioning. Hilsdale, NJ: Lawrence Erlbaum, 1993.

[7] French AW, Miller TR. Logistic regression and its use in detecting differential item functioning in polytomous items. J Educ Meas 1996; 33:315-32.

[8] Swaminathan H, Rogers HJ. Detecting differential item functioning using logistic-regrssion procedures. J Educ Meas 1990;27:361-70.
[9] Teresi JA, Kleinman M, Ocepek-Welikson K. Modern psychometric methods for detection of differential item functioning: Application to cognitive assessment measures. Stat Med 2000;19:1651-83.
[10] Hambleton RK. Principles and selected applications of item response theory. In: Linn RL, ed. Educational measurement. New York: Macmillan, 1989:143–200.
[11] Van der Linden WJ, Hambleton RK. Handbook of modern item response theory. Berlin: Springer, 1997.
[12] Petersen MA, Groenvold M, Aaronson N, Brenne E, Fayers P, et al. European Organisation for Research and Treatment of Cancer Quality of Life Group. Scoring based on item response theory did not alter the measurement ability of EORTC QLQ-C30 cales. J Clin Epidemiol 2005;58:902-8.
[13] Muraki E. A generalized partial credit model. In: van der Linden WJ, Hambleton RK, eds. Handbook of modern item response theory. Berlin: Springer; 1997:153-68.
[14] Muraki E, Bock RD. Parscale – IRT based test scoring and item analysis for graded open-ended exercises and performance tasks. Chicago: Sci Software, 1996.
[15] Bock RD, Mislevy RJ. Adaptive EAP estimation of ability in a microcomputer environment. Appl Psychol Meas 1982;6:431-44.
[16] Muraki E. Information functions of the generalized partial credit model. Appl Psychol Meas 1993;17:351-63.
[17] Du Toit M. IRT from SSI Manual. Lincolnwood: Sci Software, 2003.
[18] Petersen MA, Groenvold M, Bjorner JB, Aaronson N, Conroy T, et al. European Organisation for Research and Treatment of Cancer Quality of Life Group. Use of differential item functioning analysis to assess the equivalence of translations of a questionnaire. Qual Life Res 2003;12:373-85.
[19] Bjorner JB, Kreiner S, Ware JE, Damsgaard MT, Bech P. Differential item functioning in the Danish translation of the SF-36. J Clin Epidemiol 1998;51:1189-202.
[20] Crane K, Gibbons LE, Jolley L, Van Bell G. Differential item functioning analysis with ordinal logistic regression techniques. Med Care 2006;44(Suppl 3):S115-123.
[21] Orlando M, Sherbourne CD, Thissen D. Summed-score linking using item response theory: Application fo depression measurement. Psychol Assess 2000;12:354-59.
[22] Maydeu-Olivares A, Drasgow F, Mead AD. Distinguishing among parametric item response models for polychotomous ordered data. Appl Psychol Meas 1994;18:245-56.
[23] Badia X, Prieto L, Roset M, Diez-Perez A, Herdman M. Development of a short osteoporosis quality of life questionnaire by equating items from two existing instruments. J Clin Epidemiol 2002;55:32.40.

Section Five: Some Case Reports

In: Advanced Cancer. Pain and Quality of Life
Editors: E. Chow, J. Merrick, pp. 263-269
ISBN: 978-1-61668-207-1
© 2010 Nova Science Publishers, Inc.

Chapter XXIII

Surgical Stabilization of Severely Destructive Upper Cervical Lytic Bone Metastases

Janet Nguyen, BSc(C)[1], Matthew Chung, BSc(C)[1], Michael Ford, MD[2], Philiz Goh, BSc[1], Joel Rubenstein, MD[3], Emily Sinclair, MRT (T)[1], Gunita Mitera, MRT(T)[1] and Edward Chow, MBBS, PhD, FRCPC*[*1]

[1]Department of Radiation Oncology,
[2]Department of Orthopedics,
[3]Department of Diagnostic Radiology, Sunnybrook Health Sciences Centre,
University of Toronto, Toronto, Ontario, Canada

The spinal column is the most frequent site for skeletal metastases. Complications from spinal metastases include pain, neurological deficits, and mechanical instability – all of which may require treatment. Upper cervical metastases are rare when compared to its spinal counterparts, however when they do occur, because of anatomic characteristics of that region, instability or pathological fractures may be perceived as life-threatening. Although radiotherapy is considered the standard treatment for spinal metastases, it has a delayed effect on pain, and is not able to treat any mechanical instability a patient may have. We report a case where a breast cancer patient required surgical stabilization due to a severely destructive lesion in the upper cervical region.

[*] ***Correspondence:*** Edward Chow, MBBS, PhD, FRCPC, Department of Radiation Oncology, Odette Cancer Centre, Sunnybrook Health Sciences Centre, 2075 Bayview Avenue, Toronto, ON M4N 3M5, Canada. Tel: 416-480-4998; Fax: 416-480-6002; E-mail: Edward.Chow@sunnybrook.ca

Introduction

Skeletal metastases are very frequent in cancer patients. One out of every three patients becomes symptomatic, causing neurological deficits, biomechanical instability, and severe pain (1,2). Local pain is the prevalent symptom noted by patients. The spinal column is the most common site for skeletal metastases (3,4). Breast carcinoma has a 75% incidence of developing bone metastases (5). Primary breast cancer patients with metastases to the spine have a longer survival prognosis in comparison to other primary cancers (6), while the occurrence of metastases to the upper cervical area has a specifically shorter survival prognosis in comparison to its spinal counterparts (7). Cervical metastases may have a poorer prognosis due to a longer detection time. The cervical region is wider when compared to the thoracic, causing lesions to grow to a larger size before it can be detected (7). A late diagnosis would tend to indicate severe destruction of the vertebral body, consequently resulting in spinal instability and may be perceived as critical due to stabilizing characteristics of the upper cervical spine (8,9).

We present a case of a patient with primary breast cancer with extensive metastatic lesions to the upper cervical area of the C1 and C2 who presented with chronic neck pain.

Case Study

A 66 year-old woman was treated with a right partial mastectomy with limited lymph node resection in February 2008 and prescribed Tamoxifen. She had presented with chronic neck pain, dizziness and decreased hearing in the left ear since the beginning of that year. Investigations suggested that her chronic pain was related to degenerative changes caused by spondylosis of the C5-7. The patient was given narcotic analgesics for her pain.

With the progressive neck pain, she became bedridden. Another CT scan was performed in July 2008 which confirmed bone metastases and showed that the neck was very unstable, due to a large lytic destructive lesion involving the right C1 with minimal involvement of the upper C2 body and lateral odontoid (see figures 1 and 2). The patient was referred to an orthopedic surgeon who prompted an immediate need for fitting of a neck brace due to the severe instability of the neck, followed by a radical operation – an occipital cervical fusion from the occiput to the C3 (see figure 3). Since the C1 region had significant destructive lesion, polymethylmethacrylate (PMMA) was used as reinforcement and was placed onto the posterior portion of the spine, continuing up onto the skull. Degenerative changes were noted in the lower cervical spine, as well as first degree anterior spondylolisthesis at the levels of C5 on C6 and C6 on C7. Radiotherapy was delivered postoperatively to the neck, 2000 cGy in 5 fractions.

She recovered uneventfully and was able to move her head freely in a vertical motion and a 50-60% capability of horizontal rotation. She was able to ambulate, her pain was much improved and her pain medication was reduced.

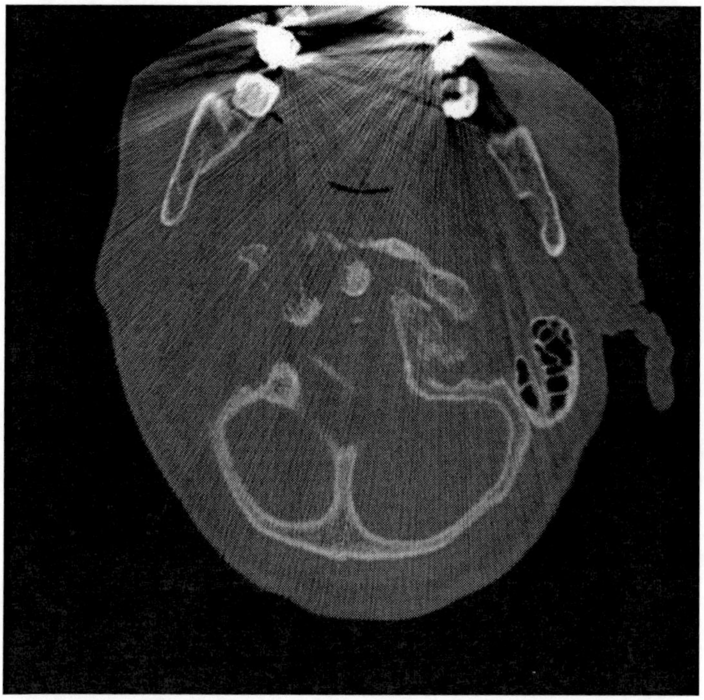

Figure 1. Axial CT image through the craniocervical junction showing extensive lytic destruction of the right lateral mass of C1 with rotation of the C1 vertebra to the left.

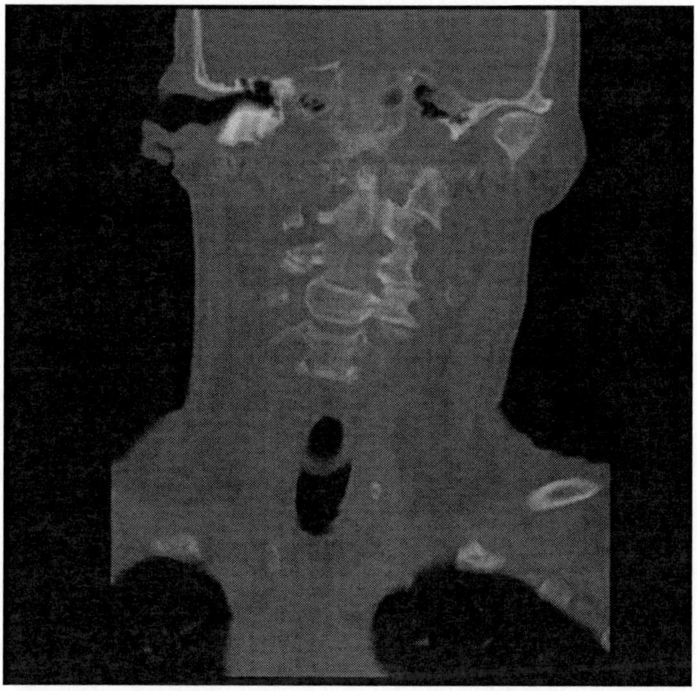

Figure 2. Coronal reformatted CT image showing lytic destruction of the right lateral mass of C1 with lateral subluxation of the left lateral mass of C1 at C1-2.

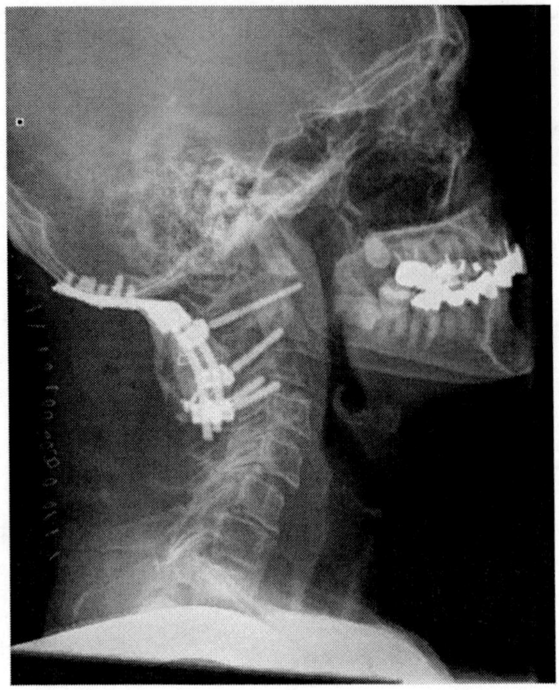

Figure 3. Postoperative lateral view of the cervical spine with posterior craniocervical instrumentation from the occiput to C3.

Discussion

The spinal column is the most common site for skeletal metastases, however it is estimated that only 5% of those spinal metastases encountered actually cause symptoms (10). Once pain and local tenderness do occur, complications such as neurological deficits are expected to occur in up to 80% of those symptomatic patients within two months. Klekamp et al. reported on the surgical outcome for spinal metastases, and found that 86% of their 105 patients claimed local pain at the affected spinal level to be the first symptom (10). Heidecke et al (8) performed a retrospective study, with 100% of their 62 patients with cervical metastases presenting with local pain as a symptom. Nakamura et al (9) had a similar finding, with 100% of their thirteen patients complaining of neck pain as a symptom for their upper cervical metastases. Two of their patients had almost their entire atlas and axis infiltrated by tumor tissue, due to being left untreated for a long period of time.

Upper cervical metastases are also rare in its occurrence in comparison to thoracic, lumbar and sacral regions (7,11). It is estimated that thoracic spine metastases tend to occur in 50-60% of all vertebral metastases, with lumbar at 30-35%, followed by the cervical spine at 10-15% 8. A delay in the diagnosis of upper cervical metastases could be the reason why it has a poorer prognosis when compared to thoracic or lumbar regions (7-9). Sciubba et al (7) did a study regarding the prognosis variables in breast cancer patients undergoing spinal surgery, and suggested that one reason for such a delay is that the upper cervical canal is wider, able to tolerate a higher degree of tumor infiltration before cord compression occurs, thereby allowing the tumor time to grow before it is detected. After the initial presentation of pain, the manifestation of neurological symptoms is rapid, within a matter of days to weeks for the lumbar spine, however in the cervical and thoracic spine it may occur over a period of weeks to months (9,12).

Treatment options for skeletal metastases include surgery, radiation, hormonal manipulation, bisphosphonates and/or chemotherapy (13). Radiation is known to be effective in treating local bone pain, however the benefits are not usually immediate, and some patients may experience a temporary period of pain flare (2,14,15). Although evidence is inconclusive as to what type of surgery should be performed for spinal metastases (13), surgical intervention and various combination modality treatments have shown improvements in ambulation and patients' quality of life (9,16). Irradiation before or after surgical intervention have had conflicting support, however, these schools of thought have both agreed upon the factors in determining the most appropriate modality on a case by case basis, which include: spinal instability, vertebral collapse, radiation resistant tumors, and the risk of neurologic deficit (15,17). Aebi (12) did mention, however, that irradiation done prior to surgery has a significantly negative effect on the outcome of the surgery, therefore it should be administered postoperatively whenever possible. The aims of surgery include stabilization, ambulatory mobility, pain reduction, and improvement in the quantity and quality of life. However, Colak et al (18) and Shehadi et al (2) stated that surgical intervention for skeletal metastases to the spine should be an available option only for palliative patients with an estimated life expectancy of at least three months. Improving quality of life is especially important considering that metastases to the spine can quickly become a major burden on the patient, due to a reduced capacity for physical activity as well as ambulation (12).

Once surgery is performed, patients are known to experience significant pain relief and improved ambulatory function (9,19). Weigel et al. did a retrospective study concerning the use of surgical intervention to manage symptomatic metastases to the spine. They found that 83% of their 72 patients were ambulatory postoperatively (19). Out of 20 patients who were non-ambulatory prior to surgery, 14 (70%) were able to walk again after surgery (19). Nakamura et al (9) reported on the treatment of metastases of the upper cervical spine, and found that 10 out of 11 patients operated on had such remarkable pain relief, they were able to ambulate as soon as a week post-surgery with a simple neck brace. In a retrospective study done by Heidecke et al., they found that spinal fusion had few complications with a good rate of permanent stabilization for the cervical spine in question (8).

Recurrence in the form of spinal metastases from a primary in breast cancer is the most common in skeletal metastases, with an overall occurrence, in the cervical area, of 10% in all spine metastases patients (2,5,20,21). Chataigner et al (14) found that administering postoperative radiotherapy did not lower the risk of local recurrence in their patients. Radiotherapy is used for palliation of pain and is recommended for those patients who are in a poor condition or those without neurological deficits (5). Radiotherapy cannot correct spinal instability (14,15). Neoplasm to the upper cervical spine are rare in comparison to cases that have been reviewed, where C3-7 is the common ground (4). There is increased mechanical risk of rotatory instability or craniocervical dislocation in cases of metastases to the atlas or axis in the spine (3). In a study by Lee (21), a relapse in the form of metastases occurred in 24% in patients with less than three positively confirmed nodules after undergoing a masectomy. Kasai et al (6) found that metastatic spine carcinoma with a primary in breast or thyroid cancer have better prognosis in an increased life expectancy as opposed to other metastatic spine cases where the primary arises elsewhere. However, Sciubba (7) determined that cervical metastases had a negative prognostic value and a shorter median survival as opposed to metastases to other areas of the spine. It is generally agreed, however, that the type of primary tumor, the degree of metastatic spread, along with the general well being of the patient is what dictates the overall survival time and long term prognosis (8).

Surgery for bone metastases in general is often reserved for palliation, and is generally only considered for those patients with neurological deficits, intractable pain, mechanical instability, or radiation resistant tumors (2,7). Surgery as a palliative treatment modality can make improvements in the quality of life, reduce pain, and improve ambulatory movement (9,16) as illustrated in our case.

Acknowledgments

This study was supported by the Michael and Karyn Goldstein Cancer Research Fund. We thank Stacy Lue for secretarial assistance.

References

[1] Raycroft JF, Hockman RP, Southwick SO. Metastatic tumors involving the cervical vertebrae: Surgical palliation. J Bone Joint Surg 1978;60(6):763-8.

[2] Shehadi JA, Sciubba DM, Suk I, Suki D, Maldaun MV, et al. Surgical treatment strategies and outcome in patients with breast cancer metastatic to the spine: A review of 87 patients. Eur Spine J 2007;16(8):1179-92.

[3] Atanasiu JP, Badatcheff F, Pidhorz L. Metastatic lesions of the cervical spine. A retrospective analysis of 20 cases. Spine 1993;18(10):1279-84.

[4] Colak A, Kutlay M, Kibici K, Demircan MN, Akin ON. Two-staged operation on C2 neoplastic lesions: Anterior excision and posterior stabilization. Neurosurg Rev 20041;27(3):189-93.

[5] Coleman RE, Rubens RD. The clinical course of bone metastases from breast cancer. Br J Cancer 1987;55(1):61-6.

[6] Kasai Y, Kawakita E, Uchida A. Clinical profile of long-term survivors of breast or thyroid cancer with metastatic spinal tumours. Int Orthop 2007;31(2):171-5.

[7] Sciubba DM, Gokaslan ZL, Suk I, Suki D, Maldaun MV, McCutcheon IE, Nader R, Theriault R, Rhines LD, Shehadi JA. Positive and negative prognostic variables for patients undergoing spine surgery for metastatic breast disease. Eur Spine J 2007;16(10):1659-67.

[8] Heidecke V, Rainov NG, Burkert W. Results and outcome of neurosurgical treatment for extradural metastases in the cervical spine. Acta Neurochir 2003;145(10):873-81.

[9] Nakamura M, Toyama Y, Suzuki N, Fujimura Y. Metastases to the upper cervical spine. J Spinal Disord 1996;9(3):195-201.
[10] Klekamp J, Samii H. Surgical results for spinal metastases. Acta Neurochir (Wien) 1998;140(9):957-67.
[11] Laus M, Pignatti G. Malaguti MC (1996) Anterior extraoral surgery to the cervical spine. Spine 1996;21(14):1687-93.
[12] Aebi M. Spinal metastasis in the elderly. Eur Spine J 2003;12(Suppl 2):S202-13.
[13] Tomita K, Kawahara N, Kobayashi T, Yoshida A, Murakami H, Akamaru T. Surgical Strategy for Spinal Metastases. Spine 2001;26(3):298-306
[14] Chataigner H, Onimus M. Surgery in spinal metastasis without spinal cord compression: Indications and strategy related to the risk of recurrence. Eur Spine J 2000;9(6):523-7.
[15] Hirabayashi H, Ebara S, Kinoshita T, Yuzawa Y, Nakamura I, et al. Clinical outcome and survival after palliative surgery for spinal metastases: Palliative surgery in spinal metastases. Cancer 2003;97(2):476-84.
[16] Thongtrangan I, Balabhadra RS, Le H, Park J, Kim DH.Vertebral body replacement with an expandable cage for reconstruction after spinal tumor resection. Neurosurg Focus 2003;15(5):E8.
[17] Sundaresan N, Rothman A, Manhart K, Kelliher K. Surgery for solitary metastases of the spine: Rationale and results of treatment. Spine 2002;27(16):1802-6
[18] Colak A, Kutlay M, Kibici K, Demircan MN, Akin ON. Two-staged operation on C2 neoplastic lesions: Anterior excision and posterior stabilization. Neurosurg Rev 2004;27(3):189-93.
[19] Weigel B, Maghsudi M, Neumann C, Kretschmer R, Muller FJ, Nerlich M. Surgical management of symptomatic spinal metastases. Postoperative outcome and quality of life. Spine 1999;24(21):2240-6.
[20] Esteva FJ, Valero V, Pusztai L, Boehnke-Michaud L, Buzdar AU, Hortobagyi GN. Chemotherapy of metastatic breast cancer: What to expect in 2001 and beyond. Oncologist 2001;6(2):133-46.
[21] Lee YT. Breast carcinoma: Pattern of recurrence and metastasis after mastectomy. Am J Clin Oncol 1984;7(5):443-9.

In: Advanced Cancer. Pain and Quality of Life
Editors: E. Chow, J. Merrick, pp. 271-277
ISBN: 978-1-61668-207-1
© 2010 Nova Science Publishers, Inc.

Chapter XXIV

Simple Bracing for the Relief of Intractable Pain

Roseanna Presutti, BSc(C)[1], Sarah Campos, BSc(C)[1], Joel Finkelstein, MD[2], Joel Rubenstein, MD[3], Emily Sinclair, MRTT[1], Gunita Mitera, MRTT[1] and Edward Chow, MBBS[*1]

[1]Department of Radiation Oncology,
[2]Department of Orthopedics,
[3]Department of Diagnostic Radiology, Sunnybrook Health Sciences Centre,
University of Toronto, Toronto, Ontario, Canada

Approximately 33% of patients with renal cell cancer develop bone metastases, most of which tend to be osteolytic in nature. Renal cell cancer is known to have a limited response to chemotherapy and radiation. In the present study, we describe a patient with renal cell cancer suffering from painful bone metastases in the left humerus. Despite surgical fixation and repeated palliative radiotherapy, the disease progressed leading to intractable pain. With no further palliative systemic, orthopedic or radiation treatments to offer as a means of pain relief, a simple brace was given to the patient. Fortunately, such bracing provided satisfactory symptom relief.

Introduction

Bone metastases are a common occurrence in patients with advanced cancer, with a prevalence of 70-85% post-mortem (1). Approximately 40% of lung, thyroid and renal cell carcinomas metastasize to the bone (2). The site of bone metastasis varies, but approximately one third occur in the appendicular skeleton (3). Only 20% develop in the upper extremities with the humerus being the most common metastatic site (4). The life expectancy of patients with bone metastases has greatly improved with recent advances in systemic therapies (5,6). As a result, skeletal complications including pain and pathological fracture (6,8) are becoming more prevalent with pathological fracture of a long bone arising in 10% (9). Such events are debilitating, and can severely reduce quality of life (QOL) in patients with metastatic cancer. In the current study, we present the case of a patient with renal cell cancer suffering from intractable pain due to bony metastasis in the left humerus.

Case study

A 62-year old gentleman, with clear cell renal cell carcinoma, initially treated with right nephrectomy in 2000, was referred to the Rapid Response Radiotherapy Program (RRRP) in December 2006 complaining of pain in the left humerus. Plain x-ray and MRI revealed a large lytic lesion with erosion of the medial cortex into the surgical neck (see figure 1). After an orthopedic consultation, the patient was considered to be at high risk for pathological fracture and was scheduled for prophylactic surgical fixation. Prior to the planned surgery, the patient suffered a pathological fracture of the left proximal humerus and received pre-operative embolization followed by an intramedullary (IM) nailing in late January 2007. A Zimmer humerus nail secured by one distal and three proximal screws was used to stabilize the extremity.

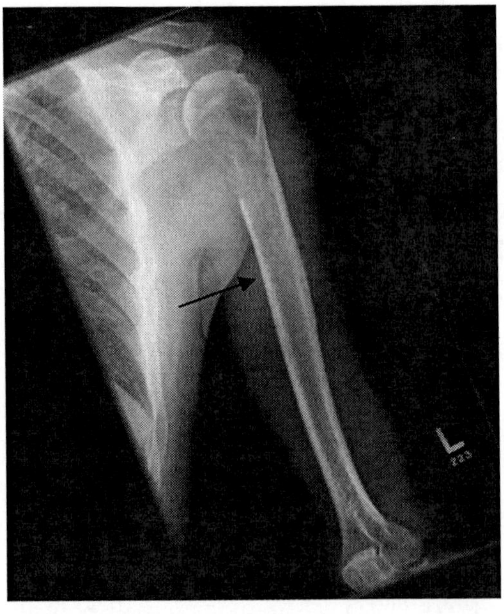

Figure 1. AP view shows a large lytic lesion in the proximal humerus with destruction of the medial cortex

* *Correspondence:* Edward Chow, MBBS, PhD, FRCPC, Department of Radiation Oncology, Odette Cancer Centre, Sunnybrook Health Sciences Centre, 2075 Bayview Avenue, Toronto, ON M4N 3M5, Canada. Tel: 416-480-4998; Fax: 416-480-6002; E-mail: Edward.Chow@sunnybrook.ca

Post-operatively, the patient was started on sunitinib. The patient was treated with palliative radiotherapy (RT), 20 Gy in five fractions, to the left humerus and shoulder in March 2007. He experienced significant pain relief post-RT. He developed cardiomyopathy with depressed cardiac function as a result of the sunitinib, and systemic therapy was therefore withheld.

In January 2008 the patient returned to the RRRP with recurring left shoulder pain. Both computed tomography (CT) and plain x-ray images showed progressive destruction of the surgical neck of the left humerus. Plain x-ray revealed stable configuration of the IM nail and therefore, further surgical intervention was not necessary. He was treated with a second course of 20Gy of RT in five fractions to the left humerus and shoulder. Post-RT, the patient continued to experience pain along the entire length of the left arm and difficulty elevating the left shoulder.

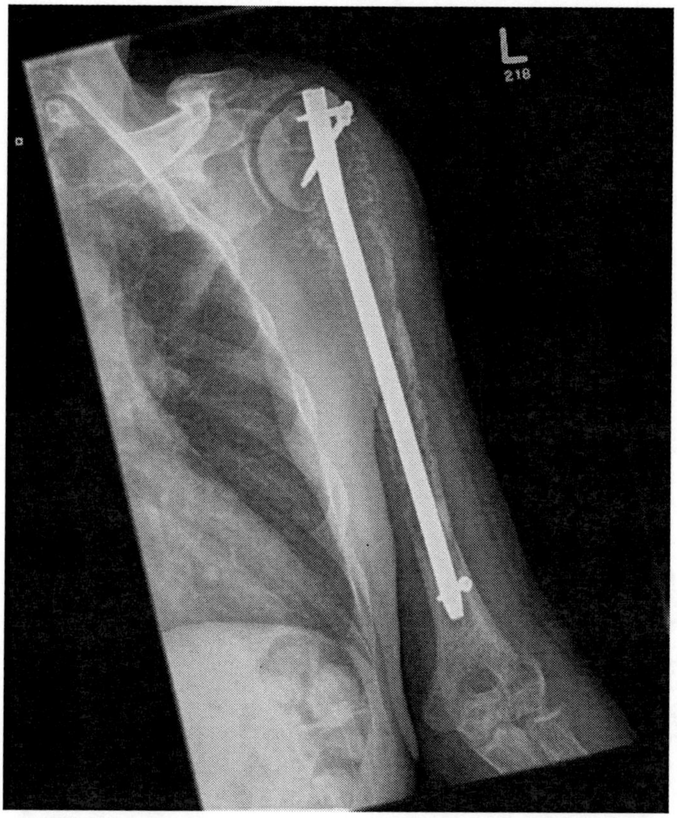

Figure 2. AP view shows fixation of the humerus with a static locking intramedullary nail and extension of the lytic destruction to involve the proximal 2/3 of the humerus

As a result of increased and unmanageable pain, the patient returned in October 2008 for consideration of further RT. Plain x-ray revealed progression of the metastatic disease with extensive lytic destruction along the entire length of the left humerus and in the left shoulder (Fig. 2). A final course of palliative RT, 20Gy in ten fractions, was delivered; however, pain relief was not experienced. Following the completion of RT, he was referred to an orthopedic surgeon for a final opinion, where it was determined that further surgery was not possible, leaving the patient with limited options for pain relief.

Thus, with the failure of palliative systemic therapy, RT and surgical intervention to relieve the patient's pain, a Sarmiento shoulder and humeral brace was prescribed (see figure 3). The brace, traditionally used by orthopedic surgeons for individuals with humeral shaft fractures, successfully provided the patient with pain relief from late October 2008 to January 2009.

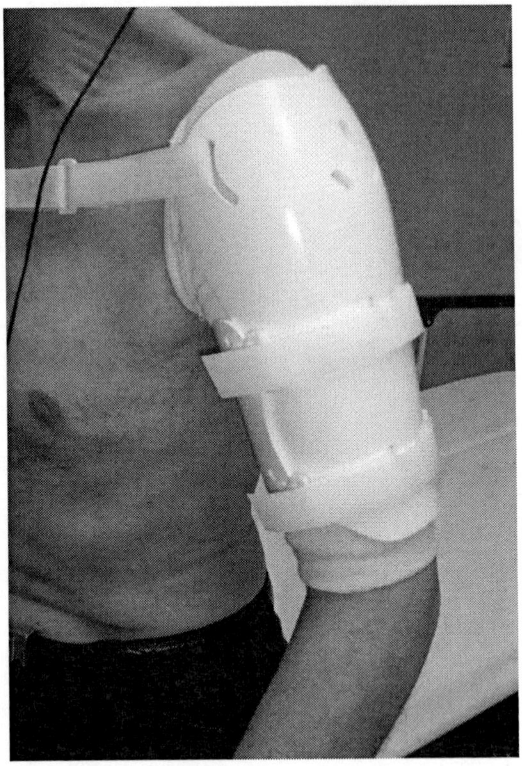

Figure 3. A Sarmiento shoulder and humeral brace was fitted and provided the patient with satisfactory pain relief where surgery, systemic therapy and palliative RT failed

Discussion

Bone lesions arising from renal cell carcinoma develop in approximately one third of patients and tend to be highly aggressive, hypervascular and osteolytic in nature (7,10-12). Osteolytic lesions involving erosion of the medial cortex are at high risk for pathological fracture, and often require surgical fixation. Due to the hypervascularity of metastatic renal cell cancer, preoperative embolization is a standard measure in order to decrease blood loss and morbidity (12,13). Furthermore, it is routine to deliver fractionated courses of palliative RT after surgical fixation of a pathological fracture (14).

The use of an interlocking IM nail for the fixation of humeral fractures is an intervention for pain relief. In a study by Sarahrudi et al (9), 11 of 27 patients with a pathological fracture of the humerus received surgical fixation by means of an IM nailing. Post operatively, all patients experienced good local pain relief (9). Tomé et al (4) found that of 12 patients with established humeral fractures treated with IM nailing, good to excellent pain relief was achieved post-operatively. Finally, in a retrospective study by Redmond et al (15), 12 out of 13 patients with humeral shaft fractures stabilized by interlocking IM nailing had good to excellent pain relief. Similar to the present study, after two-months of good function and pain relief one patient had return of pain despite receiving the conventional 20 Gy postoperative RT.

Furthermore, it is well known that metastatic renal cell carcinoma shows limited response to RT and chemotherapy (8,10,16,17). Despite reported radioresistance, RT can be a beneficial modality to relieve bony pain in renal cell cancer patients (11,18,19). In a study by Halperin et al (20), bone pain responded to RT at 77% of the irradiated sites in patients with renal cell cancer. Response was defined as a decrease in analgesic intake due to decreased pain at the treated site or patient/family reported decrease in pain at the irradiated site. In addition, Durr et al (18) reported that RT provided bony pain relief in almost all renal cell cancer patients, with up to 55% of patients experiencing complete relief. In a prospective Phase II trial by Lee et al (19), palliative RT was delivered to 31 renal cell cancer patients, 81% of whom had bone metastases. A dose of 30Gy in 10 fractions delivered to all patients was found to provide significant local pain relief for patients with bony metastases from RCC. Another study by Reichel et al (10) evaluated response to RT for 36 bony metastatic sites in renal cell cancer patients. Re-irradiation was necessary at 26% of the painful sites. However, pain returned to pre-RT levels in a median time of 2 months for all evaluable patients. Although the relief provided by palliative RT may be short lived in renal cell cancer patients, it is nevertheless a useful modality for treating bone metastases in a palliative population.

Metastatic renal cell cancer responds very poorly to many traditional cancer therapies including chemotherapy, and cytokine therapies, such as interferon-alfa (IFN-α) and interleukin-2 (IL-2), with chemotherapy and cytokines having response rates of 6% and 10-15% respectively (21,22). Sunitinib is a tyrosine kinase inhibitor that specifically targets vascular endothelial growth factor receptor 1-3 and platelet-derived growth factor α and β, and is a feasible treatment option when chemotherapy and cytokine therapies are unsuccessful (16,21-23). In patients with advanced renal cell carcinoma, sunitinib has an objective response of approximately 40% compared to 2-5% for cytokine therapy (22). Motzer et al (16) reported a similar objective response rate of 44% in patients with cytokine refractory metastatic clear cell renal cell carcinoma, with the duration of response lasting for a median of 10 months.

Despite its anti-tumor and anti-antigenic effects, sunitinib has been associated with cardiotoxicity. In a study by Telli et al (23), 15% of their patients suffered from grade 3/4 left ventricular dysfunction and symptomatic heart failure while receiving sunitinib. Similarly, Izzedine et al (22) reported incidence rates of left ventricular dysfunction and hypertension at 15% and 28% respectively in their review of sunitinib side effects in advanced metastatic renal cell carcinoma patients. Similar to these findings, in the present case, the use of sunitinib resulted in the development of cardiomyopathy resulting in the discontinuation of systemic therapy.

When no further palliative or surgical interventions were possible, a Sarmiento brace, traditionally employed for treatment of humeral shaft fractures, was prescribed to our patient. This simple, functional bracing technique was developed by Sarmiento in 1967. Muscular compression by the device forms an "inner splint" and external stabilization ensures fracture alignment and maintains limb length, allowing for mobilization of both the elbow and shoulder joint (24). In a review of 87 patients suffering from humeral shaft fractures treated with this functional bracing technique, 86% had no limitation in range of motion in the adjacent joints, with 65% of patients having no pain at follow-up assessment (24). Similarly, in a study by Rangger et al (25), all patients achieved full restoration and function in the shoulder and elbow after bracing. To our knowledge, implementation of this form of bracing has not been documented in cancer patients following surgical stabilization and post-operative RT.

The current study presented the case of a patient suffering from intractable pain due to osteolysis of the left proximal humerus. Despite surgical fixation, repeated post-operative RT and palliative systemic therapy, the patient's pain persisted. A simple brace was therefore employed in an attempt to provide symptom relief. Prior to bracing, the patient rated his worst pain as 10/10 using the Brief Pain Inventory (BPI). Immediately following implementation of the brace, the patient's worst pain was reduced to 4/10. The patient self-reported that when the brace was used, his pain was significantly reduced. Thus, when standard practice fails, and no further treatment is possible, a simple brace should be considered for the relief of intractable metastatic bony pain.

Acknowledgment

This study was supported by the Michael and Karyn Goldstein Cancer Research Fund. We would also like to thank Stacy Lue for her secretarial assistance.

References

[1] Tubiana-Hulin M. Incidence, prevalence and distribution of bone metastases. Bone 1991;12:S9-10.

[2] Pain palliation of bone metastases. Overview. InSightec.com.[homepage on the Internet]. InSightec Image Guided Treatment Ltd. 2005 1 April 2005. Available from: http://www.insightec.com/135-en-r10/BoneMetastases.aspx.

[3] Hage WD, Aboulafia AJ, Aboulafia DM. Incidence, location, and diagnostic evaluation of metastatic bone disease. Orthop Clin North Am 2000;31(4):515-28.

[4] Tome J, Carsi B, Garcia-Fernandez C, Marco F, Lopez-Duran Stern L. Treatment of pathologic fractures of the humerus with seidel nailing. Clin Orthop 1998(350):51-5.

[5] Falkmer U, Jarhult J, Wersall P, Cavallin-Stahl E. A systematic overview of radiation therapy effects in skeletal metastases. Acta Oncol 2003;42(5-6):620-33.

[6] Pavlakis N, Stockler M. Bisphosphonates for breast cancer.update in cochrane database syst rev. Cochrane Database Syst Rev 2002(1):003474 and 2005;(3):CD003474.

[7] Lipton A, Theriault RL, Hortobagyi GN, et al. Pamidronate prevents skeletal complications and is effective palliative treatment in women with breast carcinoma and osteolytic bone metastases: Long term follow-up of two randomized, placebo-controlled trials. Cancer 2000;88(5):1082-90.
[8] Kollender Y, Bickels J, Price WM, et al. Metastatic renal cell carcinoma of bone: Indications and technique of surgical intervention. J Urol 2000;164(5):1505-8.
[9] Sarahrudi K, Hora K, Heinz T, Millington S, Vecsei V. Treatment results of pathological fractures of the long bones: A retrospective analysis of 88 patients. Int Orthop 2006;30(6):519-24.
[10] Reichel LM, Pohar S, Heiner J, Buzaianu EM, Damron TA. Radiotherapy to bone has utility in multifocal metastatic renal carcinoma. Clin Orthop 2007;459:133-8.
[11] Adiga GU, Dutcher JP, Larkin M, Garl S, Koo J. Characterization of bone metastases in patients with renal cell cancer. BJU Int. 2004;93(9):1237-40.
[12] Sun S, Lang EV. Bone metastases from renal cell carcinoma: Preoperative embolization. J Vasc Interv Radiol 1998;9(2):263-9.
[13] Chatziioannou AN, Johnson ME, Pneumaticos SG, Lawrence DD, Carrasco CH. Preoperative embolization of bone metastases from renal cell carcinoma. Eur Radiol 2000;10(4):593-6.
[14] Hoegler D. Radiotherapy for palliation of symptoms in incurable cancer. Curr Problems Cancer 1997;21(3):131-83.
[15] Redmond BJ, Biermann JS, Blasier RB. Interlocking intramedullary nailing of pathological fractures of the shaft of the humerus. J Bone Joint Surg Am 1996;78(6):891-6.
[16] Motzer RJ, Rini BI, Bukowski RM, et al. Sunitinib in patients with metastatic renal cell carcinoma. JAMA 2006;295(21):2516-24.
[17] Jung ST, Ghert MA, Harrelson JM, Scully SP. Treatment of osseous metastases in patients with renal cell carcinoma. Clin Orthop 2003(409):223-31.
[18] Durr HR, Maier M, Pfahler M, Baur A, Refior HJ. Surgical treatment of osseous metastases in patients with renal cell carcinoma. Clin Orthop 1999(367):283-90.
[19] Lee J, Hodgson D, Chow E, et al. A phase II trial of palliative radiotherapy for metastatic renal cell carcinoma. Cancer 2005;104(9):1894-1900.
[20] Halperin EC, Harisiadia L. The Role of Radiation Therapy in the Management of Metastatic Renal Cell Carcinoma.Cancer 1983; 51(4):614-7.
[21] Chouhan JD, Zamarripa DE, Lai PH, Oramasionwu CU, Grabinski JL. Sunitinib (sutent): A novel agent for the treatment of metastatic renal cell carcinoma. J Oncol Pharm Pract 2007;13(1):5-15.
[22] Izzedine H, Buhaescu I, Rixe O, Deray G. Sunitinib malate. Cancer Chemother Pharmacol 2007;60(3):357-64.
[23] Telli ML, Witteles RM, Fisher GA, Srinivas S. Cardiotoxicity associated with the cancer therapeutic agent sunitinib malate. Ann Oncol 2008;19(9):1613-1618.
[24] Wallny T, Westermann K, Sagebiel C, Reimer M, Wagner UA. Functional treatment of humeral shaft fractures: Indications and results. J Orthop Trauma 1997;11(4):283-7.
[25] Rangger C, Kathrein A, Klestil T. Immediate application of fracture braces in humeral shaft fractures. J Trauma 1999;46(4):732-5.

In: Advanced Cancer. Pain and Quality of Life
Editors: E. Chow, J. Merrick, pp. 279-285
ISBN: 978-1-61668-207-1
© 2010 Nova Science Publishers, Inc.

Chapter XXV

Cemented Hemiarthroplasty, Percutaneous Acetabular Cementoplasty and Post Operative Radiation for a High Risk Lesion of the Hip

Jocelyn Pang, BSc(C)[1], Richard Jenkinson, MD[2], Gunita Mitera, MRTT[1], Andrea Donovan, MD[3], Robyn Pugash, MD[3], Maureen Trudeau, MD[4], Cindy Quinton, MD[4], Emily Sinclair, MRTT[1], Janet Nguyen, BSc(C)[1], Roseanna Presutti, BSc(C)[1] and Edward Chow, MBBS*[1]

[1]Department of Radiation Oncology,
[2]Orthopaedic Surgery,
[3]Medical Imaging,
[4]Medical Oncology, Sunnybrook Health Sciences Centre,
University of Toronto, Ontario, Canada

We present a case of a 45 year-old premenopausal patient with breast cancer who developed multiple sites of bone metastases. She presented with severe pain in her right femur and hip with inability to weight-bear. Imaging demonstrated extensive lytic destruction of the femoral neck and acetabulum. A combined approach with right hip hemiarthroplasty to treat the high risk proximal femoral lesion, cementoplasty to stabilize the acetabular lesion and palliative radiation was used. The patient suffered minimal

* ***Correspondence:*** Edward Chow, MBBS, PhD, FRCPC, Department of Radiation Oncology, Odette Cancer Centre, Sunnybrook Health Sciences Centre, 2075 Bayview Avenue, Toronto, ON M4N 3M5, Canada. Tel: 416-480-4998; Fax: 416-480-6002; E-mail: Edward.Chow@sunnybrook.ca

procedural morbidity and was discharged after a 2 day inpatient stay. She had significant pain relief and rapidly regained functional independence with full weight bearing.

Introduction

Bone metastases are a common development in breast cancer and patients (1). Nearly two thirds of patients with bone metastases will develop complications, which can include pathological fractures, severe pain, hypercalcemia, spinal cord compression, need for surgery and radiation treatment (2). Fractures are most common in long weight bearing bones, with the femur being the most frequent site. When patients present with pain related to bone metastases before a fracture has occurred, surgical intervention can decrease morbidity related to completed pathological fracture (3). Surgical reconstruction of the pelvis and acetabulum in patients with metastatic disease can be technically challenging and exposes the patient to surgical morbidity and potential complications (4). To address this problem, percutaneous cementoplasty techniques have been developed in recent years (5). We present a case of a 45 year-old woman to illustrate the potential utility of a combined treatment with arthroplasty and cementoplasty for treatment of osseous metastasis around the hip.

Case Story

A 45 year-old premenopausal female was referred in February 2007 for a second opinion regarding treatment of her breast cancer. She had undergone a left lumpectomy in December 2006 for a 1.7 cm, grade III, infiltrating ductal carcinoma. The tumor was estrogen and progesterone positive, and HER2/neu positive. Subsequent axillary lymph node dissection revealed two out of six lymph nodes positive for metastatic adenocarcinoma. The metastatic work up was negative. She was recommended Fluorouracil, Epirubicin, Cyclophosphamide, Docetaxel (FEC-D) chemotherapy followed by Tamoxifen and Herceptin as adjuvant treatment for her breast cancer. Unfortunately, her first dose of chemotherapy brought upon severe palpitations and functional decline. Her second cycle of FEC-D chemotherapy was accompanied by Neulasta because she had developed neutropenia during her treatment. The drug induced more side effects leaving her bed-ridden due to bone pain. Rather than continuing the chemotherapy treatment, the patient decided to pursue naturopathic medications. Thus, she did not receive any Tamoxifen, Herceptin, hormonal therapy or adjuvant radiation.

In March 2008, patient reported bone pain and a bone scan was performed. The scan revealed increased activity in axial and appendicular skeleton compatible with bone metastases. She received multiple treatments of palliative radiation over several months to a variety of sites. She was also prescribed various analgesics to manage her pain. Additionally, she was started on Pamidronate alongside with Zoladex and Tamoxifen; however the Zoladex caused nausea and lack of appetite. Nevertheless her illness progressed despite the hormone therapy. Therefore, in October 2008, the patient was started on Taxol chemotherapy.

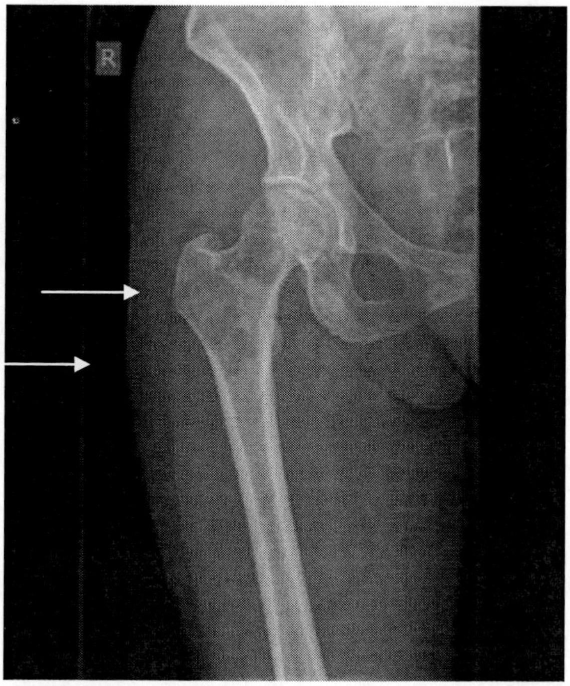

Figure 1. Right hip radiograph shows mixed lytic and sclerotic lesions in the right hemipelvis and the proximal right femur. The lytic lesion in the right femoral neck extending into the subtrochanteric femur is at high risk for a pathologic fracture (arrows)

Very soon after that, she began to report severe pain in her right thigh when bearing weight, and became wheel-chair bound. Physical examination revealed pain on internal rotation of the right hip and tenderness in the upper thigh on deep palpation. Radiographs revealed changes in the pelvis and proximal femora, and sclerotic lesions in the right distal femur (see figure 1). Destructive osteolysis in the right proximal femur was at high risk for a pathologic fracture. She was referred for an orthopedic consultation. One option was a complete pelvic reconstruction with a total hip arthroplasty. However, the relatively small, contained lesion in her right acetabulum made her a good candidate for cementoplasty. It was therefore possible to avoid the surgical morbidity associated with a pelvic reconstruction by instead performing a replacement of the proximal femur, followed by a minimally invasive cementoplasty. She underwent a long stemmed cemented bipolar hemiarthroplasty in November 2008. The procedure was tolerated well by the patient with minimal blood loss and no immediate complication. The patient was discharged two days post-operatively when mobilizing independently with minimal discomfort. The preoperative pain was decreased substantially after her proximal femoral reconstruction. She was treated with appropriate DVT prophylaxis.

Three weeks after the operation her incision had healed and her staples were removed. Her function was reported at a much higher level in comparison to pre-operation, however, she had not recovered normal endurance. After approximately 100 meters of walking she would require rest due to hip/groin pain. The patient received postoperative cementoplasty to her right acetabulum in December 2008 (Fig. 2). Further, she also received postoperative radiation therapy to her right hip in January 2009 with 2000 cGy in 5 fractions. These treatments improved her mobility to the point that it was no longer limited by hip pain.

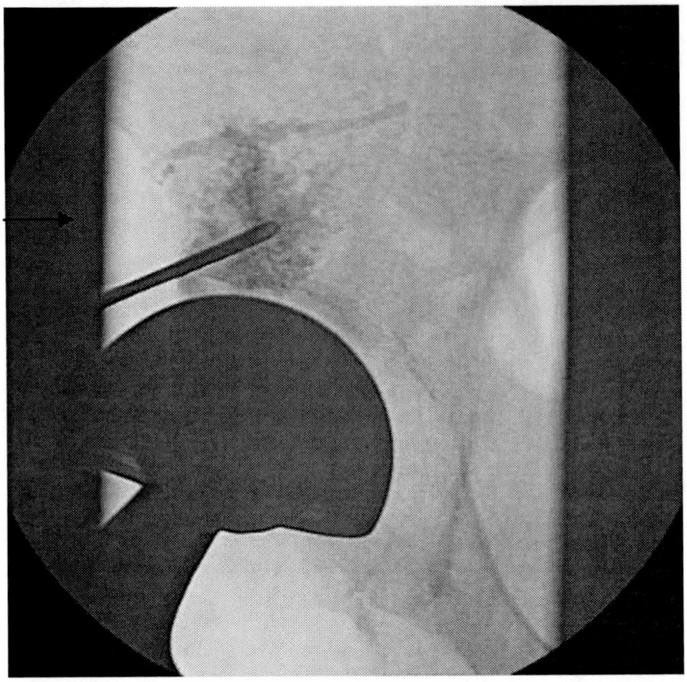

Figure 2. Fluoroscopic image of the right hip shows administration of cement via a percutaneous approach (arrow). Note right bipolar hemiarthroplasty in place

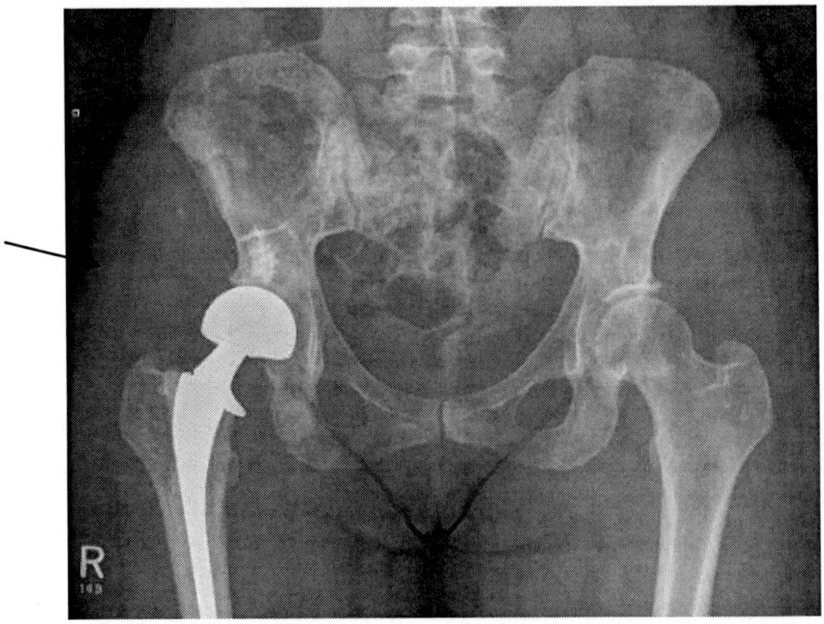

Figure 3. Radiograph of the pelvis following right bipolar hemiarthroplasty and cementoplasty of the right acetabulum.There are widespread mixed sclerotic and lytic lesions in the pelvis and proximal femora

At 8- week follow up post surgery, she did not have any leg length discrepancy and her right leg was neurovascularly intact. She had also regained a wide range of motion in her right hip. Radiographs showed hemiarthroplasty in good position and cement at the acetabulum demonstrated good filling of the lesion. There were no fractures or hardware complications (see figure 3).

Discussion

The incidence of bone metastases is highest in breast and prostate cancer patients, with breast cancer accounting for the highest frequency of pathological fracture (6). As with this patient's experience, one of the most significant symptoms of bone metastases is pain (1,2,6); if the sensation is persistent in weight bearing bones, pain can also raise suspicion of an impending pathological fracture (7). In this situation, surgical intervention should be strongly considered (6). In the hip region, impending fractures are typically stabilized through metal implants, bone cement and joint replacement; however, there are currently no evidence-based guidelines for surgical management for these lesions (4). As a result, these patients require an individualized approach to their treatment.

When considering surgical treatment for an impending fracture, both the lesion and patient are taken into consideration. This patient's lesion was lytic rather than blastic, involved a large area of the proximal femur and caused pain that precluded weight bearing. This called for immediate intervention (6). Her principal lesion involved the femoral neck which could be addressed with proximal femoral reconstruction using a hemiarthroplasty. This restored immediate independent weight bearing function to this patient with minimal surgical morbidity. Her acetabular lesion was significant but amenable to urgent outpatient treatment with percutaneous cementoplasty after her femoral surgery. This spared the patient the added surgical morbidity of a pelvic reconstruction and total hip arthroplasty.

Implant selection is affected by several factors. In general, cemented prosthesis are preferred as they provide immediate stability and allow full weight bearing. Uncemented components rely on a biological response from the surrounding bone tissue. This is often compromised by ongoing chemotherapy and radiation. A Cochrane review of the general hip fracture population revealed that pain is reported more often and with increased severity in patients who underwent arthroplasty at the proximal femur without cement. This review also reported that patients who had received bone cement regained better mobility post operation (8). These findings would likely be even more pronounced in a pathologic fracture group where failure rates of uncemented fixation would be predictably higher.

After the hemiarthroplasty, a peri-acetabular lesion underwent cementoplasty. Basile et al (5) report that cementoplasty is a safe and efficient method of managing pain associated with small lesions from bone metastases. Their entire patient group (100% of patients) reported pain relief. With respect to mobility, 80% of the treated showed improvement (5). We used radiation therapy post-surgery to minimize possible disease progression (6). As Townsend et al. showed in their study, surgery alongside radiation provides for the best possibility of reaching and maintaining a level of normal functioning (9).

While this patient has shown improvement in pain and mobility after surgery, further follow up is recommended. The short term outcome of pain and mobility from a bipolar hemiarthroplasty is more or less equal to outcomes associated with a total hip replacement. Longer term outcomes in hemiarthroplasty patients of ten years or longer reveal more complications including increased pain and occasionally a need for revision to total hip arthroplasty (10). The goal of this surgery is palliative to immediately improve mobility, decrease pain and improve quality of life (11). Currently, patients with bone metastases have a life span of approximately 2-5 years (12), the immediate advantages of the less invasive hemiarthroplasty should outweigh the future implications.

We report a successful early outcome of a multidisciplinary treatment strategy in a patient with metastatic breast carcinoma to the hip. Hemiarthroplasty was chosen as a less invasive surgical option over total hip arthroplasty with pelvic reconstruction. Post-operative cementoplasty and radiotherapy treatment were able to further improve mobility, decrease pain, and potentially limit spread of disease in this patient.

Acknowledgments

This study was supported by the Michael and Karyn Goldstein Cancer Research Fund. We would also like to thank Stacy Lue for her secretarial assistance. Conflict of interest: none.

References

[1] Solomayer E, Diel IJ, Meyberg GC, Gollan C, Bastert G. Metastatic breast cancer: Clinical course, prognosis and therapy related to the first site of metastasis. Breast Cancer Res Treat 2000;59(3):271-8.

[2] Coleman RE, Rubens RD. The clinical course of bone metastases from breast-cancer. Br J Cancer 1987;55(1):61-6.

[3] Johnson SK, Knobf MT. Surgical interventions for cancer patients with impending or actual pathologic fractures. Orthop Nurs 2008;27(3):160-71.

[4] Kreder HJ. Factors affecting outcome after surgical treatment of acetabular and femoral metastatic lesions. Tech Orthop 2004;19(1):38-44.

[5] Basile A, Giuliano G, Scuderi V, Motta S, Crisafi R, Coppolino F, et al. Cementoplasty in the management of painful extraspinal bone metastases: Our experience. Radiol Med 2008;113(7):1018-28.

[6] Swanson KC, Pritchard DJ, Sim FH. Surgical treatment of metastatic disease of the femur. J Am Acad Orthop Surg 2000;8(1):56-65.

[7] Riccio AI, Wodajo FM, Malawer M. Metastatic carcinoma of the long bones. Am Fam Physician 2007;76(10):1489-94.

[8] Parker MJ, Gurusamy KS. Arthroplasties (with and without bone cement) for proximal femoral fractures in adults (review). Cochrane DB Syst Rev. 2006;3:1.

[9] Townsend PW, Smalley SR, Cozad SC, Rosenthal HG, Hassanein RES. Role of postoperative radiation therapy after stabilization of fractures caused by metastatic disease. Int J Radiat Oncol 1995;31(1):43-9.

[10] Muraki M, Sudo A, Hasegawa M, Fukuda A, Uchida A. Long-term results of bipolar hemiarthroplasty for osteoarthritis of the hip and idiopathic osteonecrosis of the femoral head. J Orthop Sci 2008;13(4):313-7.

[11] Stephen D. Management of metastatic osseous lesions of the lower extremity. Tech Orthop. 2004;19(1):15-24.

[12] Chow E, Hoskin P, van der Linden, Y., Bottomley A, Velikova G. Quality of life and symptom end points in palliative bone metastases trials. Clin Oncol 2006(18):67-9.

In: Advanced Cancer. Pain and Quality of Life
Editors: E. Chow, J. Merrick, pp. 287-294
ISBN: 978-1-61668-207-1
© 2010 Nova Science Publishers, Inc.

Chapter XXVI

Remineralization of an Impending Fracture from an Osteolytic Metastasis in a Breast Cancer Patient from Palliative Radiotherapy and Bisphosphonate

***Gunita Mitera, BSc, MRT(T)*[1], *Joel Rubenstein, MD*[2], *Joel Finkelstein, MD*[3], *Melanie TM Davidson, PhD*[4] and *Edward Chow, MBBS*[*1]**

[1]Rapid Response Radiotherapy Program, Department of Radiation Oncology,
[2]Department of Radiology,
[3]Department of Orthopedic Surgery,
[4]Department of Physics, Sunnybrook Health Sciences Centre,
University of Toronto, Toronto, Ontario, Canada

Metastatic disease to the bone is a common manifestation of breast cancer. A skeletally related event (SRE) may occur in up to two-thirds of patients with bone metastases. An SRE may include pathological fractures, severe pain, hypercalcemia, spinal cord compression, need for surgery and radiation treatment. This case report highlights the management for an impending pathological fracture that most frequently presents in the femur, a weight-bearing area. This case study presents a patient with an osteolytic lesion within the intertrochantic region of the right femur. She was offered prophylactic fixation of the right hip and femur and post-operative radiotherapy, but she refused surgical intervention. Given the heightened concern for an impending pathological fracture, we managed her using radiotherapy with Clodronate, a bisphosphonate to stabilize and

* Correspondence: Gunita Mitera BSc, MRT(T), Department of Radiation Therapy, Odette Cancer Centre, Sunnybrook Health Sciences Centre, 2075 Bayview Avenue, Toronto, ON, Canada M4N 3M5. Tel: 416-480-6100 ext 7543; Fax: 416-480-6002; E-mail: Gunita.Mitera@sunnybrook.ca

promote bone growth in the metastatic area. Based on our case study, we confirm radiotherapy in addition to bisphophonates may help to stabilize an osteolytic impending fracture from breast histology if patient is not a surgical candidate or refuses surgery if offered.

Introduction

Metastatic disease to the bone is a common manifestation of breast cancer (1). A skeletally related event (SRE) may occur in up to two-thirds of patients with bone metastases. An SRE may include pathological fractures, severe pain, hypercalcemia, spinal cord compression, need for surgery and radiation treatment (2). This case report highlights the management for an impending pathological fracture that most frequently presents in the femur, a weight-bearing area (3). This case study presents a patient with an osteolytic lesion within the intertrochantic region of the right femur. She was offered prophylactic fixation of the right hip and femur and post-operative radiotherapy; however, she refused surgical intervention. Given the heightened concern for an impending pathological fracture, we managed her using radiotherapy with Clodronate, a bisphosphonate to stabilize and promote bone growth in the metastatic area.

Case Study

A 55-year old female was diagnosed with a stage I, Estrogen-receptor equivocal and Progesterone-receptor positive left-sided breast cancer in 1997. Her treatment included breast conserving surgery with axillary node dissection and radiotherapy. Subsequently, her oncologist followed her on an annual basis for her breast cancer. In 2003 she suffered from local recurrence and was treated with a mastectomy, four cycles of doxorubicin and cyclophosphamide (AC) chemotherapy and Tamoxifen.

In January of 2008, she complained of right hip pain. Bone scan revealed an intense uptake in the right intertrochanteric region. Plain x-rays of the right pelvis and femur revealed an extensive mixed osteolytic and osteosclerotic focus within the right femoral neck and intertrochanteric area, along with cortical permeation. Furthermore, a computed tomography (CT) volumetric scan showed an extensive irregular lytic, permeative lesion in the proximal femoral diaphysis, extending to the lesser tuberosity and femoral neck, consistent with metastasis. It also confirmed extensive cortical permeation at the posterolateral femoral head, encompassing approximately 25% of the circumference. There was an additional focal cortical permeation at the anterior aspect of the mid-femoral neck. Radiographically, this was concerning for a significantly high risk of fracture (see figure 1).

Based on the imaging studies, the patient was immediately referred to the orthopedic surgeon for consideration of prophylactic fixation of the right hip and femur prior to radiotherapy. Prophylactic surgery was offered to the patient; however, she refused surgery. Hence, it was recommended that the patient walk with a cane to avoid the possibility of a fracture. Due to the high risk of fracture, as an alternative option the patient was offered palliative radiotherapy to the right hip and femur with 3000 cGy in 10 fractions. During a response assessment at three weeks, the patient reported reduced pain level and no longer walked with a limp, and discontinued the use of a cane. At two and four weeks post-radiotherapy, plain x-rays of the right hip and femur revealed no significant changes. Two months post-radiotherapy, the patient reported the pain to have resolved and was able to walk comfortably.

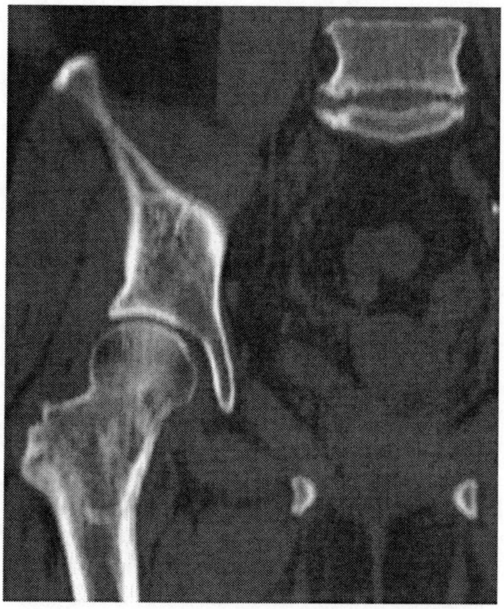

Figure 1.CT of right hip and femur before radiotherapy treatment showing permeative lytic destruction of bone in the proximal femur

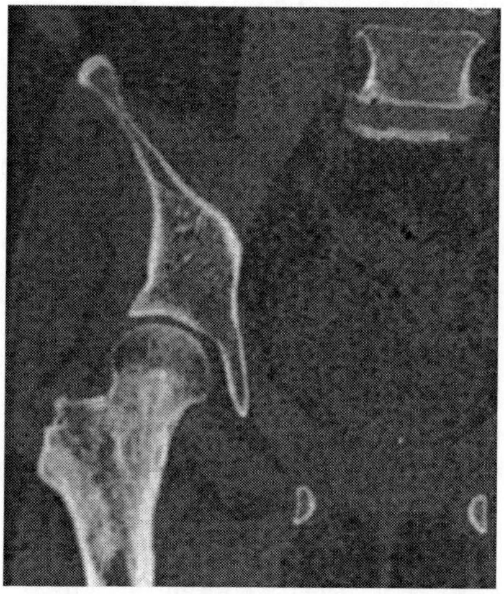

Figure. 2.CT of right hip and femur 14-months after radiotherapy treatment showing sclerotic new bone formation in the region of previous lytic destruction

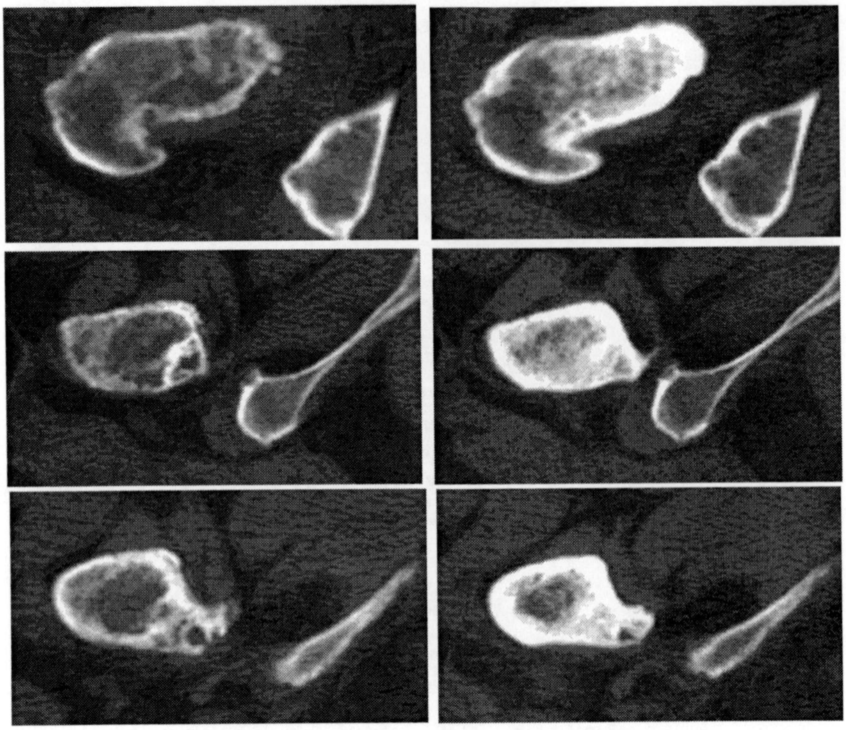

Figure 3. An enhanced view of the pre-radiation lytic destruction and post-radiation sclerosis within the right hip and femur

On her four-month follow-up, the patient still had complete relief of her pain and her activity level had increased such that she was able to dance again. X-rays reveal evidence of bone filing and no pathological fracture. Consequently, the surgeon declared the risk of fracture of the right femur to be minimal. The patient had also been prescribed Femara 2.5mg daily and Clodronate. Almost one-year post-radiotherapy treatment, the patient reported excellent range of motion of her right hip. X-rays continued to report no pathological fracture, with minimal changes. However, at this time there were two new noted sclerotic foci in the supraacetabular ilium. Since they were clinically asymptomatic, they were not treated with radiotherapy. Finally, 14-months post-radiotherapy, follow-up CT scan revealed sclerotic lesions in the radiated right hip and femur, compatible with treatment related response with significant improvement (figures 2 and 3).

Discussion

Approximately 75% of breast cancer patients with recurrent disease will develop bone metastases during the course of their disease, and for one third of patients this is the first sign of recurrence (4). Breast cancer patients with bone metastases alone have a life expectancy of several years. This is longer when compared with patients who have visceral metastases from the same primary histology (5-8). Hence, it is important to evaluate the long-term efficacy of any offered treatment regimen in order to promote an improved quality of life for our patients (9).

Osteolytic bony metastases from breast histology may result in intractable pain and a high risk of pathologic fracture. Once bone has lost its structural integrity and is not yet fractured, they may be unable to support weight-bearing function for months. Under these circumstances, quality of life may be directly related to intact limb function that is necessary for ambulatory ability and activities of daily living (10).

When either patient dysfunction or pain is rated as severe, a treatment option that provides quick resolve of pain as well as quality of life should be considered. Treatment options in the management of metastatic bone disease are not mutually exclusive. Hence, an upfront multi-disciplinary approach is imperative for appropriate and timely decision-making. For example, surgical stabilization may revive functionality, while post-operative radiotherapy or chemotherapy may be required for pain relief and tumor control (10).

For impending pathological fractures routine follow-up with imaging and physical examination is recommended in order to prevent a fracture. The morbidity associated with a pathological fracture is not only devastating for the patient; moreover, it also narrows the range of treatment options, mitigates against full functional restoration, and demands a rehabilitation hiatus (10).

For clinicians to determine the risk of pathological fracture, Mirels (11) developed an objective scoring system that is governed by both clinical and radiographic evidence for each patient. It was developed with the intent to be used as an objective measure to help determine the risk of pathological fracture, and hopefully to prevent it from happening at all.

This system allots one, two, or three points to each risk factor based on both clinical and radiographic evidence for each patient. The maximum obtainable score is 12 points and the summation of these factors equips a clinician with an individualized accuracy for a given risk of fracture, as compared to evaluating any individual factor alone. A score of 9 suggests a 33% chance of fracture and is considered to the most accurate in Mirels' study (11) due to the 0% false positive rate. However, scores of 7 and 8 were associated with a smaller risk of fracture, but were confounded with a higher false positive rate within the study. Mirels (11) recommended that lesions with scores of 8 or higher require prophylactic internal fixation prior to radiotherapy, and lesions that obtain scores of 7 or lower can be safely irradiated without a risk of fracture. Table 1 demonstrates this scoring system.

Table 1. Scoring system for risk of pathological fracture

SCORE			
VARIABLE	1	2	3
Site	Upper limb	Lower limb	Peritrochanter
Pain	Mild	Moderate	Functional (Severe)
Lesion	Blastic	Mixed	Lytic
Size	<1/3	1/3 – 2/3	>2/3

Using Mirel's criteria (11), our patient would be assigned a score of 10, and this would equate to a high risk for pathological fracture. Surgical stabilization is recommended to be the first line of treatment for such clinical scenarios, however, beyond the scoring criteria, other considerations should include the location of the metastasis, primary tumor, ability to withstand general anesthesia, life expectancy and expected clinical response to non-operative therapy (10,12).

Radiotherapy is an established treatment for metastatic bone pain (10,14); however, its role in remineralization of osteolytic lesions as an upfront therapy for high-risk bony metastases remains unclear. While the literature recommends post-operative radiotherapy (11,12,14), there is a paucity of evidence to determine the optimal radiotherapy dose fractionation schedule to promote bone healing and prevent fracture (12-14).

We previously reviewed 25 breast cancer patients with osteolytic metastases who had CT scans before and three months after palliative radiotherapy. The median percent density change following a single 8 Gy, 20 Gy in 5 treatments, and 30 Gy in 10 treatments were demonstrated to be 128 (range 98–255), 141 (range 79–342), and 145 (range 65–235), respectively. It was feasible to evaluate remineralization of osteolytic lesions with palliative radiotherapy using CT imaging (13). However, beyond its feasibility the appropriate dose fractionation scheme is still controversial.

A study by the Radiation Therapy Oncology Group (RTOG) observed an increased risk of pathological fracture after 40.5 Gy as compared with after 25 Gy (12). In contrast, there has been a randomized study that has evaluated the effects of pain relief and remineralization for patients with histologically proven breast, lung, prostate or kidney cancer and radiologically confirmed bone metastases. These patients were randomized to either a single 8 Gy or 30 Gy in 10 fractions. Pain relief was determined using pain score, analgesic usage and subjective perception of pain. Remineralization was measured using CT imaging. Results were captured prior to radiotherapy, the day after, 6 weeks, 3 and 6 months post-treatment. Of 107 patients, there was no significant difference in overall (81% versus 78%) and complete (33% versus 31%) pain response for the use of 8 Gy versus 30 Gy respectively. However, the remineralization rate proved to be significantly different between patients in the fractionated group (173%) and the single dose group (120%, $p < 0.0001$). Specifically, this trend was highly significant for patients with a primary breast histology ($p < 0.001$) (15).

Another treatment modality, bisphosphonates, has demonstrated promise within in vivo studies to prevent or delay SREs. More interestingly, Krempien demonstrate that the use of early bisphosphonates administration in conjunction with radiotherapy improves remineralization and restabilization of osteolytic bone metastases in animal tumor models (16). For example, in a mouse model of tumor-induced osteolysis, concurrent administration of zoledronic acid with radiation therapy was found to improve bone density, biomechanical strength and microarchitecture (17). Particularly, there is in vitro evidence for synergistic effects between zoledronic acid and radiation when demonstrated on breast cancer cells (18). Furthermore, a pilot study conducted by Vassiliou et al (19), delivered 30-40 Gy of radiotherapy delivered over 3 - 4.5 weeks combined with 10 cycles of monthly intravenous ibandronate. This was demonstrated to provide substantial bone pain relief and increased bone density for patients. The majority of these patients had primary breast (29%), lung (29%), or prostate (13%) cancers. Therefore, these studies support the idea that under circumstances where surgical intervention is either technically not feasible or the patient does not wish to have surgery for an impending fracture, perhaps these combined treatment interventions may be less invasive alternative options to help stabilize an osteolytic impending fracture from a breast histology.

Comprehensive management of patients with metastatic bone disease requires the participation of an orthopedic surgeon early in the clinical course. Early consultation and mutual follow-up will benefit the patient in maintaining independent function and avoid a possible fracture that may be devastating to the patient (10). When a pathological fracture has occurred, the primary goal is to provide pain relief. Secondary intentions are to achieve stability and to restore function. Unless medical contraindications exist, or unless life expectancy is extremely short, surgery is usually recommended. Based on our case study, we confirm radiotherapy in addition to bisphophonates may help to stabilize an osteolytic impending fracture from breast histology if patient is not a surgical candidate or refuses surgery if offered.

References

[1] Solomayer E, Diel IJ, Meyberg GC, et al. Metastatic breast cancer: Clinical course, prognosis and therapy related to the first site of metastasis. Breast Cancer Res Treat 2000;59(3):271-8.

[2] Coleman RE, Rubens RD. The clinical course of bone metastases from breast-cancer. Br J Cancer 1987;55(1): 61-6.

[3] Johnson SK, Knobf MT. Surgical interventions for cancer patients with impending or actual pathologic fractures. Orthop Nurs 2008;27(3):160-71.

[4] Stoll B. Natural history, prognosis and staging of bone metastasis. In: Stroll BA, Parbhoo S, eds. Bone metastasis: Monitoring and treatment. New York: Raven Press, 1983:1-20.

[5] Perez JE, Machiavelli M, Leone BA, et al. Bone-only versus visceral-only metastatic pattern in breast cancer: analysis of 150 patients. A GOCS study. Am J Clin Oncol 1990;13(4):294-8.

[6] Toma S, Venturino A, Sogno G, et al. Metastatic bone tumors. Nonsurgical treatment. Outcome and survival. Clin Orthop 1993;295:246-51.

[7] Brown JE, Coleman RE. The present and future role of bisphosphonates in the management of patients with breast cancer. Breast Cancer Res 2002;4(1):24-9.

[8] Coleman RE. Skeletal complications of malignancy. Cancer 1997;80(8 Suppl):1588-94.

[9] Rasmussen B, Vejborg I, Jensend AB, et al. Irradiation of bone metastases in breast cancer patients: a randomized study with 1 year follow-up Radiother Oncol 1995;34:179-84.

[10] Colyer RA. Surgical stabilization of pathological neoplastic fractures Curr Probl Cancer 1986;10(3):117-68.

[11] Mirels H. Metastatic disease in long bones A proposed scoring system for diagnosing impending pathologic fractures Clin Orthop Relat Res 2003;415S: S4-13.

[12] Andreson PR, Coia LR. Fractionation and outcomes with palliative radiation therapy Semin Radiat Oncol 2000;10(3):191-9.

[13] Chow E, Holden L, Rubenstein J, et al. Computed tomography (CT) evaluation of breast cancer patients with osteolytic bone metastases undergoing palliative radiotherapy—a feasibility study. Radiother Oncol 2004;70:291-4.

[14] Chow E, Harris K, Fan G, et al. Palliative radiotherapy trials for bone metastases: a systematic review. J Clin Oncol 2007;25(11):1423-36.

[15] Koswig S, Budach V. Recalcification and pain relief following radiotherapy for bone metastases: A randomized trial of 2 different fractionation schedules (10 X 3 Gy vs. 1 X 8 Gy). Strahlenther Onkol 1999;175:500-8. [German]

[16] Krempien R, Huber P, Hrms W, et al. Combination of early bisphosphonate administration and irradiation leads to improved remineralization and restabilization of osteolytic bone metastases in an animal tumor model. Cancer 2003;98(6):1318-24.

[17] Arrington SA, Damron TA, Mann KA, et al. Concurrent administration of zoledronic acid and irradiation leads to improved bone density, biomechanical strendgth and microarchitecture in a mouse model of tumor-induced osteolysis. J Surg Oncol 2008;97(3):284-90.

[18] Ural AU, Avcu F, Candir M, et al. In vitro synergistic cyroreductive effects of zoledronic acid and radiation on breast cancer cells, Breast Cancer Res 2006;8(4): R52.

[19] Vassiliou V, Kalogeropoulou C, Christopoulos C, et al. Combination ibandronate and radiotherapy for the treatment of bone metastases: clinical evaluation and radiologic assessment. Int J Radiat Oncol Biol Phys 2007;67(1):264-72.

Section Six: Acknowledgments

In: Advanced Cancer. Pain and Quality of Life
Editors: E. Chow, J. Merrick, pp. 297-298
ISBN: 978-1-61668-207-1
© 2010 Nova Science Publishers, Inc.

Chapter XXVII

About the Editors

Edward Chow MBBS, MSc, PhD, FRCPC, is professor of radiation oncology at the University of Toronto in Canada. He is the chairperson of the Rapid Response Radiotherapy Program and Bone Metastases Site Group at Odette Cancer Centre, Sunnybrook Health Sciences Centre, Toronto, Canada and also a clinician scientist at Sunnybrook Research Institute. He has published in the area of palliative radiotherapy and end of life care issues. E-mail: Edward.Chow@sunnybrook.ca

Joav Merrick, MD, MMedSci, DMSc, is professor of pediatrics, child health and human development affiliated with Kentucky Children's Hospital, University of Kentucky, Lexington, United States and the Zusman Child Development Center, Division of Pediatrics, Soroka University Medical Center, Ben Gurion University, Beer-Sheva, Israel, the medical director of the Division for Mental Retardation, Ministry of Social Affairs, Jerusalem, the founder and director of the National Institute of Child Health and Human Development. Numerous publications in the field of pediatrics, child health and human development, rehabilitation, intellectual disability, disability, health, welfare, abuse, advocacy, quality of life and prevention. Received the Peter Sabroe Child Award for outstanding work on behalf of Danish Children in 1985 and the International LEGO-Prize ("The Children's Nobel Prize") for an extraordinary contribution towards improvement in child welfare and well-being in 1987. E-Mail: jmerrick@zahav.net.il; Website: www.nichd-israel.com; Home-page: http://jmerrick50.googlepages.com/home

Acknowledgments

The editors wants to acknowledge Stacy Lue BA, CMS, Sunnybrook Health Sciences and Odette Cancer Centre, Department of Radiation Oncology, Toronto, Canada and administrative assistant to Edward Chow for her dedication, effective work and handling of the logistic work around the creation of this book.

In: Advanced Cancer. Pain and Quality of Life
Editors: E. Chow, J. Merrick, pp. 299
ISBN: 978-1-61668-207-1
© 2010 Nova Science Publishers, Inc.

CHAPTER XXVIII

About the Department of Radiation Oncology, Sunnybrook Health Sciences Centre, Canada

The Odette Cancer Centre, the comprehensive cancer program of Sunnybrook Health Sciences Centre is a leading regional cancer centre in Toronto, Ontario, Canada. It is the sixth largest cancer centre in North America in terms of number of new cancer patients seen per year. The Department of Radiation Oncology at Sunnybrook is an academic unit fully affiliated with the University of Toronto. Palliative radiotherapy is one of the key research foci in the Department of Radiation Oncology.

Contact

Edward Chow, MBBS, PhD, FRCPC, Department of Radiation Oncology, Odette Cancer Centre, Sunnybrook Health Sciences Centre, 2075 Bayview Avenue, Toronto, Ontario, Canada M4N 3M5. Tel: 416-480-4998; Fax: 416-480-6002; E-mail: Edward.Chow@sunnybrook.ca

In: Advanced Cancer. Pain and Quality of Life
Editors: E. Chow, J. Merrick, pp. 301-303
ISBN: 978-1-61668-207-1
© 2010 Nova Science Publishers, Inc.

Chapter XXIX

About the National Institute of Child Health and Human Development in Israel

The National Institute of Child Health and Human Development (NICHD) in Israel was established in 1998 as a virtual institute under the auspicies of the Medical Director, Ministry of Social Affairs and Social Services in order to function as the research arm for the Office of the Medical Director. In 1998 the National Council for Child Health and Pediatrics, Ministry of Health and in 1999 the Director General and Deputy Director General of the Ministry of Health endorsed the establishment of the NICHD.

Mission

The mission of a National Institute for Child Health and Human Development in Israel is to provide an academic focal point for the scholarly interdisciplinary study of child life, health, public health, welfare, disability, rehabilitation, intellectual disability and related aspects of human development. This mission includes research, teaching, clinical work, information and public service activities in the field of child health and human development.

Service and academic activities

Over the years many activities became focused in the south of Israel due to collaboration with various professionals at the Faculty of Health Sciences (FOHS) at the Ben Gurion University of the Negev (BGU). Since 2000 an affiliation with the Zusman Child Development Center at the Pediatric Division of Soroka University Medical Center has resulted in collaboration around the establishment of the Down Syndrome Clinic at that center. In 2002 a full course on "Disability" was established at the Recanati School for Allied Professions in the Community, FOHS, BGU and in 2005 collaboration was started with the Primary Care Unit of the faculty and disability became part of the master of public health course on "Children and society". In the academic year 2005-2006 a one semester course on "Aging with disability" was started as part of the master of science program in gerontology in our collaboration with the Center for Multidisciplinary Research in Aging.

Research activities

The affiliated staff have over the years published work from projects and research activities in this national and international collaboration. In the year 2000 the International Journal of Adolescent Medicine and Health and in 2005 the International Journal on Disability and Human development of Freund Publishing House (London and Tel Aviv), in the year 2003 the TSW-Child Health and Human Development and in 2006 the TSW-Holistic Health and Medicine of the Scientific World Journal (New York and Kirkkonummi, Finland), all peer-reviewed international journals were affiliated with the National Institute of Child Health and Human Development. From 2008 also the International Journal of Child Health and Human Development (Nova Science, New York), the International Journal of Child and Adolescent Health (Nova Science) and the Journal of Pain Management (Nova Science) affiliated and from 2009 thw International Public Health Journal (Nova Science) and Journal of Alternative Medicine Research (Nova Science).

National collaborations

Nationally the NICHD works in collaboration with the Faculty of Health Sciences, Ben Gurion University of the Negev; Department of Physical Therapy, Sackler School of Medicine, Tel Aviv University; Autism Center, Assaf HaRofeh Medical Center; National Rett and PKU Centers at Chaim Sheba Medical Center, Tel HaShomer; Department of Physiotherapy, Haifa University; Department of Education, Bar Ilan University, Ramat Gan, Faculty of Social Sciences and Health Sciences; College of Judea and Samaria in Ariel and recently also collaborations has been established with the Division of Pediatrics at Hadassah, Center for Pediatric Chronic Illness, Har HaZofim in Jerusalem.

International collaborations

Internationally with the Department of Disability and Human Development, College of Applied Health Sciences, University of Illinois at Chicago; Strong Center for Developmental Disabilities, Golisano Children's Hospital at Strong, University of Rochester School of Medicine and Dentistry, New York; Centre on Intellectual Disabilities, University of Albany, New York; Centre for Chronic Disease Prevention and Control, Health Canada, Ottawa; Chandler Medical Center and Children's Hospital, Kentucky Children's Hospital, Section of Adolescent Medicine, University of Kentucky, Lexington; Chronic Disease Prevention and

Control Research Center, Baylor College of Medicine, Houston, Texas; Division of Neuroscience, Department of Psychiatry, Columbia University, New York; Institute for the Study of Disadvantage and Disability, Atlanta; Center for Autism and Related Disorders, Department Psychiatry, Children's Hospital Boston, Boston; Department of Paediatrics, Child Health and Adolescent Medicine, Children's Hospital at Westmead, Westmead, Australia; International Centre for the Study of Occupational and Mental Health, Düsseldorf, Germany; Centre for Advanced Studies in Nursing, Department of General Practice and Primary Care, University of Aberdeen, Aberdeen, United Kingdom; Quality of Life Research Center, Copenhagen, Denmark; Nordic School of Public Health, Gottenburg, Sweden, Scandinavian Institute of Quality of Working Life, Oslo, Norway; Centre for Quality of Life of the Hong Kong Institute of Asia-Pacific Studies and School of Social Work, Chinese University, Hong Kong.

Targets

Our focus is on research, international collaborations, clinical work, teaching and policy in health, disability and human development and to establish the NICHD as a permanent institute at one of the residential care centers for persons with intellectual disability in Israel in order to conduct model research and together with the four university schools of public health/medicine in Israel establish a national master and doctoral program in disability and human development at the institute to secure the next generation of professionals working in this often non-prestigious/low-status field of work. For this project we need your support. We are looking for all kinds of support and eventually an endowment.

Contact

Joav Merrick, MD, DMSc
Professor of Pediatrics, Child Health and Human Development
Medical Director, Division for Mental Retardation, Ministry of Social Affairs and Social Services, POB 1260, IL-91012 Jerusalem, Israel.
E-mail: jmerrick@inter.net.il

In: Advanced Cancer. Pain and Quality of Life
Editors: E. Chow, J. Merrick, pp. 305-306
ISBN: 978-1-61668-207-1
© 2010 Nova Science Publishers, Inc.

Chapter XXX

About the Book Series "Health and Human Development"

Health and human development is a book series with publications from a multidisciplinary group of researchers, practitioners and clinicians for an international professional forum interested in the broad spectrum of health and human development.

- Merrick J, Omar HA, eds. Adolescent behavior research. International perspectives. New York: Nova Science, 2007.
- Kratky KW. Complementary medicine systems: Comparison and integration. New York: Nova Science, 2008.
- Schofield P, Merrick J, eds. Pain in children and youth. New York: Nova Science, 2009.
- Greydanus DE, Patel DR, Pratt HD, Calles Jr JL, eds. Behavioral pediatrics, 3 ed. New York: Nova Science, 2009.
- Ventegodt S, Merrick J, eds. Meaningful work: Research in quality of working life. New York: Nova Science, 2009.
- Omar HA, Greydanus DE, Patel DR, Merrick J, eds. Obesity and adolescence. A public health concern. New York: Nova Science, 2009.
- Lieberman A, Merrick J, eds. Poverty and children. A public health concern. New York: Nova Science, 2009.
- Goodbread J. Living on the edge. The mythical, spiritual and philosophical roots of social marginality. New York: Nova Science, 2009.
- Bennett DL, Towns S, Elliot E, Merrick J, eds. Challenges in adolescent health: An Australian perspective. New York: Nova Science, 2009.
- Schofield P, Merrick J, eds. Children and pain. New York: Nova Science, 2009.
- Sher L, Kandel I, Merrick J. Alcohol-related cognitive disorders: Research and clinical perspectives. New York: Nova Science, 2009.
- Anyanwu EC. Advances in environmental health effects of toxigenic mold and mycotoxins. New York: Nova Science, 2009.
- Bell E, Merrick J, eds. Rural child health. International aspects. New York: Nova Science, 2009.

- Dubowitz H, Merrick J, eds. International aspects of child abuse and neglect. New York: Nova Science, 2010.
- Shahtahmasebi S, Berridge D. Conceptualizing behavior: A practical guide to data analysis. New York: Nova Science, 2010.
- Wernik U. Chance action and therapy. The playful way of changing. New York: Nova Science, 2010.
- Omar HA, Greydanus DE, Patel DR, Merrick J, eds. Adolescence and chronic illness. A public health concern. New York: Nova Science, 2010.
- Patel DR, Greydanus DE, Omar HA, Merrick J, eds. Adolescence and sports. New York: Nova Science, 2010.
- Shek DTL, Ma HK, Merrick J, eds. Positive youth development: Evaluation and future directions in a Chinese context. New York: Nova Science, 2010.
- Shek DTL, Ma HK, Merrick J, eds. Positive youth development: Implementation of a youth program in a Chinese context. New York: Nova Science, 2010.
- Omar HA, Greydanus DE, Tsitsika AK, Patel DR, Merrick J, eds. Pediatric and adolescent sexuality and gynecology: Principles for the primary care clinician. New York: Nova Science, 2010.
- Chow E, Merrick J, eds. Advanced cancer. Pain and quality of life. New York: Nova Science, 2010.

Contact

Professor Joav Merrick, MD, MMedSci, DMSc
Medical Director, Division for Mental Retardation
Ministry of Social Affairs, POBox 1260
IL-91012 Jerusalem, Israel
E-mail: jmerrick@internet-zahav.net
Website: www.nichd-israel.com

Index

B

C

I

N

Q

R

S

W

X

Z